10.00

Recent Advances in
ANAESTHESIA AND ANALGESIA

C. LANGTON HEWER MB BS(Lond) MRCP(Lond) Hon.FFARCS(Eng)
Consulting Anaesthetist to St Bartholomew's Hospital and to the Hospital for Tropical Diseases, London. Late Anaesthetist to the Brompton Chest Hospital. Editor Emeritus, 'Anaesthesia'

R. S. ATKINSON MA MB BCHIR FFARCS
Consultant Anaesthetist, Southend General Hospital, Essex

Recent Advances in
ANAESTHESIA AND ANALGESIA

EDITED BY
C. LANGTON HEWER
and
R. S. ATKINSON

NUMBER THIRTEEN

CHURCHILL LIVINGSTONE
EDINBURGH LONDON AND NEW YORK 1979

CHURCHILL LIVINGSTONE
Medical Division of Longman Group Limited

Distributed in the United States of America by
Longman Inc., 19 West 44th Street, New York,
N.Y. 10036, and by associated companies,
branches and representatives throughout
the world.

First published 1979

ISBN 0 443 01944 4 (cased)
ISBN 0 443 01795 6 (limp)

British Library Cataloguing in Publication Data
Recent advances in anesthesia and analgesia.
    No. 13
    1. Anesthesia   2. Analgesia
    617'.96   RD81   78–40777

Printed in Great Britain by Bell and Bain, Glasgow

Preface

The last volume of *Recent Advances in Anaesthesia and Analgesia* was published in 1976, but already sufficient material is available to warrant production of a new one. The subjects chosen are different to those considered last time and to some extent the two volumes are complementary. Topics of current interest have been included and it has been our aim to provide, with the help of expert contributors, readable accounts informative to the clinical anaesthetist who does not have time to go to the original sources himself.

The newer anaesthetic agents, enflurane and etomidate, are considered in some depth as is the concept of total intravenous anaesthesia, though the last is not yet, in our opinion, a satisfactory replacement for conventional methods.

There is current interest in the use of rebreathing systems and co-axial circuits, while recent accidents with flexible pipelines for medical gases and their connection to anaesthetic apparatus have indicated the need for improved safety precautions. One Chapter of this volume is devoted to both these aspects of the delivery of medical gases to patients.

The scope of cardiac surgery has increased greatly in recent years. The low mortality rate that now exists is a compliment to both the surgical technique itself and the excellent peri-operative care that patients receive. It is therefore appropriate that those aspects of interest to the anaesthetist are considered.

Avoidable maternal deaths still occur in obstetric practice associated with general anaesthesia, while perfect pain relief is not available to all mothers in labour. There is therefore a Chapter devoted to obstetric anaesthesia and analgesia.

Concern continues with regard to anaesthesia for the ambulant dental patient. Controversy exists with regard to clinical techniques and there are organisational problems to be overcome in the future if this work is to continue in premises outside the main hospital building. This subject is reviewed.

Sodium nitroprusside is considered in a separate Chapter. Though not a new drug, the indications and methods of use have only recently been evaluated. Toxic effects can also occur and their avoidance depends on an understanding of the metabolism of the compound.

Controlled ventilation in the intensive care unit is never without potential problems and complications. Mechanical ventilators are expensive items of equipment and it is not easy to advise on a best buy. Nor are the pros and cons of positive and expiratory pressure and intermittent mandatory ventilation easy to evaluate in a particular clinical situation. Monitoring is another area where economic constraints are operative since without this there would be no limit to the possible development of electronic expertise. Both these topics are therefore considered.

Postoperative care is a field which often receives less attention than it deserves. The patient may be in a critical condition in the few hours following completion of surgery and in all but the simplest case pain relief is necessary and arterial hypoxaemia may occur.

The anaesthetist is often involved in the acute management of the trauma patient whether this be in the accident centre, the operating theatre or the intensive care unit. Aspects of care which are the proper concern of the anaesthetist are reviewed.

Patients suffering from deliberate self-poisoning or accidental overdose form a significant percentage of those admitted to intensive care units. The availability of an ever widening range of potentially toxic substances means that the pattern of attempted suicide has changed greatly in recent years. It is no longer sufficient just to maintain lung ventilation and cardiac output and wait for the effects of the drug to wear off. We have therefore considered it appropriate to include a review of this subject.

In the last volume we noted that so many contributors had used abbreviations that an index of these was added at the end of the book. Since that date, the proliferation of abbreviations has become so enormous that a *Dictionary of Abbreviations in Medicine and the Health Sciences* (price over £14) is now available containing no fewer than 12 000 items. It is therefore inevitable that identical capital letter sequences may have two or more meanings which may lead to bizarre or even dangerous conclusions. An example of the former can be quoted from a most respected medical journal which carried a leading article entitled 'VIP and watery diarrhoea'. A physician interested in the effects of emotion on gastro-intestinal motility found to his annoyance that the writer was not discussing a member of the 'top brass' but vasoactive intestinal peptide. We must therefore point out that the new appendix refers only to abbreviations used *in this book*.

We thank the contributors who all met a rather tight schedule to ensure that there were no delays in publication. We also thank the publishers for their help and forbearance.

C.L.H.
R.S.A.

London 1978

Since the first *Recent Advances in Anaesthesia and Analgesia* was published in 1932, the developments in this progressing field have been examined in depth in twelve further volumes in the series, published respectively in 1937, 1939, 1943, 1944 (reprinted 1946), 1948, 1953, 1957 (reprinted 1958), 1963, 1967, 1972 and 1976, culminating in the publication of the present volume, number thirteen, in 1979.

Contributors

A. P. ADAMS MB BS FFARCS
Consultant Anaesthetist and Clinical Lecturer, Nuffield Department of
Anaesthetics, Radcliffe Infirmary, Oxford

R. S. ATKINSON MB BChir FFARCS
Consultant Anaesthetist, Southend General Hospital, Essex

DONALD CAMPBELL MB ChB FFARCS
Professor of Anaesthesia, University of Glasgow; Honorary Consultant
Anaesthetist, Royal Infirmary, Glasgow

PETER COLE MB ChB FFARCS
Consultant Anaesthetist, St Bartholomew's Hospital, London

C. B. FRANKLIN MB ChB FFARCS
Consultant Anaesthetist, Wythenshawe Hospital, Manchester

ALAN GILSTON MB ChB FFARCS
Consultant Anaesthetist, National Heart Hospital, London

J. D. HENVILLE MB BS FFARCS
Consultant Anaesthetist, Nuffield Department of Anaesthetics, Radcliffe
Infirmary, Oxford

J. R. KRAPEZ MB BS FFARCS DRCOG
Consultant Anaesthetist, St Bartholomew's Hospital, London

DONALD D. MOIR MD FFARCS DRCOG
Consultant Anaesthetist, Queen Mother's Hospital, Glasgow; Hon. Clinical
Lecturer, University of Glasgow

T. M. SAVEGE MB BS FFARCS
Assistant Director, Anaesthetics Unit, The London Hospital

J. C. STODDART MD FFARCS
Consultant Anaesthetist; Consultant in Charge, Intensive Therapy Unit,
Royal Victoria Infirmary, Newcastle on Tyne

J. A. THORNTON MD FFARCS
Professor and Head of Department of Anaesthetics, University of Sheffield
Medical School

Contents

1. New anaesthetic drugs and techniques—enflurane, etomidate and total intravenous anaesthesia

T. M. Savege

In this Chapter recent research on two new anaesthetic agents are reviewed, one a volatile anaesthetic, the other an intravenous agent.

Techniques of continuous intravenous anaesthesia have recently been modified and refurbished under the term 'Total Intravenous Anaesthesia'. The application of this technique, its advantages and disadvantages will be discussed.

ENFLURANE

Enflurane has been an established anaesthetic agent for a number of years. However, it is still the subject of intense investigation.

Although it is said that enflurane is not flammable this is not strictly correct. High percentages of either halothane or enflurane in oxygen can be ignited. The addition of nitrous oxide reduces the percentage of volatile agent required to make the mixture flammable. 30 per cent oxygen in nitrous oxide can be ignited in the presence of 5.75 per cent enflurane. A reduction to 20 per cent oxygen in nitrous oxide allows the critical enflurane concentration to be reduced to 4.25 per cent whilst the mixture's flammability is retained. Fortunately, these concentrations of enflurane are not commonly used, furthermore a static discharge would not have sufficient energy to ignite the mixture. However, electro cautery used in the upper airway in the presence of high concentrations of enflurane could be dangerous.[1]

Earlier studies on enflurane reported that the agent was capable of inducing electroencephalographic (EEG) seizure activity often associated with tonic and/or clonic movements.[2] In addition, work in animals demonstrated that seizure activity could be detected on the EEG in the postoperative period and might persist for up to 16 days.[3] Subsequently two case reports of unexplained motor seizures occurring, one at six days and the other at eight days after anaesthesia, have been published.[4] Neither patient had had previous motor seizures but one had a family history of epilepsy.[4] Recently the EEG changes following prolonged exposure to enflurane (9.6 MAC hours) have been studied.[5] Two-thirds of the subjects developed spontaneous seizure activity revealed by the EEG during anaesthesia. In five of these subjects increased tone and clonic movements of the extremities developed at the same time. After anaesthesia all the EEG records showed diffuse slowing of α activity at one and two days, the trace becoming normal at the sixth day. Eight subjects showed minor changes on the EEG lasting from 6 to 30 days but none showed evidence of post anaesthetic seizure activity. It has been postulated that enflurane might precipitate seizure activity in patients with a pre-existing epileptic focus or in those with a clinical condition that could in itself lead to convulsions.[5] Consequently, enflurane is probably best avoided in patients of this type. Treatment of clonic movements by administration of thiopentone may exacerbate the EEG signs of seizure at light levels of anaesthesia and suppress them at deep levels.[6]

Enflurane increases cerebral blood flow[7] but to a lesser extent than halothane.[8] Studies of cerebral blood flow using a specially adapted goat model show that both enflurane and halothane at 1 MAC abolish autoregulation of cerebral blood flow under conditions of normocarbia.[9] For each change in mean arterial blood pressure there was a parallel variation in cerebral blood flow. Hypocarbia exerted some residual effect in that both the magnitude of cerebral blood flow and the rate of change of flow in response to variation in mean arterial pressure were less marked.

It has also been shown that the quantity of water that collects in the tissues round an artificially induced cerebral lesion in an animal model is greater following enflurane and other halogenated volatile agents than after either barbiturate or fentanyl-droperidol-nitrous oxide anaesthesia. The volume of water could be directly correlated to the percentage change in cerebral blood flow.[10]

Initial reports on the cardiovascular effects of enflurane suggested that it only induced small changes at 1 MAC.[11] Recently, work undertaken on intact dogs has shown that enflurane depresses the cardiovascular system by as much if not more than does halothane when administered in comparable doses.[12,13,14] The depressant effect is dose related,[12,14] at 2.3 per cent enflurane mean systemic arterial pressure fell by 23 per cent, cardiac output by 18 per cent and LV dp/dt by 19 per cent compared with awake values.[12] Systemic vascular resistance was little changed and heart rate increased by over 30 per cent.[12] At higher doses (3.6–3.8 per cent) mean systemic arterial pressure, cardiac output and LV dp/dt fell by some 50 per cent[12,13] and left atrial pressure rose.[12] Some of these changes may have been exacerbated by the failure of heart rate to rise with the increased concentration of enflurane. These cardiovascular effects were accompanied by comparable falls in myocardial blood flow[12] but there was no evidence to suggest that the heart became anoxic. Myocardial oxygen consumption also fell, by over 50 per cent,[12,13] and oxygen consumption to other tissues was reduced but by a lesser amount.[13] Animal studies seem to reflect fairly accurately the changes in man.[14] However, different species do show variations, for example heart rate does not progressively rise in dogs,[12,14] whereas it does in man.[15] In contrast, it falls progressively in monkeys which consequently show more marked cardiovascular depression.[16]

The effects of enflurane were compared with those of halothane when administered with nitrous oxide to a group of unpremedicated volunteers breathing spontaneously.[17] Enflurane at approximately 1 MAC depressed mean systemic arterial pressure by 22 per cent, more than twice the fall induced by halothane. Myocardial contractility as measured by pre-ejection period and its derivatives was also depressed by enflurane but to a lesser extent than by halothane. However, this might not reflect the true action of enflurane on the myocardium for the mean Pa_{CO_2} measured in that group was approximately 1 kPa (7.5 mmHg) greater than in the halothane group.

Evidence of myocardial depression during anaesthesia is not necessarily a bad sign; under certain circumstances the reduction in heart work can be beneficial. Furthermore, in the animal studies, despite myocardial depression there was no evidence to suggest that the oxygen supply to the heart[12] or to other tissues was inadequate and the oxygen tension in venous blood remained either normal or raised.[13] However, blood lactate did significantly increase and no adequate explanation for this is available at present.[12] Although myocardial depression might not in itself be harmful it is important to establish whether or not the cardiovascular system is capable of responding effectively to stress. The evidence both in man and animals suggests that the cardiovascular system does respond to hypercarbia[11] and to hypovolaemia[14] but that the response to the latter is impaired.

The large fall in mean systemic arterial pressure that is so consistently reported is a disadvantage because this could reduce critically coronary artery perfusion.

Enflurane may be a safer drug to use in the presence of raised blood catecholamines than halothane. The application of a solution containing adrenaline to mucous membranes and other tissues is less likely to induce dysrhythmias.[18,19] Although the administration of 2–20 ml adrenaline (1 in 100 000 dilution) either to mucous membranes or as a subcutaneous infiltration during enflurane anaesthesia increased blood pressure and heart rate in 20 per cent of patients, only 1.2 per cent developed premature ventricular contractions. These never exceeded five per minute. Additional doses of 20 ml solution could be injected hourly without inducing arrhythmias.[20] The evidence suggests that up to three times more adrenaline may be administered safely during enflurane anaesthesia compared with halothane anaesthesia.[18]

Enflurane depresses pulmonary ventilation in animals and man.[21] Recent studies in unpremedicated dogs have shown that enflurane, like halothane, did not result in increased $Paco_2$ when administered at 1 MAC but did so at 2 MAC.[22] Pulmonary ventilation is increased as a consequence of a raised $Paco_2$[22,23] but the response is not as effective as that in the awake animal. Furthermore, the ventilatory response to hypoxia is also reduced.[22] Normally if hypercarbia occurs at the same time as hypoxia the ventilatory response is augmented. This effect is abolished by both halothane and enflurane at 1 MAC.[22]

Enflurane dilates the bronchoconstriction induced by hypocapnia in an isolated denervated canine lung preparation. The dilatation is not as marked as that induced by halothane. This action does not seem to be mediated through the β receptor as β blockade does not affect it.[24] These findings may have some clinical significance. Morr-Strathmann and colleagues have shown that although enflurane slightly reduces lung compliance it also reduces airway resistance in healthy volunteers, the change being very similar to those measured with halothane.[25] The two drugs have been compared when used as the main anaesthetic agent in patients with chronic obstructive pulmonary disease.[26] The quality of anaesthesia was comparable between the two agents but there was a slightly higher incidence of coughing, wheezing, production of secretions and hypotension with enflurane.[26]

Clinical studies suggest that enflurane enhances muscle relaxation provided by muscle relaxant drugs.[27,28] Waud and Waud have shown in isolated guinea pig muscle that most volatile anaesthetic agents depress carbachol-induced depolarisation of the end plate region at a site distal to the acetyl choline-receptor complex.[29,30] In man enflurane has been shown to depress the ability of muscle to sustain contracture in response to tetanic stimulation. Furthermore, with increasing doses it progressively augments the twitch depression induced by tubocurarine and prolongs the recovery time of twitch response.[31] Less non-depolarising muscle relaxant is required during enflurane anaesthesia than during halothane anaesthesia to depress the twitch response by 50 per cent.[31] However, this finding relates to very small doses of relaxant drug, and, judging from the slope of the dose response curves, may not apply to doses used in clinical anaesthesia.

Enflurane has been used in small concentrations (0.5–0.8 per cent) prior to delivery during anaesthesia for Caesarean section.[32] This did not significantly depress the Apgar score of the infants and was apparently not associated with excessive uterine haemorrhage. There was no evidence of maternal awareness during the procedure or recall afterwards.

Most enflurane is excreted through the lungs and less than 3 per cent is metabolised to inorganic fluoride.[34] This is less than that reported for other fluorinated anaesthetic drugs and probably reflects the greater chemical stability of the enflurane molecule.[34] It may also reflect the more rapid excretion of the drug which occurs as a result of its relatively low tissue solubility.[34,35] Rapid elimination reduces the time available for metabolism. Consequently the serum inorganic fluoride level does not remain elevated for as long after enflurane as it does after methoxyflurane. The mean peak level is normally less than $25~\mu\text{M/l}$[35,36] which is about half the concentration that is likely to cause renal damage.[37,38] There is no evidence to suggest that enflurane impairs renal function in otherwise healthy patients undergoing routine surgery and anaesthesia[35,36] or in volunteers undergoing prolonged anaesthesia (9.6 MAC hours).[39] However, high serum inorganic fluoride levels have been measured in a few instances[35,36] and are probably due to a delay in excretion of either enflurane, for example in obese patients, or of inorganic fluoride, for example in patients with impaired glomerular filtration. Some support for this suggestion comes from reports of nephrotoxicity following enflurane anaesthesia and surgery in patients with impaired preoperative renal function.[40,41] Another cause of raised serum inorganic fluoride might be its increased production as a result of induction of hepatic microsomal enzymes by drugs.[35,36] Enflurane itself has been shown to induce hepatic enzymes[42] so that previous exposure to the agent might lead to increased production of inorganic fluoride. Such a mechanism may have contributed to the renal failure reported following six hours of surgery and anaesthesia with enflurane in a patient with moderately severe heart disease who had been exposed to enflurane six weeks previously.[43] Urinary output returned spontaneously after three days and renal function gradually improved. The peak level of serum inorganic fluoride was not measured but the level two days post-anaesthesia was $93~\mu\text{M/l}$ far in excess of the toxic threshold. It seems advisable to avoid enflurane in patients who have impaired glomerular function (i.e. raised blood urea or impaired creatinine clearance) or who have recently taken drugs that are known to induce liver enzymes. For the present this must include recent exposure to enflurane.

Apart from inorganic fluoride other biochemical variables have been measured following routine anaesthesia[35,36] and after prolonged anaesthesia without surgery.[39] There was no evidence to suggest in either group of studies that liver function was impaired. However, SGOT was increased by three times the control value following prolonged anaesthesia and elevated significantly after routine anaesthesia.[35,39] This change is unexplained at present. Hepato-cellular dysfunction and jaundice have been reported in isolated cases after enflurane anaesthesia[44,45] but there is insufficient evidence to confirm that the anaesthetic agent was responsible.

Other small changes in serum electrolytes and other blood variables have been reported but are thought to be related to changes associated with stress.[35]

A marked and very variable increase in creatinine phosphokinase has also been measured in four volunteers following prolonged enflurane anaesthesia.[39] The clinical significance of this is not known at present. However, two cases of malignant hyperpyrexia have been attributed to enflurane.[46,47] In both of these patients suxamethonium was administered and therefore cannot be excluded as the responsible agent.

Enflurane administered in the absence of surgery does not significantly depress the immune response as measured by the ability of a volunteer's lymphocytes to transform in response to phytohaemagglutinin. It does induce a modest leucocytosis that persists until the first postoperative day.[48] In vitro studies have shown that enflurane has no mutagenic effect.[49]

The volatile anaesthetic enflurane has the advantage of inducing anaesthesia rapidly and allowing a fast recovery afterwards. It augments the action of non-depolarising muscle relaxants. It is a safer drug to use than halothane in the presence of raised blood catecholamines. It may induce seizure activity on the EEG and could under adverse conditions exacerbate and even induce renal failure. So far it has not been shown to cause liver damage. Otherwise many of its properties are similar to those of halothane.

ETOMIDATE

Etomidate is a potent rapidly acting intravenous hypnotic agent first introduced into clinical anaesthesia by Doenicke[50] in 1973 after animal studies by Janssen et al.[51] It is an ethyl-imidazole carboxylate derivative and consequently not related to any previous intravenous induction agent. It is a white crystalline powder, soluble in a wide range of solvents including water, ethanol and propylene glycol. The pH of the aqueous solution is 3.46 and its osmolality 254 mOs/kg.[52] Dissolving the drug in propylene glycol (the current solvent) increases the pH to 8.1 and the osmolality to 4640 mOs/kg.[52] Following intravenous administration, the plug is distributed approximately equally between red blood cells and plasma. Plasma binding in man is 76.5 per cent.[53] The dose is rapidly redistributed from the blood to other tissues. Animal studies show that only 2.5 per cent of the original dose remains in the circulation two minutes after intravenous administration.[54] In contrast peak levels are measured in the brain, heart, lungs, liver and kidney at that time and by 28 min only fat contains a high concentration of drug.[54] In man the fall in plasma concentration has been shown to fit a three compartment model with half times of the three phases being 2.8 min, 32.1 min and nearly four hours.[55] Studies in Wistar rats suggest that etomidate is metabolised in the liver probably by capacity limited hydrolysis of the methylated ester. Peak blood level of metabolites were measured at 7 min though these had no anaesthetic activity.[54] The biological half life of the drug was shown to be 40 min.[54] About 50 per cent of a tritium labelled dose was excreted in the urine within four hours and 10 per cent of the dose excreted in the bile.

Studies in man of the renal excretion of labelled drug gave similar results; nearly 50 per cent of the administered dose was recovered within four hours and nearly 80 per cent by 24 hours.[56]

Etomidate rapidly induces hypnosis. Consciousness is lost within 10–65 seconds of administration, depending on the rate of injection, dose of hypnotic and type of premedication.[57,58] The time to loss of consciousness is similar to that after thiopentone.[59] The optimum dose that has been recommended for induction is 0.3 mg/kg.[50] This induces effective hypnosis for approximately 4–5 min with minimum cardiovascular changes.[60] Smaller doses within the range 0.12/0.16 mg/kg induce drowsiness but not necessarily hypnosis.[60]

Within the clinical range, the duration of unconsciousness depends on the dose of etomidate. 0.2 mg/kg induces sleep for 2–3 min whereas 0.4 mg/kg induces sleep for 6–7 min.[60,61] Premedication with narcotics increases the duration of hypnosis.[60,61] If etomidate 0.1 mg/kg is administered each time a patient awakes over a period of 30 minutes the duration of anaesthesia is not prolonged as the total dose rises.[62] However, cumulation, as judged by prolonged recovery time, has been noted when larger quantities of etomidate are administered as the principal anaesthetic.[61,63] Delayed recovery, i.e. more than 30 minutes after surgery, was recorded in 15 per cent of patients during an early study which used a continuous intravenous infusion of etomidate.[63]

Little work has been carried out to establish the relative potency of etomidate compared with other agents. However, using the criterion of duration of abolition of eyelash reflex 0.2 mg/kg etomidate is equivalent to 0.036 mg/kg Althesin (Table 1.1). This comparison was carried out double blind and in the same group of patients having repeated electro-convulsive therapy.[64] It is interesting to note that in a previous study carried out in a similar manner 50 mg methohexitone abolished eyelash reflex for the same period of time.[65]

Some studies have also been undertaken into the time to long-term recovery. Ten unpremedicated volunteers given 30 mg etomidate were asked to perform a vigilance test involving the recognition of numbers on a board. The mean time from induction to the achievement of a comparable performance with control was 24 min.[66] Kay has shown that ocular movements as measured by the Maddox wing had returned to control values some 30 min after the administration of etomidate 0.2 mg/kg.[62] Out-patients induced with either etomidate 0.3 mg/kg or propanidid 7 mg/kg and kept anaesthetised with nitrous oxide and halothane for minor surgical procedures woke at approximately the same time—some 6–8 min afterwards. They were able to stand and walk steadily within 17–20 min, the etomidate group taking slightly longer.[67] The quality of recovery after a single dose of etomidate is good with no 'hangover'.[68]

The EEG changes that occur during anaesthesia with etomidate (0.3 mg/kg) are broadly similar to those that occur with thiopentone or Althesin.[59,69,70,71] There is an initial increase in the overall energy level and then a progressive decrease with burst suppression becoming established in some cases.[69] Frequency analysis shows that there is less fast β activity than is normally associated with intravenous anaesthesia.[59,70] Etomidate is similar to Althesin and different from the barbiturates in that slow activity (<2 Hz) persists after induction.[70] This probably reflects the persistence of muscle activity that is characteristic of both these drugs.[70,72] The addition of diazepam or fentanyl at induction increases the rate of development of deep cortical depression and prolongs its duration.[69] The high incidence of myoclonic movements that occurs with etomidate anaesthesia is not associated with specific EEG changes or epileptiform discharges.[59,69,71] Furthermore, the drug has been administered to a group of patients with epilepsy and no specific

Table 1.1   Mean time from administration of drug to return of eyelash reflex (seconds). Adapted from O'Carroll, T. M., Blogg, C. E., Hoinville, E. A. & Savege, T. M. (1977);[64] Foley, E. I., Walton, B., Savege, T. M., Strunin, L. & Simpson, B. R. (1972)[65]

		S.D.
Etomidate (0.2 mg/kg)	252 s	(± 87)
Althesin (0.36 mg/kg)	253 s	(± 106)
Methohexitone (50 mg)	251 s	

adverse effects resulted.[73] It is presumed therefore that these movements originate in deep cerebral structures or in the brain stem.[59,69] The cerebral function monitor, which derives a trace from the EEG signal, indicates changes following etomidate that are similar to those induced by the barbiturates and Althesin.[74] However, the changes during a continuous infusion of etomidate are less obvious than those noted following Althesin. This makes control of the infusion less precise.

Although etomidate is an effective hypnotic it will not prevent movement in response to relatively minor stimulation.[59,62,75] Furthermore, the increase in blood pressure that is characteristically seen at the time of intubation is if anything more marked following etomidate than after methohexitone.[76] Anaesthesia with nitrous oxide, muscle relaxant and repeated bolus doses of etomidate does not suppress obvious clinical signs of increased autonomic activity during the noxious stimulation of surgery.[61] The paradox that deep cortical depression, as shown by burst suppression on the EEG, can be demonstrated at the same time as the patient responds with movement or autonomic changes to noxious stimulation has been reported previously with Althesin.[77,78] It emphasises the error of equating depth of cortical depression with adequacy of anaesthesia. Althesin and etomidate are potent depressants of the cerebral cortex but are far less effective at obtunding reflex responses to noxious stimulation. The administration of more hypnotic in an attempt to prevent autonomic changes or movement will merely depress the cortex further thus tending to prolong recovery without improving the quality of anaesthesia.[78]

There is wide agreement that etomidate exerts very little effect on the cardiovascular system of healthy patients.[57,58,67,79,80,81,82,83] Occasional dysrhythmias have been reported,[75,84] the incidence being approximately 1 per cent in adults and rather higher in children.[75,84] It is unlikely that this is a specific effect of etomidate, the incidence being comparable to that following thiopentone.[75,84] In healthy patients premedicated with atropine only, etomidate in doses between 0.15–0.3 mg/kg induces a small increase in heart rate, either no change or a small fall in systemic and pulmonary arterial pressure, a fall in systemic vascular resistance and either no change or a small rise in cardiac output.[82,85] Myocardial contractility, measured indirectly, is either unchanged[82] or slightly increased.[80] Myocardial blood flow, measured in five patients, rose, yet myocardial oxygen consumption only increased by a small amount which suggests that etomidate dilates coronary vessels.[82] A feature of many reports is that patients move during induction of anaesthesia with etomidate and may develop marked myoclonia. In the cardiovascular study of Kettler and colleagues,[82] measurements became difficult because of movement, and four out of five patients had to be held down. Rifat and colleagues[85] also noted muscle movement and myoclonia in 9/14 patients in their study. It is noticeable that the only other intravenous anaesthetic that does not overtly depress the cardiovascular system is ketamine which also induces increased muscle tone and movement. It is presumably to be expected that when patients become unconscious the cardiovascular system will show reduced activity unless the drug administered induces specific pharmacological stimulation. One suspects that central stimulation, with or without muscle movement and myoclonia, is the price that must be paid if 'depression' of the cardiovascular system is to be avoided at induction of anaesthesia. The tachycardia and movement following etomidate has been related to the incidence of pain that often accompanies intravenous administration of the drug[84] but it would be wrong to conclude that these effects are caused by pain; narcotic analgesics, which prevent these clinical signs, could do so by separate mechanisms. Whatever the mechanism, narcotic premedication is known to modify the incidence of myoclonia and movement[68] and as a result probably modifies the cardiovascular effects. In this context it is interesting to note that the cardiovascular changes following the administration of etomidate to heavily premedicated patients with heart disease were indistinguishable from those measured following Althesin 0.05 ml/kg.[86] In none of that group was there any complaint of pain on injection and no evidence of movement or myoclonia.

Comparison of the effect of etomidate with other agents is difficult because there is no agreed equipotent dose range. In general, etomidate alters cardiovascular activity less than all the other commonly used induction agents except ketamine and possibly methohexitone.[80,82,87] It is doubtful if the doses of different induction agents against which etomidate has been compared are always appropriate. In one study 0.15 mg/kg etomidate was compared with 1.5 mg/kg methohexitone.[80] Similarly in two other studies 0.3 mg/kg etomidate was compared with 0.075 ml/kg Althesin.[82,87] The doses used for comparison are probably of critical importance because the cardiovascular effects of the barbiturates and Althesin are dependent on the quantity administered per unit of time. Thiopentone was originally used in much larger doses which frequently had catastrophic effects on the cardiovascular system.[88] However, all these agents, if administered slowly, in small doses, will induce hypnosis with little reduction in cardiovascular variables.

Changes in cerebral blood flow following the administration of intravenous induction agents have been measured in a group of healthy premedicated patients anaesthetised with propanidid, nitrous oxide and 0.1–0.4 per cent halothane and ventilated, using intermittent suxamethonium, to keep $Paco_2$ within the normal range. Etomidate 0.2 mg/kg reduced cerebral blood flow by 37 per cent, 30 sec after administration, but flow had returned to control value by 5 min. In contrast, the barbiturates and propanidid depressed flow by a greater percentage at 30 sec. By 10 min cerebral blood flow had returned to control values following both propanidid (5 mg/kg) and methohexitone (1 mg/kg) whereas after thiopentone (4 mg/kg) cerebral blood flow remained reduced and close to minimum values.[89] It is difficult to assess the clinical significance of such an investigation where so many other factors that alter cerebral blood flow were operating.

Famewo[90] has shown that etomidate 0.3 mg/kg reduced intraocular pressure in a group of premedicated patients by 33 per cent, a rather surprising finding in the face of the drug's minimum effect on the cardiovascular system and the high incidence of myoclonia and increased muscle tone that etomidate induces.

Etomidate slows respiratory rate for a short period following induction[61] and then increases it slightly.[58,59,81,91] Tidal volume increases for a brief period shortly after injection of the drug[59,81,91] and is followed by a short period of shallow ventilation.[91] Apnoea may occur but is less common than after thiopentone.[84] Its incidence is between 16–50 per cent[68,79,83,84,91] and is short lived.[79] Respiratory changes do not seem to be influenced much by pre-medication.[68,79,83] A fall in Pao_2 to a mean value of 66 mmHg was measured in a group of patients with heart disease breathing air and induced with etomidate (0.3 mg/kg) but this fall was less than that measured after Althesin (0.05 ml/kg).[92] $Paco_2$ and pH were not altered. However, in a similar group of patients pre-medicated with papaveretum and hyoscine, the $Paco_2$ increased by a mean maximum of nearly 1 kPa (7.5 mmHg) over the 10 minutes following the administration of etomidate 0.3 mg/kg.[86] Coughing, hiccough, and stridor seldom occur[64,68] and are not more frequent than after thiopentone.[84]

No consistent and marked changes have been detected in liver function tests, renal function tests or in plasma electrolytes at 24 hours and 7 days after etomidate.[93]

The principal complications of etomidate are muscle movement and pain at the site of intravenous administration. Much has been written about muscle movement and this has even been broken down into sub-headings such as myoclonus—mild or severe, spontaneous movement in response to noxious stimulation and generalised increase in muscle tone. Mild myoclonus is reported in 18–70 per cent of patients following induction.[57,59,64,68,67,75,79,81,83,84,90,91,93,94] Severe myo-clonus or a generalised increase in muscle tone is less common (6–12 per cent).[68,79,81,84] The incidence of movement is far higher than after thiopentone (7.4 per cent),[84] Althesin (3.0 per cent)[64] or propanidid (0 per cent).[67] Movement is increased if the patient is stimulated and decreased by premedication especially if it contains narcotic analgesics.[68,79,83] Holdcroft and colleagues[68] demonstrated that papaveretum and hyoscine premedication reduced the incidence of movement by approximately 40 per cent. Muscle movement is probably the result of two factors:

1. Central stimulation by etomidate at a level somewhere below the cortex.[59,69]
2. A reflex response to noxious stimulation.

The latter may be relatively mild, such as holding up the chin or placing a mask on the face. Pain on injection may also be a cause for movement.[84] It is difficult to assess how much the muscle movement limits the use of etomidate. Provided anaesthesia is effectively maintained movement rapidly subsides and so it is probably no more than an irritation for the anaesthetist. It also seems quite likely that this increased activity at induction is responsible for maintaining cardiovascular 'stability'.

The incidence of pain at the site of injection during the administration of etomidate is high, but there is wide variation in the reported incidence (15–81 per cent);[51,68] however, most studies describe an incidence of between 25–50 per cent.[59,67,75,79,83,94] The severity of pain can be modified according to the site of injection, the solvent used and the type of premedication.[95] Fast injection may be less painful[67,95] as is injection into a vein in the antecubital fossa compared with a vein on the back of the hand.[59,79] The aqueous solution of etomidate induces most pain and the solution made up in polyethylene glycol the least[52,94] the incidence of pain falling from 30 per cent to 4 per cent.[52] It is suggested that the improvement is due to the more physiological pH and osmolality of the latter solution.[52] Propylene glycol is the solvent currently used with etomidate and the incidence of pain during injection is slightly greater than that for the polyethylene glycol solutions.[94]

The occurrence of local reactions at the site of injection does not reflect the high incidence of pain. In 5–6 per cent of patients there is a local skin flush[64,83] and in several studies phlebitis has been reported in one or two patients.[68,79] Venous thrombosis observed three days after etomidate occurs in 8 per cent of cases.[95]

The incidence of nausea and vomiting is apparently rather higher than that following other induction agents. In a series of patients undergoing general surgical procedures the incidence was around 25 per cent with premedication making only small differences.[68] In a group of gynaecology patients, notorious for postoperative vomiting, the incidence was between 35–53 per cent varying slightly with the speed of injection and the solvent used.[94]

Doenicke and colleagues[96] demonstrated that etomidate does not release histamine when administered to volunteers unlike other commonly used induction agents.[96,97] In their study changes in plasma histamine also failed to develop in at least half of the subjects following the administration of Althesin or propanidid. It would therefore be useful to have the results for etomidate confirmed in a series larger than the eight subjects originally studied. Histamine release is initiated by a wide range of drugs used in anaesthesia without the development of clinical signs.[97] Another factor must be present to explain the severe clinical reactions that have been reported following the administration of other induction agents.[98] At this stage one cannot conclude that etomidate will never induce such a reaction. However, none has been reported to date despite many thousands of etomidate anaesthetics.

Etomidate is an effective short acting hypnotic drug which has little adverse effect on the cardiovascular or respiratory system. It is compatible with all other drugs routinely administered in anaesthesia. It does not prevent reflex response to noxious stimulation when used in normal induction doses. A relatively high incidence of pain on injection and muscle movement following administration has been reported and these two effects have influenced a number of anaesthetists adversely. The significance of these two side effects remains to be established. Their incidence could probably be much reduced by simple modification of the anaesthetic technique.

Clearly any general anaesthetic agent will have a number of unique properties so that learning to use it to its best advantage will take time. Different techniques and combinations of drugs may have to be developed. It would be very unfortunate if new anaesthetic agents were rejected before suitable techniques had been developed for their use and their full potential explored.

A NEW TECHNIQUE—TOTAL INTRAVENOUS ANAESTHESIA

From time to time attempts have been made to use intravenous induction agents as a sole anaesthetic. Initial experiences in war casualties were disastrous and led to thiopentone being described as an ideal form of euthanasia.[99] Subsequently intravenous anaesthesia either by continuous infusion or intermittent administration has been used from time to time, usually for some specific purpose, for example in certain neurosurgical procedures[100,101] or in the treatment of grand mal epilepsy.[102]

Techniques did not develop further because conventional methods of anaesthesia have proved both safe and effective. Recently there has been growing concern that some techniques of anaesthesia might not be satisfactory, for two reasons. Firstly, during nitrous oxide relaxant anaesthesia many more patients than the quoted 2 per cent might be awake during the procedure.[103,104] Secondly, that anaesthetic gases and vapours might harm operating room personnel if inhaled over a long period of time.

It is possible that 20 per cent of patients or more are awake during nitrous oxide relaxant anaesthesia and subsequently forget the event. This would not diminish the terror of being aware at the time of surgery nor the pain that is felt and reported by 50 per cent of patients who do recall the event.[105] Furthermore, there is evidence to suggest that the forgotten experience is stored in the subconscious memory and may adversely affect the patient.[106,107]

Recent fears that pollution of the operating room with anaesthetic gases and vapours may be harmful to health have already led to recommendations that the concentration of anaesthetic agents in the air should be reduced to minimum detectable levels.[108] The only long term solution to these two problems is the development of a safe effective, intravenous anaesthetic technique. At present no intravenous anaesthetic drug possesses all the characteristics of an ideal agent. It seems sensible therefore to use the concept of balanced anaesthesia first suggested by Rees and Gray[109] and build a technique that uses separate drugs to provide hypnosis, muscle relaxation and suppression of the reflex responses to noxious stimulation. In this way each modality of balanced anaesthesia can be provided independently of the other.

The hypnotic needs to be an effective agent, simple to administer, as safe as is compatible with its action and rapidly redistributed and eliminated so that cumulation is unlikely to occur. The time to awakening after the end of surgery should compare with other conventional techniques. Du Cailer reported that continuous infusion of Althesin provided effective hypnosis and a rapid recovery.[110] This agent formed the basis of the technique used at The London Hospital[111] and subsequently adopted and modified elsewhere.[112,113] However, there is no reason to believe that other intravenous anaesthetic agents could not be used in the same manner. Methohexitone, ketamine or etomidate might be particularly suitable.

The analgesic agent is required to suppress the reflex response to noxious stimulation, induction agents being relatively ineffective in this respect.[75,78] The response to noxious stimulation embraces a wide range of physiological changes, simple limb movement as the result of the surgical incision at one end of the spectrum and all the changes associated with the stress response at the other. Narcotic drugs can modify and even eliminate all these responses if administered in sufficiently large doses.[78,114,115] Their great disadvantage is their respiratory depressant action which may be prolonged.[116] It is difficult to titrate the dose of narcotic agent so that the responses to noxious stimulation are effectively reduced and spontaneous respiration remains adequate. Once muscle relaxant drugs are used and ventilation is controlled excellent operating conditions can be assured and the anaesthetist is free to select whatever dose of narcotic agent he considers most appropriate, although large dose regimens may result in respiratory depression postoperatively just as they do in other techniques. The response to noxious stimulation can also be blocked by local analgesic techniques and these are particularly suitable for use with a continuous infusion of intravenous anaesthetic.

The third modality of balanced anaesthesia, muscle relaxation is provided by muscle relaxant drugs, using the same criteria adopted for other types of anaesthesia.

The technique of total intravenous anaesthesia may be less complicated than other methods that use anaesthetic gases and volatile agents, but does require some reorganisation of the anaesthetic room. An infusion set with an in-line 100 ml burette is prepared and used for successive patients. The burette allows relatively accurate assessment of the quantity of anaesthetic administered and increases the safety of the technique by limiting the dose of drug that could be administered inadvertently. The intravenous anaesthetic is diluted either in the burette or in the infusion bottle, the diluent being any conventional intravenous electrolyte solution. Althesin is usually mixed as 10 ml drug with 90 ml diluent directly into the burette. This concentration allows good control of the level of anaesthesia and simple calculation of the total dose administered. Etomidate is conveniently made up as a solution containing 1 mg drug per ml.

The infusion set is connected to a fine extension tube and a three-way tap. The extension tube is required to prevent accidental contamination of the main infusion system by the patient's blood and the tap is necessary for the administration of other drugs.

The patient is usually premedicated and normally a narcotic drug is included although experience has shown that the combination of papaveretum for pre-medication and fentanyl at induction is likely to cause a short period of apnoea. On arrival in the anaesthetic room a needle is inserted into a vein on the arm or hand and connected to the infusion system. A separate infusion for the administration of intravenous fluids is set up after induction of anaesthesia if it is required.

The patient is preoxygenated according to the anaesthetists' usual practice and the initial dose of narcotic is administered intravenously. Fentanyl 1 μg/kg or pentazocine 0.25 mg/kg[112] have been recommended. Anaesthesia is induced with Althesin, administered as a small bolus dose (2 ml) or by a rapid infusion of the dilute solution (100 drops/min using a Travenol Buretrol system). Larger doses of induction agent are not normally necessary, are more likely to cause cardiovascular depression, and may prolong the recovery time after short procedures.

Once the patient is anaesthetised and it is evident that respiration is not obviously depressed, a second dose of narcotic drug is administered before surgical incision. Thereafter analgesic agents are administered at appropriate intervals, the dose depending upon whether ventilation is spontaneous or controlled. Patients will normally continue to breathe adequately if increments of fentanyl 1 μg/kg are administered every 15 min.

Anaesthesia is maintained by the constant infusion of Althesin. The infusion rate is varied to maintain unconsciousness and precise control is greatly facilitated by the use of an infusion pump. Deepening anaesthesia by increasing the drip rate does not usually prevent a patient responding to noxious stimulation,[75,78] it merely prolongs recovery time. The infusion may be set to drip at 100 drops/min until the time of the surgical incision, provided there is no undue delay. Thereafter, an infusion rate of 50–75 drops/min will maintain unconsciousness although there will be individual variation in the depth of cortical depression. This rate may be reduced to 25 drops/min during final closure of the wound. Normally the infusion is discontinued some 5–10 minutes before the completion of surgery. The mean infusion rate for the last 120 patients anaesthetised in this manner at The London Hospital was 3.4 ml/min of diluted solution (10 per cent v.v.). The total mean dose of Althesin required for induction and 30 minutes of anaesthesia was approximately 11 ml of undiluted drug. Bolus doses of Althesin may also be administered but these can depress markedly the level of cortical activity[74] and prolong recovery time. However, a successful technique using bolus doses without an infusion has been described for short procedures. A mean total dose of 6.9 ml Althesin provided anaesthesia for a mean time of 13.4 min.[112]

Patients breathing spontaneously may be given humidified air with added oxygen to breathe using, for example, the East Radcliffe blower humidifier. When controlled ventilation is required the ventilator used should be capable of administering air with added oxygen. A theoretical inspired oxygen concentration of just less than 30 per cent can be provided by the addition of oxygen at a flow in litres equivalent to 10 per cent of the expired minute volume.[111]

If unconsciosness is not required immediately, for example because an epidural block is to be performed, an infusion of Althesin may be used to provide sedation, the drip rate being adjusted to achieve the desired level.[117] However, patients should always be prepared as for anaesthesia because studies in volunteers have shown that as soon as consciousness is lost the larynx becomes incompetent and radio-opaque dye, placed on the back of the tongue is inhaled into the lung (unpublished findings).

At the end of the procedure the infusion set is disconnected from the three-way tap and extension tubing, capped with a blind hub and subsequently connected to the next patient. The extension tube and tap are discarded.

The quality of anaesthesia was found to be good or satisfactory in over 80 per cent of patients. The main difficulty was some limb movement in response to surgery; the mean incidence in the most recent group of 120 patients was 13 per cent. Movement is now seldom a serious problem and only once in this group of patients was the technique abandoned. Shallow ventilation becomes more common as the dose of fentanyl is increased. Other complications during anaesthesia are rare and have not been serious. However, there is always the possibility that a patient may develop a reaction to Althesin characterised by hypotension and sometimes accompanied by bronchospasm.[118] This is thought to be a reaction induced either as a direct pharmacological effect or as an immune mediated hypersensitivity[120] and has been estimated to occur once every 11 000–19 000 administrations.[119]

The mean recovery time, measured as time from end of surgery to the patient opening eyes on command, following 32 minutes of anaesthesia was some 11 min in the most recent group of 120 patients anaesthetised by this method. Some 30 per cent of the total time the patient was unconscious was spent in the recovery area. However, individuals show marked variation, some being awake at completion of surgery, others remaining unconscious for 30 min or more. It is likely that the technique will improve as experience increases, but for patients breathing spontaneously it is not yet as good as other conventional methods. However, in ventilated patients the technique has considerable potential advantages.

Postoperatively, no specific complication was noticeable but restlessness, weeping, nausea, vomiting and shallow respiration have been noted in a few cases. The incidence is not apparently worse than that after conventional techniques.

The long term adverse effects of Althesin are not known but large doses of the agent have been associated with a significant rise in serum bilirubin. However, this was not more marked than the rise seen with other anaesthetics used for similar procedures.[121] At present there is no evidence to suggest that other anaesthetic agents would be more suitable than Althesin. Initial experience with an etomidate infusion was satisfactory although pain on injection and muscle movement were noted. The mean time to awakening after 35 min of surgery was 15.8 min although in 14 per cent of patients this was more than doubled. The mean dose used for infusion was 114 mg, that is 2.3 mg/min.[63] This may have been an excessive infusion rate and it is likely that the dose will be reduced as experience is gained.

A number of groups have suggested the use of a continuous infusion of dilute ketamine (1 mg/ml) for the maintenance of anaesthesia both during cardiac surgery and other routine procedures.[127–131] Premedication usually includes diazepam and induction of anaesthesia is started by the administration of diazepam 0.3 mg/kg intravenously and supplemented with ketamine 1–1.5 mg/kg. Muscle relaxants are given and anaesthesia is maintained by a slow infusion of ketamine 0.5–0.75 mg/min and nitrous oxide 50 per cent. Although this is not a total intravenous anaesthetic technique it will probably only be a matter of time before the nitrous oxide is replaced by intravenous analgesic drugs.

The technique of intravenous anaesthesia has highlighted a problem that also applies to other techniques. How is it possible to assess depth of anaesthesia so that the patient is unconscious and not aware but at the same time ensure that he is not unnecessarily deeply anaesthetised. The latter is not only potentially dangerous in terms of central nervous system depression but it also indicates that excessive drug has been administered, and will therefore prolong recovery.

The conventional signs of depth of anaesthesia are unreliable and all signs of inadequate anaesthesia can be abolished by drugs that have no anaesthetic potency.[122] The EEG can show changes that reflect the effect of increasing dose of anaesthetic agent[123] but it is impractical to use because it is difficult to interpret, difficult to use, expensive and easily affected by interference. The cerebral function monitor (CFM) developed by Maynard[124] produces a signal derived from the EEG via two biparietal scalp electrodes. The equipment is relatively simple, less expensive, less subject to interference and easier to interpret.[74] The instrument measures voltage between the electrodes and this varies both with amplitude and frequency of cerebral waves. The variation in voltage is plotted with respect to time on a semi-logarithmic scale so that wide variation in cerebral activity can be contained on one trace. The position of the trace on the paper gives an indication of the overall cerebral energy. When used with intravenous anaesthetic agents a characteristic pattern of change is observed and this is most obvious with the barbiturates and Althesin.[74] At induction of anaesthesia the cerebral function monitor trace moves sharply upwards to reach a peak. As anaesthesia becomes effective the trace moves over the peak and is progressively depressed by increasing doses of anaesthetic until the trace becomes flat along the baseline representing absence of cortical activity and very deep anaesthesia.

Studies with slow intravenous infusion show that the patient is not unconscious at the stage of the initial peak on the CFM but is drowsy and amnesic. As the trace is depressed below the peak by more anaesthetic the patient becomes unconscious. The trace moves towards the baseline with increasing depth of anaesthesia becoming broader—an indication of greater variation in energy across the cortex. These changes are suggestive of burst suppression—a stage which has been associated with relatively deep anaesthesia.[125] On discontinuing the intravenous anaesthetic the trace moves up and narrows to reach a second less clearly defined peak, usually lower than the first. At this point the patient is lightly unconscious. Finally, the trace moves from the second peak down towards the original control values and the patient awakes during this final descent.

Some of the landmarks are illustrated in the Figure 1.1. Three doses of Althesin were administered. After the first the typical peak is shown and thereafter the trace is slightly depressed suggesting light anaesthesia. It moves up to a second less defined peak and then descends to the point of awakening which is indicated. A second dose of drug, given when the patient is conscious but before the trace has fully returned to control values, produces similar changes. This time the trace becomes broader and lower suggesting deeper cortical depression and some cumulation of drug effect. Before the patient has time to wake up again, a third dose of anaesthetic is given. Now no peak is seen, merely further depression of the trace to reach an even lower position on the scale. The increased width of the trace suggests burst suppression. It is not difficult to imagine that one could infuse the anaesthetic to maintain a stable level of anaesthesia at some as yet unspecified distance below the initial peak but above the level of burst suppression. In practice this instrument has been found to be an effective method of preventing awareness on the one hand and unnecessary depth of anaesthesia on the other.

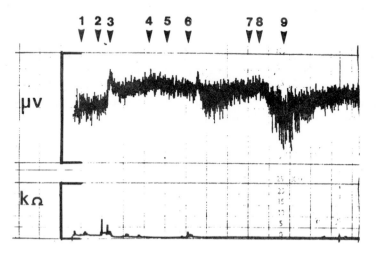

Fig. 1.1   Changes in cerebral function monitor trace following three bolus doses of Althesin (3.0 ml). (1) Awake trace; (2) Induction dose of Althesin (3 ml); (3) First peak; (4) Second peak; (5) Opening eyes and talking; (6) Second dose of Althesin (3 ml); (7) Patient still unconscious; (8) Third dose of Althesin (3 ml); (9) Burst suppression.

An example is illustrated in Figure 1.2. A patient was anaesthetised with an infusion of Althesin and became deeply anaesthetised according to criteria taken from the CFM. Clinically there was no evidence to suggest that anaesthesia was deep and the dose administered was not unusually large. The infusion was discontinued and this led to an upward movement of the trace. When this was thought to reach the appropriate level the infusion was restarted and controlled to keep the CFM trace stable (Fig. 1.2).

A further observation can be made on Figure 1.1. Change from the conscious state to the unconscious state following a dose of intravenous anaesthetic is associated with a peak of increased cerebral activity. In contrast, change from unconsciousness to deeper anaesthesia following a bolus dose is associated with a downward movement of the trace. These two different responses to a dose of anaesthetic drug might be used to distinguish between a patient who is aware during intravenous anaesthesia and a patient who is unconscious.

With the cerebral function monitor one can adjust the dose of intravenous anaesthetic to guarantee unconsciousness something that has not been possible with nitrous oxide anaesthesia. The changes in the CFM during inhalational anaesthesia are probably similar in principle but the variation in the cerebral energy is much less marked and more difficult to follow when using a logarithmic scale. This aspect of the CFM has not yet been properly evaluated. An extra advantage of the cerebral function monitor is that it can indicate the rare catastrophic events such as hypoxia, when cortical activity is suddenly and markedly depressed.[126]

The advantages of total intravenous anaesthesia are indisputable and a technique that is satisfactory for the majority of patients is now being developed. However it has not yet found a place in routine anaesthesia and more work needs to be undertaken to improve the technique and ensure it does not introduce new unwanted complications into anaesthesia.

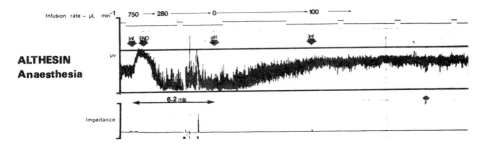

Fig. 1.2 Change in cerebral function monitor during induction and maintenance of anaesthesia with an infusion of Althesin. Note initial peak, deep depression of trace subsequently, movement of trace upwards following discontinuation of infusion and point of restarting infusion. Inf = Infusion of Althesin; ENO = not opening eyes on command

REFERENCES

1. Leonard, P. F. (1975) The lower limits of flammability of halothane, enflurane, and isoflurane. *Anesthesia and Analgesia, Current Researches,* **54,** 238–240.
2. Burchiel, K. J., Stockard, J. J., Myers, R. R. et al (1975) Metabolic and electrophysiologic mechanisms in the initiation and termination of enflurane-induced seizures in man and cats. *Electroencephogr Clin Neurophysiol,* **38,** 555.
3. Julien, R. M. & Kavan, E. M. (1972) Electrographic studies of a new volatile anesthetic agent: enflurane (Ethrane). *Journal of Pharmacology and Experimental Therapeutics,* **183,** 393–403.
4. Ohm, W. W., Cullen, B. F., Amory, D. W. & Kennedy, R. D. (1975) Delayed seizure activity following enflurane anesthesia. *Anesthesiology,* **42,** 367–368.
5. Burchiel, K. J., Stockard, J. J., Calverley, R. K. & Smith, N. Ty. (1977) Relationship of pre- and postanesthetic EEG abnormalities to enflurane-induced seizure activity. *Anesthesia and Analgesia, Current Researches,* **56,** 509–514.
6. Furgang, F. A. & Sohn, J. J. (1977) The effect of thiopentone on enflurane-induced cortical seizures. *British Journal of Anaesthesia,* **49,** 127–132.
7. Michenfelder, J. D. & Cucchiara, R. F. (1974) Canine cerebral oxygen consumption during enflurane anesthesia and its modification during induced seizures. *Anesthesiology,* **40,** 575–580.
8. McKay, R. D., Sundt, T. M., Michenfelder, J. D., Gronert, G. A., Messick, J. M., Sharbrough, F. W. & Piepgras, D. G. (1976) Internal carotid artery stump pressure and cerebral blood flow during carotid endarterectomy. *Anesthesiology,* **45,** 390–399.
9. Miletich, D. J., Ivankovich, A. D., Albrecht, R. F., Reimann, C. R., Rosenberg, R. & McKissic, E. D. (1976) Absence of autoregulation of cerebral blood flow during halothane and enflurane anesthesia. *Anesthesia and Analgesia, Current Researches,* **55,** 100–105.
10. Smith, A. L. & Marque, J. J. (1976) Anesthetics and cerebral edema. *Anesthesiology,* **45,** 64–72.
11. Marshall, B. E., Cohen, P. J., Klingenmaier, C. H., Neigh, J. L. & Pender, J. W. (1971) Some pulmonary and cardiovascular effects of enflurane (Ethrane) anaesthesia with varying $Paco_2$ in man. *British Journal of Anaesthesia,* **43,** 996–1002.

12. Merin, R. G., Kumazawa, T. & Luka, N. L. (1976) Enflurane depresses myocardial function, perfusion, and metabolism in the dog. *Anesthesiology*, **45**, 501–507.
13. Theye, R. A. & Michenfelder, J. D. (1975) Whole-body and organ $\dot{V}o_2$ changes with enflurane, isoflurane, and halothane. *British Journal of Anaesthesia*, **47**, 813–817.
14. Horan, B. F., Prys-Roberts, C., Hamilton, W. K. & Roberts, J. G. (1977) Haemodynamic responses to enflurane anaesthesia and hypovolaemia in the dog, and their modification by propranolol. *British Journal of Anaesthesia*, **49**, 1189–1197.
15. Calverley, R. K., Smith, N. T., Prys-Roberts, C., Eger, E. I., Jones, C. W. & Ramme, F. B. (1975) Cardiovascular effects of prolonged enflurane anesthesia in man. Abstracts of Scientific Papers, American Society of Anesthesiologists Annual Meeting, 57.
16. Ritzman, J. R., Erickson, H. H. & Miller, E. D. (1976) Cardiovascular effects of enflurane and halothane on the rhesus monkey. *Anesthesia and Analgesia, Current Researches*, **55**, 85–91.
17. Kaplan, J. A., Miller, E. D. & Bailey, D. R. (1976) A comparative study of enflurane and halothane using systolic time intervals. *Anesthesia and Analgesia, Current Researches*, **55**, 263–268.
18. Johnston, R. R., Eger, E. I. & Wilson, C. (1976) A comparative interaction of epinephrine with enflurane, isoflurane, and halothane in man. *Anesthesia and Analgesia, Current Researches*, **55**, 709–712.
19. Reisner, L. S. & Lippmann, M. (1975) Ventricular arrhythmias after epinephrine injection in enflurane and in halothane anesthesia. *Anesthesia and Analgesia, Current Researches*, **54**, 468–470.
20. Zarbalian, A., Naraghi, M. & Adriani, J. (1976) The compatibility of exogenous epinephrine with enflurane during surgical anesthesia. *Anesthesiology Review*, August, 16–17.
21. Egilmez, A. & Dobkin, A. B. (1972) Enflurane in man. A clinical evaluation. *Anaesthesia*, **27**, 171.
22. Hirshman, C. A., McCullough, R. E., Cohen, P. J. & Weil, J. V. (1977) Depression of hypoxic ventilatory response by halothane, enflurane and isoflurane in dogs. *British Journal of Anaesthesia*, **49**, 957–963.
23. Dobkin, A. B., Byles, P. H., Africa, B. F. & Levy, A. A. (1976) A comparison of eleven general anaesthetics administered with 7.5 per cent carbon dioxide during spontaneous breathing. *Canadian Anaesthetists' Society Journal*, **23**, 408–424.
24. Coon, R. L. & Kampine, J. P. (1975) Hypocapnic bronchoconstriction and inhalation anesthetics. *Anesthesiology*, **43**, 635–641.
25. Morr-Strathmann, U., Welter, J. & Lawin, P. (1976) The effect of enflurane and halothane on normal values of pulmonary function. Proceeding Belgian Congress of Anaesthesiology, p. 262.
26. Rodriguez, R. & Gold, M. I. (1976) Enflurane as a primary anesthetic agent for patients with chronic obstructive pulmonary disease. *Anesthesia and Analgesia, Current Researches*, **55**, 806–809.
27. Lebowitz, M. H., Blitt, C. D. & Dillon, J. B. (1970) Clinical investigations of compound 347 (Ethrane). *Anesthesia Analgesia (Cleveland)*, **49**, 1–10.
28. Botty, C., Brown, B., Stanley, V. et al (1968) Clinical experience with compound 347, a halogenated anesthetic agent. *Anesthesia Analgesia (Cleveland)*, **47**, 499–505.
29. Waud, B. E. & Waud, D. R. (1975) The effects of diethyl ether, enflurane, and isoflurane at the neuromuscular junction. *Anesthesiology*, **42**, 275–280.
30. Waud, B. E. & Waud, D. R. (1975) Comparison of the effects of general anesthetics on the end-plate of skeletal muscle. *Anesthesiology*, **43**, 540–547.
31. Fogdall, R. P. & Miller, R. D. (1975) Neuromuscular effects of enflurane, alone and combined with d-tubocurarine, pancuronium, and succinylcholine, in man. *Anesthesiology*, **42**, 173–178.
32. Coleman, A. J. & Downing, J. W. (1975) Enflurane anesthesia for cesarean section. *Anesthesiology*, **43**, 354–357.
34. Chase, R. E., Holaday, D. A., Fiserova-Bergerova, V., Saidman, L. J. & Mack, F. E. (1971) The biotransformation of ethrane in man. *Anesthesiology*, **35**, 262–267.
35. Corall, I. M., Knights, K. & Strunin, L. (1977) Enflurane anaesthesia in man. Metabolism and effects on biochemical and haematological variables. *British Journal of Anaesthesia*, **49**, 881.
36. Cousins, M. J., Greenstein, L. R., Hitt, B. A. & Mazze, R. I. (1976) Metabolism and renal effects of enflurane in man. *Anesthesiology*, **44**, 44–53.
37. Cousins, M. J. & Mazze, R. I. (1973) Methoxyflurane nephrotoxicity: a study of dose-response in man. *Journal of the American Medical Association*, **225**, 1611–1616.
38. Cousins, M. J., Mazze, R. I., Kosek, J. C. et al (1974) The etiology of methoxyflurane nephrotoxicity. *Journal Pharmacology & Experimental Therapeutics*, **190**, 530–541.
39. Eger, E. I., Calverley, R. K. & Smith, N. T. (1976) Changes in blood chemistries following prolonged enflurane anesthesia. *Anesthesia and Analgesia, Current Researches*, **55**, 547–549.
40. Loehning, R. & Mazze, R. I. (1974) Renal dysfunction following enflurane anesthesia: report of a case. *Anesthesiology*, **40**, 203–205.
41. Hartnett, M. N., Lane, W. & Bennett, W. M. (1974) Non-oliguric renal failure and enflurane. *Annals of Internal Medicine*, **81**, 560.

42. Berman, M. L., Green, O. C., Calverley, R. K., Smith, N. T. & Eger, E. I. (1976) Enzyme induction by enflurane in man. *Anesthesiology*, **44**, 496–500.
43. Eichhorn, J. H., Hedley-Whyte, J., Steinman, T. I., Kaufmann, J. M. & Laasberg, L. H. (1976) Renal failure following enflurane anesthesia. *Anesthesiology*, **45**, 557–560.
44. Denlinger, J. K., Lecky, J. H. & Nahrwold, M. L. (1974) Hepatocellular dysfunction without jaundice after enflurane anesthesia. *Anesthesiology*, **41**, 86–87.
45. Reis, L. V. D., Askin, S. J., Frecker, G. N. & Fitzgerald, W. J. (1974) Hepatic necrosis after enflurane anesthesia. *Journal of the American Medical Association*, **227**, 76.
46. Caropreso, P. R., Gittleman, M. A., Reilly, D. J. & Patterson, L. T. (1975) Malignant hyperthermia associated with enflurane anesthesia. *Archives of Surgery*, **110**, 1491–1493.
47. Pan, T.-H., Wollack, A. R. & DeMarco, J. A. (1975) Malignant hyperthermia associated with enflurane anesthesia: a case report. *Anesthesia and Analgesia, Current Researches*, **54**, 47–49.
48. Duncan, P. G., Cullen, B. F., Calverly, R., Smith, N. T., Eger, E. I. & Bone, R. (1976) Failure of enflurane and halothane anesthesia to inhibit lymphocyte transformation in volunteers. *Anesthesiology*, **45**, 661–665.
49. Sturrock, J. E. (1977) No mutagenic effect of enflurane on cultured cells. *British Journal of Anaesthesia*, **49**, 777–779.
50. Doenicke, A., Kugler, J., Penzel, G., Laub, M., Kalmar, L., Killian, J. & Bezecny, H. (1973) Hirnfunktion und toleranzbreite nach etomidate, einen neuer barbituratfreien i.v. applizierbaren hypnoticum. *Anaesthesist*, **22**, 357–366.
51. Janssen, P. A. J., Niemegeers, C. J. E., Schellekens, R. H. L. & Lenaerts, F. M. (1971) Etomidate, R-(+)-ethyl-1-1-(a-methyl-benzyl)-immidazole-5-carboxylate (R 16 659), a potent, short-acting, relatively atoxic intravenous hypnotic agent in rats. *Arzneimittelforschung (Drug Res.)*, **21**, 1234.
52. Hendry, J. G. B., Miller, B. M. & Lees, N. W. (1977) Etomidate in a new solvent. *Anaesthesia*, **32**, 996–999.
53. Meuldermans, W. & Heykants, J. (1975) The plasma protein binding and distribution of etomidate in dog, rat and human blood. *Biological Research Report R26490/14*, Janssen Pharmaceuticals.
54. Heykants, J. J. P., Meuldermans, W. E. G., Michiels, L. J. M., Lewi, P. J. & Janssen, P. A. J. (1975) Distribution, metabolism and excretion of etomidate, a short-acting hypnotic drug, in the rat. Comparative study of (R)-(+) and (S)-(−)-etomidate. *Archives internationales de Pharmacodynamie et de Thérapie*, **216**, 113–124.
55. Ambre, J. J., Hamme, M. J. V., Ghoneim, M. M. & Gross, E. G. (1977) Pharmacokinetics of etomidate, a new intravenous anesthetic. *Federation Proceedings*, **36**, 997.
56. Heykants, J., Brugmans, G. & Doenicke, A. (1973) On the pharmacokinetics of etomidate (R26490) in human volunteers: plasma levels, metabolism and excretion. *Clinical Research Report*. Janssen Pharmaceuticals.
57. Morgan, M., Lumley, J. & Whitwam, J. G. (1975) Etomidate, a new water-soluble non-barbiturate intravenous induction agent. *The Lancet*, **1**, 955.
58. Famewo, C. E. & Odugbesan, C. O. (1977) Clinical trial of etomidate. Preliminary observations on a new non-barbiturate induction agent. *Canadian Anaesthetists' Society Journal*, **24**, 35–38.
59. Ghoneim, M. M. & Yamada, T. (1977) Etomidate: a clinical and electroencephalographic comparison with thiopental. *Anesthesia and Analgesia, Current Researches*, **56**, 479–485.
60. Brückner, J. B., Marquandt, B., Rahmann, M. K., Passian, J. & Weymar, A. (1974) Induction of anaesthesia with etomidate. Results of clinical tests. Institute for Anaesthesiology of the Free University of Berlin.
61. Van de Walle, J., Lauwers, P., Adriaensen, H. & Demeyere, R. (1976) Clinical study on etomidate. *Acta Anaesthesiologica Belgica*, **27**, Suppl., 139–142.
62. Kay, B. (1976) A dose-response relationship for etomidate, with some observations on cumulation. *British Journal of Anaesthesia*, **48**, 213–216.
63. O'Carroll, T. M. (1977) Total intravenous anaesthesia with etomidate and fentanyl. March 1977. Annual Scientific Meeting for Junior Anaesthetists, Cambridge.
64. O'Carroll, T. M., Blogg, C. E., Hoinville, E. A. & Savege, T. M. (1977) Etomidate in electroconvulsive therapy. *Anaesthesia*, **32**, 868–872.
65. Foley, E. I., Walton, B., Savege, T. M., Strunin, L. & Simpson, B. R. (1972) A comparison of recovery times between althesin and methohexitone following anaesthesia for electro-convulsive therapy. *Postgraduate Medical Journal*, June Supplement, 112–115.
66. Rombout, N., De Cree, J., Jageneau, A. (1975) *Clinical Research Report, R26490/6*. Janssen Pharmaceuticals.
67. Lees, N. W. & Hendry, J. G. B. (1977) Etomidate in urological outpatient anaesthesia. *Anaesthesia*, **32**, 592–602.
68. Holdcroft, A., Morgan, M., Whitwam, J. G. & Lumley, J. (1976) Effect of dose and

premedication on induction complications with etomidate. *British Journal of Anaesthesia*, **48**, 199–204.

69. Kugler, J. & Doenicke, A. (1973) The EEG after etomidate. Departments of Neurophysiology and Anaesthesia, The Surgical Polyclinic, Munich University.

70. Ingram, G. S., Payne, J. P. & Perry, I. R. (1976) Electroencephalographic patterns during anaesthetic induction with etomidate. *British Journal of Clinical Pharmacology*, **3**, 2.

71. Mol, J. H. F. & Lelkens, J. P. M. EEG evaluation during sleep induced by etomidate or thiopental. *Clinical Research Report R26490/13*, Janssen Pharmaceuticals.

72. Scott, D. F. & Virden, S. (1972) Comparison of the effect of Althesin with other induction agents on electroencephalographic patterns. *Postgraduate Medical Journal*, June Suppl. 93–96.

73. Sabathié, M. & Renou, A. (1975) Induction and maintenance of anaesthesia with etomidate in 34 patients with epilepsy. Hôpital Saint-André, Bordeaux, France.

74. Dubois, M., Savege, T. M., O'Carroll, T. M. & Frank, M. (1978) General anaesthesia and changes on the cerebral function monitor. *Anaesthesia*, **33**, 157–164.

75. Kay, B. (1976) A clinical assessment of the use of etomidate in children. *British Journal of Anaesthesia*, **48**, 107–211.

76. Thomas, B., Meirlaen, L., Rolly, G. & Weyne, L. (1976) Clinical use of etomidate. *Acta Anaesthesiologica Belgica*, **27**, Suppl., 167–174.

77. Savege, T. M., Foley, E. I., Coultas, R. J., Walton, B., Strunin, L., Simpson, B. R. & Scott, D. F. (1971) CT1341: some effects in man. Cardiorespiratory, electroencephalographic and biochemical measurements. *Anaesthesia*, **26**, 402–413.

78. Savege, T. M., Dubois, M., Frank, M. & Holly, J. M. P. (1978) Preliminary investigation into a new method of assessing the quality of anaesthesia: the cardiovascular response to a measured noxious stimulus. *British Journal of Anaesthesia*, **50**, 481.

79. Gooding, J. M. & Corssen, G. (1976) Etomidate: an ultrashort-acting nonbarbiturate agent for anesthesia induction. *Anesthesia and Analgesia, Current Researches*, **55**, 286–289.

80. Doenicke, A., Gabanyi, D., Lemcke, H. & Schurk-Bulich, M. (1974) Circulatory behaviour and myocardial function after the administration of three short-acting I.V. hypnotics Etomidate, Propanidid and Methohexital. *Anaesthetist*, **23**, 108–115.

81. Fragen, R. J., Caldwell, N. & Brunner, E. A. (1976) Clinical use of etomidate for anesthesia induction: a preliminary report. *Anesthesia and Analgesia, Current Researches*, **55**, 730–733.

82. Kettler, D., Sonntag, H., Donath, U., Regensburger, D. & Schenk, H. D. (1974) Haemodynamics, myocardial function, oxygen requirement and oxygen supply of the human heart after the administration of etomidate. *Anaesthesist*, **23**, 116–121.

83. Dubois-Primo, J., Bastenier-Geens, J., Genicot, C. & Rucquoi, M. (1976) A comparative study of etomidate and methohexital as induction agents for analgesic anesthesia. *Acta Anaesthesiologica Belgica*, **27**, 187–195.

84. Schuermans, V., Dom, J., Dony, J., Scheijgrond, H. & Brugmans, J. (1977) Multinational evaluation of etomidate for anesthesia induction conclusions and consequences. *Anaesthesist*, **26**, 1.

85. Rifat, K., Gamulin, Z. & Gemperle, M. (1976) Etomidate: effets cardio-vasculaires du nouvel agent anesthesique intraveineux. *Canadian Anaesthetists' Society Journal*, **23**, 492–503.

86. Colvin, M. P., Savege, T. M., Newland, P., Weaver, E. J. M., Waters, A., Innis, R. & Brookes, J. (1978) The cardiorespiratory effects of etomidate in patients with cardiac disease. In preparation.

87. Patschke, D., Brückner, J. B., Eberlein, H. J., Hess, W., Tarnow, J. & Weymar, A. (1977) Effects of althesin, etomidate and fentanyl on haemodynamics and myocardial oxygen consumption in man. *Canadian Anaesthetists' Society Journal*, **24**, 57–69.

88. Dundee, J. W. (1978) Total intravenous anaesthesia. *British Journal of Anaesthesia*, **50**, 89–90.

89. Herrschaft, H., Schmidt, H. et al (1975) The response of humans' cerebral blood flow to anaesthesia with thiopentone, methohexitone, propandid and etomidate. *Advances in Neurosurgery*, 3rd edition, p. 120, Springer-Verlag.

90. Famewo, C. E., Odugbesan, C. O. & Osuntokun, O. O. (1977) Effect of etomidate on intra-ocular pressure. *Canadian Anaesthetists' Society Journal*, **24**, 712–716.

91. Morgan, M., Lumley, J. & Whitwam, J. G. (1977) Respiratory effects of etomidate. *British Journal of Anaesthesia*, **49**, 233–236.

92. Hempelmann, G., Hempelmann, W., Piepenbrock, S., Oster, W. & Karlinzek, G. (1974) Blood gas analyses and haemodynamic studies on heart surgery patients using etomidate. *Acta Anaesthesiologica Belgica*, **23**, 423–429.

93. Admiraal, P., Schellenberger, A., Doenicke, A., Spiess, K., Bruckner, J., Popescu, D. & Bergmann, H. (1975) Induction of anaesthesia with etomidate. Analysis and tabulation of 1,000 case records of clinical studies. *Report*. Janssen Pharmaceuticals.

94. Zacharias, M., Clarke, R. S. J., Dundee, J. W. & Johnston, S. B. (1978) An evaluation of three preparations of etomidate. *British Journal of Anaesthesia*, in press.

95. Zacharias, M., Dundee, J. W. & Clarke, R. S. L. (1978) Evaluation of etomidate. *British Journal of Anaesthesia*, **50,** 633.
96. Doenicke, A., Lorenz, W., Beigl, R., Bezecny, H., Uhlig, G., Kalmar, L., Praetorius, B. & Mann, G. (1973) Histamine release after intravenous application of short-acting hypnotics. A comparison of etomidate, althesin (CT 1341) and propanidid. *British Journal of Anaesthesia*, **45,** 1097–1104.
97. Lorenz, W., Doenicke, A., Meyer, R., Reimann, H. J., Kusche, J., Barth, H., Geesing, H., Hutzel, M. & Weissenbacker, B. (1972) Histamine release in man by propanidid and thiopentone: pharmacological effects and clinical consequences. *British Journal of Anaesthesia*, **44,** 355.
98. Fisher, M. McD. (1975) Severe histamine mediated reactions to intravenous drugs used in anaesthesia. *Anaesthesia and Intensive Care*, **3,** 180–197.
99. Halford, F. J. (1943) A critique of intravenous anesthesia in war surgery. *Anesthesiology*, **4,** 67.
100. Hunter, A. R. (1972) Thiopentone supplemented anaesthesia for intracranial surgery. *British Journal of Anaesthesia*, **44,** 506.
101. Fletcher, R. (1976) A method of anaesthesia for fractional coagulation of the Gasserian ganglion. Intermittent anaesthesia with propanidid. *Anaesthesia*, **31,** 1280–1284.
102. Browne, O'D. (1950) The treatment of eclampsia. *Journal of Obstetrics and Gynaecology British Empire*, **57,** 573.
103. Bourne, J. G. (1960) *Nitrous Oxide in Dentistry, Its Danger and Alternatives.* London: Lloyd-Luke (Medical Books) Ltd.
104. Tunstall, M. E. (1977) Detecting wakefulness during general anaesthesia for caesarean section. *British Medical Journal*, **1,** 1321.
105. Utting, J. E. (1975) Phillip Gett memorial lecture. Awareness in anaesthesia. *Anaesthesia and Intensive Care*, **3,** 334–340.
106. Cheek, D. B. (1964) Further evidence of persistence of hearing under chemo-anesthesia: detailed case report. *American Journal of Clinical Hypnosis*, **7,** 55.
107. Cheek, D. B. (1966) The meaning of continued hearing sense under general chemo-anesthesia: a progress report and report of a case. *American Journal of Clinical Hypnosis*, **8,** 275.
108. *Criteria for a recommended standard-occupational exposure to waste anaesthetic gases and vapours.* Report published by National Institute of Occupational Safety and Health, United States of America, March, 1977.
109. Rees, G. J. & Gray, T. C. (1950) Methyl-n-propyl ether. *British Journal of Anaesthesia*, **22,** 83.
110. Cailar, J. Du. (1972) The effects in man of infusions of Althesin with particular regard to the cardiovascular system. *Postgraduate Medical Journal*, June Suppl. 72–79.
111. Savege, T. M., Ramsay, M. A. E., Curran, J. P. J., Cotter, J., Walling, P. T. & Simpson, B. R. (1975) Intravenous anaesthesia by infusion. A technique using alphaxolone/alphadolone (Althesin). *Anaesthesia*, **30,** 757–764.
112. Jago, R. H. & Restall, J. (1977) Total intravenous anaesthesia. A technique based on alphaxalone/alphadolone and pentazocine. *Anaesthesia*, **32,** 904–907.
113. Dechêne, J. P. (1977) Alfathesin by continuous infusion supplemented with intermittent pentazocine. *Canadian Anaesthetists' Society Journal*, **24,** 702.
114. Hall, G. M., Young, C., Holdcroft, A. & Alaghband-Zadeh, J. (1978) Substrate mobilisation during surgery. A comparison between halothane and fentanyl anaesthesia. *Anaesthesia*, in press.
115. George, J. M., Reier, C. E., Lanese, R. R. & Rower, M. J. (1974) Morphine anesthesia blocks cortisol and growth hormone response to surgical stress in humans. *Journal of Clinical Endocrinology and Metabolism*, **38,** 736.
116. Adams, A. P. & Pybus, D. A. (1978) Delayed respiratory depression after use of fentanyl during anaesthesia. *British Medical Journal*, **1,** 278.
117. Ramsay, M. A. E., Savege, T. M., Simpson, B. R. J. & Goodwin, R. (1974) Controlled sedation with alphaxalone-alphadolone. *British Medical Journal*, **2,** 656–659.
118. Clarke, R. S. J., Dundee, J. W., Garrett, R. T., McArdle, G. K. & Sutton, J. A. (1975) Adverse reactions to intravenous anaesthetics. A survey of 100 reports. *British Journal of Anaesthesia*, **47,** 575.
119. Dundee, J. W. (1976) Hypersensitivity to intravenous anaesthetic agents. *British Journal of Anaesthesia*, **48,** 57.
120. Watkins, J., Udnoon, S., Appleyard, T. N. & Thornton, J. A. (1976) Identification and quantitation of hypersensitivity reactions to intravenous anaesthetic agents. *British Journal of Anaesthesia*, **48,** 457.
121. Clarke, R. S. J., Dundee, J. W., Doggart, J. R. & Lavery, T. (1974) The effects of single and intermittent administrations of althesin and other intravenous anesthetic agents on liver function. *Anesthesia and Analgesia, Current Researches*, **53,** 461.
122. Robson, J. G. (1969) Measurement of depth of anaesthesia. *British Journal of Anaesthesia*, **41,** 785.

123. Marshall, M., Longley, B. P. & Stanton, W. H. (1965) Electroencephalography in anaesthetic practice. *British Journal of Anaesthesia*, 37, 845.
124. Maynard, M., Prior, P. F. & Scott, D. F. (1969) Device for continuous monitoring of cerebral activity in resuscitated patients. *British Medical Journal*, 4, 545–546.
125. Faulconer, A. & Bickford, R. G. (1960) *Electroencephalography in Anaesthesia*. C. C. Thomas, Springfield, Illinois, U.S.A.
126. Schwartz, M. S., Colvin, M. P., Prior, P. F., Strunin, L., Simpson, B. R., Weaver, E. J. M. & Scott, D. F. (1973) The cerebral function monitor. *Anaesthesia*, 28, 611–618.
127. Chodoff, P. & Stella, J. G. (1966) Use of CI 581. *Anesthesia and Analgesia, Current Researches*, 45, 527.
128. Hatano, S., Keane, D. M., Boggs, R. E., El-Naggar, M. A. & Sadone, M. S. (1976) Diazepam-ketamine anesthesia for open heart surgery. A 'micro-mini' drip administration technique. *Canadian Anaesthetists' Society Journal*, 23, 648.
129. El-Naggar, M., Letcher, J., Middleton, E. & Levine, H. (1977) Administration of ketamine or innovar by the microdrip technic: a double blind study. *Anesthesia and Analgesia, Current Researches*, 56, 279.
130. Steen, S. N., Lippman, M. & Mok, M. S. (1978) Continuous drip low dose ketamine in general anaesthesia. V European Congress of Anaesthesiology. International Congress Series 452, abstract 253. Excerpta Medica, Amsterdam.
131. O'Dwyer, H. S. (1978) An assessment of ketamine hydrochloride by continuous intravenous infusion for elective intra-abdominal surgery. V European Congress of Anaesthesiology. International Congress Series 452, abstract 248. Excerpta Medica, Amsterdam.

2. Anaesthetic circuits and flexible pipelines for medical gases

A. P. Adams   J. D. Henville

This chapter is concerned with the delivery of anaesthetic gases to patients. The co-axial and circle systems have been the subject of recent interest, partly because of their possible advantages in relation to theatre pollution, and they are considered in some detail here. Flexible pipelines and their connections to anaesthetic machines is another important subject in the light of accidents which have been reported and a discussion on safety aspects and testing is included.

CO-AXIAL CIRCUITS

The Bain circuit

The Bain circuit (Fig. 2.1) was described by Bain and Spoerel of the University of Western Ontario in 1972. The circuit is a lightweight streamlined breathing attachment nearly 2 m long and was designed to facilitate general anaesthesia for head and neck surgery or in situations where the anaesthetic machine is remote from the patient.

The principle of the Bain system was used by Macintosh and Pask during the Second World War to administer ether-air anaesthesia delivered from an Oxford Vaporiser by an Oxford Inflating Bellows to a spontaneously breathing subject during experiments designed to assess the buoyant qualities of various life-jackets used by Allied forces. The design of life-jackets at that time was such that an unconscious airman who 'ditched' would not always be self-righted by his jacket so that the face was not clear of the water.[1,2]

A dummy could not be used for these tests because of the difference in density from a man. Accordingly, the anaesthetist E. A. Pask was repeatedly anaesthetised and acted as the 'subject'.[3] The testing conditions also required that the anaesthetic attachment did not disturb the buoyancy of the anaesthetised man in his life-jacket. A lightweight single-limb co-axial breathing system of up to 20 feet long was devised which did not affect the buoyancy of the subject or cause drag and which provided venting of expired gases remotely from the subject without permitting rebreathing. The experiments were conducted in the swimming pool of an Oxford school and later in a tank at Ealing Film Studios, London. An airman was set on guard at the point of exit of waste gases; he had a large notice around his neck 'Danger—No Smoking'![4]

The Bain circuit (i.e. the North American version of the circuit described by Bain and Spoerel) comprises a 1.8 m length of corrugated plastic tubing 22 mm in diameter, through whose length runs a small-bore tube of approximately 7 mm o.d. which delivers fresh gases from the anaesthetic machine to the patient (distal) end of the circuit.[5] The system is therefore a form of T-piece and may be regarded as a form of Mapleson E circuit.[6] Attachment of an expiratory valve and a reservoir bag to the non-patient end of the circuit converts it into a Mapleson D system (Fig. 2.1). It must be emphasised that the inner tube of the Bain circuit is purely a means of delivering the fresh gases directly to the patient's mouth. The patient breathes through the annular space or outer tube. The Bain circuit thus differs fundamentally from the Lack co-axial circuit (vide infra) in which the inner tube provides the route for expiration and the outer tube that for inspiration.

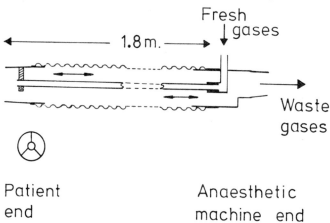

Fig. 2.1   Diagram of the Bain circuit distributed by Respiratory Care Inc., U.S.A. The anaesthetic machine end of the circuit is connected to a reservoir bag and a spill valve.

The outer tube of the Bain circuit was made of an electrically conductive opaque plastic material but a transparent non-conductive version later became available; this was an important development because it allowed some inspection of the inner tube within the circuit. Disconnection of the inner tube from its mount at the non-patient or proximal end of the circuit created a greatly increased apparatus deadspace. The Bain circuit uses a 15 mm ISO taper at this end of the circuit. A combined adaptor (Canox Ltd.) can be used to accommodate the reservoir bag and expiratory valve as well as to mount the proximal end of the circuit onto a rail fitted on the front of the anaesthetic machine.[7]

The Penlon Company has introduced a modified version of the Bain circuit called the Penlon co-axial circuit.[8] The inner tube of the Penlon co-axial circuit is made of antistatic material with electrical continuity at both ends of the circuit; the outer tube is transparent. The advantage of the Penlon circuit is that it can be fitted directly to the outlet of the anaesthetic machine by means of a co-axial circuit valve (Fig. 2.2). Fresh gases are passed straight through the valve unit via a metal tube to which is connected the inner tube of the co-axial breathing circuit. The expiratory valve is of the shrouded type for connection to a waste or scavenging system and is used to spill excess gas from the outer tube of the circuit. The original Bain circuit can be used with this Penlon co-axial valve by simply cutting off the 15 mm adaptor at the proximal end of this circuit and making the appropriate connections of the tubing to the valve. Original versions of the Penlon co-axial valve were made of metal but later versions were made of transparent plastic so that the movement of the valve could be observed during spontaneous ventilation. These valves are cumbersome and some have too-high a resistance; an improved version is currently being developed. Other forms of valve and means of conducting the fresh gases from the anaesthetic machine to the inner tube of the circuit have been described.[9,10]

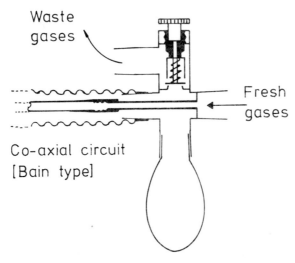

Waste gases

Fresh gases

Co-axial circuit [Bain type]

Fig. 2.2   Diagram of the Penlon co-axial circuit. The valve connector (a) directs the flow of gases, (b) forms a spill valve, (c) forms an attachment for the reservoir bag, and (d) forms a taper to connect with the fresh gas outlet from the anaesthetic machine.

Advantages of the Bain and Penlon co-axial circuits
Mapleson originally described five semi-closed anaesthetic circuits and the economy of fresh gas flow in them.[6] The D system is-first choice for controlled ventilation and is second choice for spontaneous ventilation. The A system (Magill attachment) is the last choice for controlled ventilation and is first choice for spontaneous ventilation. The Bain system can be used for children as well as for adults. Because of these overall considerations the Bain (D/E) system appears to justify consideration as a universal circuit.[11,12]

The Bain circuit is especially useful where access to the patient is limited (e.g. head and neck surgery, risks from procedures involving radiation), it causes minimal drag on the endotracheal tube or mask and it facilitates the scavenging of expired gases from the anaesthetic machine (proximal) end of the circuit. Interchange between spontaneous and controlled ventilation is easily made because the valve is situated at the anaesthetic machine end of the circuit. A further advantage during head and neck surgery is that exhaled gases are not spilled near the surgical site thus reducing the risk of flash fires. The humidity delivered by the Bain circuit in laboratory tests is satisfactory and is consistently above that delivered from the circle absorber at comparable flow rates and minute volumes.[13]

An important development following the introduction of the Bain circuit into anaesthesia has been the use of small inexpensive lung ventilators to provide controlled ventilation.[14-17] The ventilator and Bain circuit are connected by a standard 1 m length of corrugated anaesthetic breathing hose (Fig. 2.3). The interposition of this length of hose prevents the driving gas of the ventilator (air or oxygen) from diluting the anaesthetic gas mixture breathed by the patient.[18]

Another advantage of the Bain system with IPPV is that it permits the use of large tidal volumes, e.g. up to 15 ml/kg body weight, without concomitant hypocapnia. Hence the functional residual capacity of the lung and arterial oxygenation are maintained without the washout of CO_2 from the body which leads to depression of cardiac output during operations[19] and respiratory inadequacy in the post-operative period.[20]

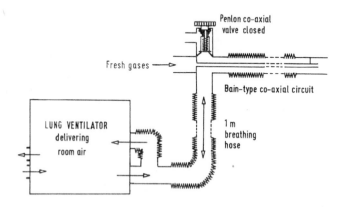

Fig. 2.3   Diagram showing the mode of connexion of a conventional lung ventilator to the Penlon co-axial circuit. The twin patient breathing hose from the ventilator has been shortened to avoid unnecessary tubing. Note the interposition of a length of standard 'elephant hose' between the co-axial circuit and the lung ventilator to prevent the air delivered to the ventilator from reaching the patient (see text).

The resistance of the Penlon co-axial circuit at 30 litres/min is less than 0.5 cm H_2O; that of the Bain circuit at a comparable flow rate is less than 0.7 cm H_2O.[21] Both these figures refer to tests without consideration of the resistance of the expiratory valve. The resistance of these expiratory valves varies considerably according to manufacturer and usage. Some of the original valves supplied with the Penlon co-axial circuit were of unduly high resistance. The main factor causing this resistance is the mass of the spring; using the valve in an inverted position overcomes the problem. However, recent improvements in manufacture have reduced the resistance of these valves.[22]

Hazards of the Bain circuit

Mention has already been made of the risk of accidental disconnection of the inner gas supply tube from its connector at the anaesthetic machine end of the circuit. This fault was especially likely to arise in the Bain circuit because of repeated cleansing and stretching of an item originally intended to be disposable.[23] Early versions of the Bain circuit were prone to weakness of the attachments of the outer tube at either end of the circuit. This problem was accentuated by attempts to investigate the construction of the circuit or to check the integrity of the joint on the inner tube. Improved manufacturing methods have reduced this problem and the circuits can withstand repeated cleaning and sterilizing processes.

The use of the Canox attachment[7] (*vide supra*) has led to a hazard in which the supply of fresh gas has been accidentally connected to the outer tube instead of the inner tube, hence creating a large apparatus deadspace.[24]

Another problem which can occur is that the inner gas delivery tube can become doubled-back on itself (Z-effect) so causing total obstruction to the delivery of fresh gases to the patient.[25] This can happen if the inner tube is too long relative to the outer tube; the fault may also occur if the outer tube of a Penlon co-axial circuit has been deliberately shortened. A double-length version (4 m long) of the Penlon co-axial circuit is produced for special situations; particular care should be taken with these special circuits as the Z-effect is more likely to occur. For this reason these 4 m length circuits are not advised for routine use but should be kept for the special situations for which they are intended (e.g. radiation hazards).

The high resistance of the inner delivery tube in the circuit 'can lead to problems. Frequent disconnection and reconnection of the inner tube to the metal mount of the Penlon co-axial valve unit may eventually cause a weakness in the hose at this junction. A small leak may be produced at this point with the effect that the flow of fresh gas reaching the patient through the length of high-resistance narrow tube is reduced. A similar problem occurs if there is a leak at connections between the anaesthetic flowmeters and the proximal end of the circuit. Some anaesthetic machines are fitted with a pressure-relief valve on the backbar;[26] if this valve is set at low values, operation of the emergency oxygen switch can lead to loss of some of this supply through the relief-valve in the face of the downstream resistance offered by the inner hose of the Bain circuit. A similar consideration applies to other circuits fed by narrow-bore tubing, e.g. the Water's to-and-fro system, children's T-piece circuits and some forms of the circle.

Co-axial circuits should not be used with intermittent-flow anaesthetic machines, e.g. those used for dental anaesthesia. The sub-atmospheric pressure generated by the patient's inspiratory efforts cannot be transmitted through the high resistance of the inner tube of the circuit to the demand valve of the machine and so no fresh gases are delivered to the circuit. Adjustment of the anaesthetic machine to provide a continuous and adequate flow of fresh gases overcomes this problem; such adjustment should preferably be permanent and the adequacy of flow periodically checked.

Testing of Bain and Penlon co-axial circuits
The test suggested by Pethick for the Bain circuit aims to prove the integrity of connection of the inner tube by operating the oxygen bypass and observing whether the reservoir bag deflates or inflates.[27] Deflation of the bag suggests that the continuity of the inner tube is intact, i.e. the high flow through the inner tube lowers the pressure in the outer tube by a venturi effect. The bag inflates if the connection is broken. However, we have not found this test to be reliable and do not recommend it. The following checks for the Penlon co-axial circuit are suggested:

1. The connections to the fresh gas outlet from the flowmeters and the anaesthetic machine must be secure and free of leaks
2. The inner tube of the co-axial circuit must be secure at both ends
3. The complete assembly (valve and circuit) should be fitted to the anaesthetic machine and the valve closed.

The outer tube is detached at the anaesthetic machine (proximal) end, and a flow of oxygen, e.g. 4 litre/min, is turned on. The flow of gas at the patient end of the circuit should be confirmed by holding this end close to the skin. The outer tube is then securely refitted and the inner tube then checked internally along its whole length for kinks or excessive twisting; re-check that oxygen still flows from the patient end of the circuit. The outer tube (not the inner tube) at the patient end of the circuit is then blocked and the oxygen bypass control operated, so allowing the reservoir bag to inflate. The circuit valve is then opened to discharge the oxygen and the supply then turned off.

I.P.P.V. with the Bain system

During controlled ventilation mathematical and experimental analysis shows that system D is the most efficient and system A the least efficient of the original five systems described by Mapleson.[6] The patient's $Paco_2$ is entirely determined by the flow rate of fresh gases into the Bain circuit provided that this flow rate is exceeded by the minute volume of ventilation. A fresh gas flow rate of 70 ml/kg body weight/min has been found to achieve normocapnia, and a flow rate of 100 ml/kg body weight/min achieves mild hyperventilation.[11,28,29,30] A 70 kg adult would therefore receive a total flow of almost 5 litres/min; in practice the flow is set to the nearest convenient marks on the anaesthetic flowmeters, say, 2 litres/min O_2 and 4 litres/min N_2O on modern machines (Fig. 2.4).

This relation between fresh gas inflow to the Bain circuit and $Paco_2$ holds for patients above a weight of 40 kg.[11] Below this weight the metabolic rate and therefore the amount of CO_2 produced in proportion to body weight is higher. Bain and Spoerel recommended a minimum fresh gas inflow of 3.5 litres/min for patients weighing less than 50 kg because of the difficulty in setting accurate flows below this level. A minimum flow of about 3 litres/min has been found necessary with small children and babies. However, flows of this magnitude convert the system into a non-rebreathing system and thus minute ventilation, and not fresh gas flow, determines the $Paco_2$. Rayburn and Graves used the Bain circuit to predict $Paco_2$ from fresh gas flow in babies and children of weights 5–50 kg. A ventilation of three times the predicted alveolar ventilation provided good mixing in the exhalation limb of the Bain circuit thereby giving a constant concentration of mixed expired carbon dioxide.[31] Under these conditions these authors found that a fresh gas flow rate which was approximately equal to the alveolar ventilation appeared sufficient to maintain near-normal $Paco_2$. The alveolar ventilation in these experiments was calculated as equal to twenty times the CO_2 production (Vco_2 at S.T.P.D.), where Vco_2 was assumed to be about 100 ml/m^2 surface area/min.

Spontaneous ventilation with the Bain system

It is unfortunate that some authors have confused the flow rates of 70 ml/kg body weight/min recommended for the Bain circuit using controlled ventilation with the flow rates required for spontaneous breathing.[32] It has long been established that higher flow rates of fresh gas are necessary during spontaneous breathing than with controlled ventilation with the D and E circuits.[6] Recent work suggests that rebreathing does not occur with the Rees modified T-piece until the fresh gas inflow is reduced to twice the patient's minute volume.[33,34] A recent study of the Bain circuit recommends a fresh gas flow of at least three times the minute volume; this study refers to only a few awake volunteers and does not consider any effect of the ratio of inspiration to expiration (I:E ratio).[35] It might be expected that a high I:E ratio would favour the use of lower fresh gas

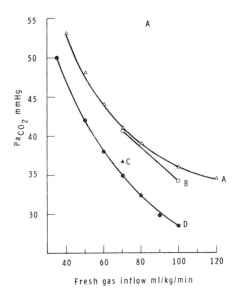

Fig. 2.4   Graph of the relation between arterial carbon dioxide tension and fresh gas flow delivered to the Bain circuit and Mapleson 'E' circuit during controlled ventilation. Curve A from Baraka, 1969; curve B from Henville and Adams, 1976; point C from Bain and Spoerel, 1973; curve D from Bain and Spoerel, 1975.

flows because the longer the pause following expiration the greater the volume of fresh gas which accumulates in the annular limb of the circuit near the patient. Furthermore, the situation in anaesthetised patients is different as minute volume depends on the degree of respiratory depression established by premedication, the depth of anaesthesia, the pattern and frequency of breathing and the amount of reflex respiratory stimulation provoked by the surgeon. A patient who has had no narcotic premedication, who is lightly anaesthetised, who exhibits tachypnoea, and who is undergoing a stimulating part of the operation will have an increased minute volume and hence require an increased fresh gas flow rate. This is the case whether the Magill circuit or the Bain circuit is used. However, it is important not to use too low a fresh gas flow with the Bain circuit to avoid establishing a vicious circle. Fresh gas flows of about $7\frac{1}{2}$ litres/min (5 litres/min N_2O and $2\frac{1}{2}$ litres/min O_2) i.e. about 105 ml/kg/body weight/min appear satisfactory in the majority of adult patients anaesthetised with halothane in nitrous oxide and oxygen. These flow rates should be adjusted in the light of the depth of anaesthesia, the size of the patient, the breathing pattern and the type of surgery. Figure 2.5 shows the change in fresh gas flow requirement at different levels of anaesthesia during spontaneous breathing at comparable levels of surgical stimulation.

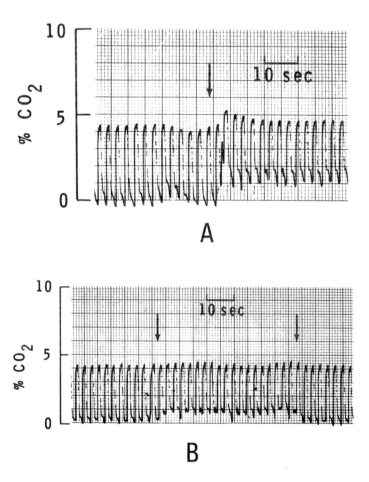

Fig. 2.5   Spontaneous breathing through a Bain circuit during an abdominal operation (colectomy) in an 84-year-old lady weighing 52.6 kg. The recording shows the concentration of CO_2 sampled from a catheter placed inside the tracheal portion of the endotracheal tube and measured by a mass spectrometer. The anaesthetic was 3 per cent enflurane vaporized by a mixture of 33 per cent oxygen in nitrous oxide.
(A)   Fresh gas inflow to the Bain circuit was 4.5 litres/min. At the arrow, the flow was reduced to 3 litres/min and CO_2 appeared in the inspired gas together with an increase in end-tidal CO_2 concentration.
(B)   The anaesthetic was 1.5 per cent enflurane vaporized by a mixture of 33 per cent oxygen in nitrous oxide. Fresh gas inflow to the circuit was 6 litres/min except for the period between the arrows when the flow was reduced to 4.5 litres/min; this led to the appearance of CO_2 in the inspired gas. The amount of surgical stimulation was the same as in (A) but note that the lighter level of anaesthesia and expected increase in minute volume due to the reduction in enflurane concentration in (B) requires a higher fresh gas flow to avoid rebreathing.

A recent study of patients breathing spontaneously during operations for craniotomy using fresh gas inflows ranging from 90 to 160 ml/kg body weight/min showed a mean $Paco_2$ of 39 ± 6 mmHg.[36] There was no difference between a group of patients receiving a flow of 93 ml/kg body weight/min and a group receiving 143 ml/kg body weight/min. The Bain circuit supplied with a fresh gas flow rate of 100 ml/kg body weight/min was also found to be as efficient as the Magill circuit supplied with a fresh gas flow rate of 70 ml/kg body weight/min in a series of 101 unpremedicated young adults undergoing oral surgery under endotracheal anaesthesia with halothane or enflurane in nitrous oxide and oxygen.[36]

Sterilisation of the Bain circuit
Sterilisation of Bain circuits by activated glutaraldehyde is reported to be unsatisfactory, although ethylene oxide sterilisation is effective without producing adverse physical or chemical alterations of the circuit.[37] We have found low pressure autoclaving satisfactory for the Penlon co-axial circuit but the use of hypochlorite solutions is not recommended because of the damage caused to the electroplating of the Penlon co-axial valves.

The Lack circuit
This co-axial system was described in 1976 as an anaesthetic circuit 1.05 m long which formed part of an operating theatre pollution control system.[38] The Lack circuit (Fig. 2.6) was designed to function as a co-axial version of the Magill (Mapleson A) circuit in which the expiratory valve is resited at the anaesthetic machine end of the circuit. The Lack circuit differs from the Bain circuit in several important respects. In the Lack circuit the patient breathes through both the inner and the outer tubes. The outer tube permits inspiration from the reservoir bag and the patient exhales through the inner tube and valve.

The original Lack circuit has been studied during experiments on conscious volunteers and has been critised on two counts.[39] First, the resistance to gas flow is unacceptably high, and second, the system does not in fact behave as a Magill circuit. The nominal internal volume of the standard length of corrugated 22 mm diameter breathing hose, used as the outer tube, is 500 ml; however, this volume is reduced to about 250 ml because of the presence of the inner (exhalation) tube. The efficiency of the circuit deteriorates if the patient's tidal volume exceeds 350 ml and in order to avoid the onset of CO_2 rebreathing a fresh gas inflow of 150 per cent of the patient's minute volume is required. Previous studies have already established that the Magill circuit requires a fresh gas flow of only 70 per cent of the patient's minute volume.[40,41]

The commercial version of the Lack circuit has been improved.[42,43] The length is 1.5 m, the internal diameter of the outer tube 30 mm and the dimensions of the inner tube are 14 mm internal and 18 mm external diameter. The inventor states that the capacity of the inspiratory limb is increased to 500 ml and the resistance to flow at 30 litres/min is reduced to 1.63 cm H_2O.[44] Slightly better figures (570 ml inspiratory capacity and 1.34 cm H_2O resistance at 30 litres/min) have been reported.[45] We have found that this improved version of the Lack circuit gives satisfactory performance in clinical use. Further improvements on these figures would require a much bulkier circuit in order to accommodate two breathing tubes of adequate bore in the co-axial mode. However, the main disadvantage of the Lack circuit is that, unlike the Bain circuit, it does not permit the use of anaesthetic ventilators to provide controlled ventilation.

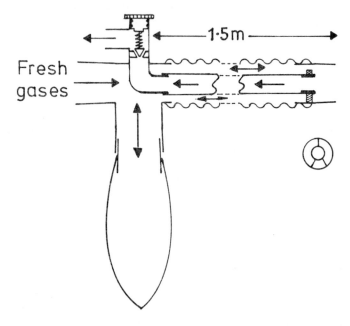

Fig 2.6   Diagram of the Lack circuit. Note the different direction of gas flows compared with the Bain circuit. The patient has to breathe through *both* tubes. Note the encroachment on the volume of the inspiratory limb by the presence of the inner, expiratory, tube.

HAFNIA MODIFICATIONS OF MAPLESON CIRCUITS

Modifications of the Mapleson semi-closed circuits A, B, C and D have been described with the aim of preventing atmospheric pollution by using suction directly from the circuit.[46] The usual expiratory valve is replaced by a suction port, and the rate of flow through this is measured with an ejector flowmeter.[47] The advantage claimed is that respiratory resistance is reduced, compared with the standard circuits, if the rate of gas removal equals the fresh gas inflow rate. A high-pressure expiratory valve is also incorporated and an air-inlet (dumping) valve may be used in case significant sub-atmospheric pressures develop.[48] There is no difference in the fresh gas inflow required to prevent rebreathing between the Hafnia modifications and the standard circuits, with the exception of system A, which appears to require a considerably higher inflow in the Hafnia version.[49]

THE CIRCLE WITH ABSORBER

The concept of a rebreathing circuit with absorption of CO_2 was first advocated by D. E. Jackson and sodalime was introduced into clinical anaesthesia by

Ralph Waters in 1922, using a to-and-fro system.[50] The circle system with flow-directing valves was devised by Brian Sword in 1926 and has since remained the system of choice.[51] The to-and-fro system, though portable and compact, has several practical disadvantages: bulky apparatus needs to be balanced close to the patient's head, restricting surgical access and making use of in-circuit vaporisers difficult; the size of the sodalime charge must be matched to the tidal volume; apparatus deadspace steadily increases with time and inhalation of sodalime dust is possible. The circle with absorber has been much less in evidence in recent years though it has always been more popular in the USA than in Britain. Its period of decline started in the 1950s when cyclopropane gradually fell out of use because the introduction of potent fluorinated volatile anaesthetic agents together with accurately-calibrated vaporisers, allowed the delivery in high-flow circuits of concentrations which, it could be predicted, would produce the required level of anaesthesia. However, with recent concern over environmental levels of anaesthetic gases and vapours in operating areas, interest has been rekindled in the circle absorber as a practical method of reducing pollution and providing economical use of inhalational anaesthetics.

A conventional circle system contains two uni-directional valves, a spill or overflow valve, a reservoir bag, a sodalime canister and a fresh gas port, connected by tubing. The number of different ways in which these components could be arranged is legion. Which is the best? The first essential is to ensure that rebreathing of CO_2-containing gas cannot occur. The function of the uni-directional valves is to direct CO_2-containing gas through the sodalime absorber before it is reinhaled, so any arrangement which compromises this function is pointless. This will happen if exhalation can occur into the inspiratory limb or inhalation occurs from the expiratory limb. Eger gives three rules which must be followed to prevent this happening:[52]

1. There must be a valve between the reservoir bag and patient on both the inspiratory and expiratory sides of the circuit
2. Fresh gas must not enter between the expiratory valve and the patient
3. The overflow must not be placed between the patient and the inspiratory valve.

Unfortunately some commercially-available circle absorbers violate these rules. The Hafnia circle absorber[53] uses an Ambu-E valve as combined inspiratory and expiratory valves and would appear to violate rule 3 above, although tests using a fresh gas inflow of 2 litres/min or more showed a satisfactory performance. Placing the overflow between the Ambu valve and the reservoir bag would restore satisfactory function.

Given a functionally competent circuit, the aims to be considered in arrangement of components are:

1. Conservation of fresh gas
2. Maintenance of inspired concentrations of oxygen and anaesthetics
3. Economical use of sodalime
4. Practical convenience
5. Accurate respirometer readings
6. Maximal humidity and warming of inspired gases.

The differing requirements of spontaneous and controlled ventilation must also be considered. There is no single arrangement which will accommodate all purposes with equal effect.

A circuit which preferentially ejects alveolar gas and retains deadspace and fresh gas will also best preserve inspired concentrations. If alveolar gas is ejected before the absorber is reached, sodalime usage will be prolonged. Several authors have recently studied circuits in detail with regard to these functions. Systems with high CO_2 elimination in general will have the greatest economy of anaesthetic utilization. However, absorption of volatile anaesthetics by rubber and sodalime may reduce the anaesthetic economy to half the CO_2 economy in the same system.[54]

The order in which components are arranged is of greatest importance with low fresh gas flows from about 1 to 4 litres/min. With high inflows of fresh gas rebreathing will diminish until eventually the circuit behaves as a semi-closed non-rebreathing circuit and sodalime is unnecessary: with basal inflows rebreathing is total and all expired CO_2 is absorbed. Under both these circumstances the positions of the components become much less critical.

Eger and Ethans examined several circuits to determine which arrangement of unidirectional valves, fresh gas inflow and expired gas overflow provided the greatest economy of sodalime and anaesthetic gases at various levels of fresh gas inflow, ventilation and deadspace.[55] This extended work previously reported by Brown and his colleagues.[56] Circuits were divided into groups according to the arrangement of fresh gas inflow and inspiratory and expiratory valves; group subdivisions were determined by position of the overflow valve. During spontaneous respiration and with a given inflow of fresh gas, the system which ejected the most alveolar gas through the overflow valve had this valve sited next to the patient; when the overflow valve was distant from the patient the economy was minimal. During controlled ventilation the economy of the system with adjacent overflow fell to zero, with one exception, whereas the system with distant overflow remained unchanged. The exception was a system with the unidirectional valves in the Y-piece and the overflow immediately downstream of the expiratory valve. This arrangement prevents loss of fresh gas when system pressure is raised during controlled respiration and was the most economical of all during both spontaneous and controlled ventilation.

Economy (of sodalime) increased directly with fresh gas inflow and indirectly with alveolar ventilation. Increases in deadspace with constant alveolar ventilation reduced economy in systems with distant overflow but produced no change when the overflow was adjacent to the patient. Replacement of the standard overflow valve with a low-pressure relief valve which closes with sudden increase in system pressure enabled the circuit with Y-piece overflow to retain its economy on changing from spontaneous to controlled ventilation. This type of valve requires constant attention, however, to ensure that it does not jam.

It might be supposed that the circuit with the valved Y-piece and adjacent expiratory valve would be the 'best buy' on the basis of this assessment. Practical considerations would suggest otherwise. Valves in the Y-piece add bulk to an already heavy piece of apparatus, cannot be seen working, are more liable to stick and have a higher resistance than disc valves mounted on the absorber body. In addition, should a valved Y-piece be used inadvertently with a valved absorber unit there is an even chance of producing opposed valves and a totally obstructed circuit.[57] Another possible error would be to assemble a completely unvalved circuit which would produce profound hypercapnia. The valved Y-piece is an uncommon item in Britain: most circle absorbers have all the components, with the exception of the tubing, Y-piece and optional overflow, mounted onto the absorber body.

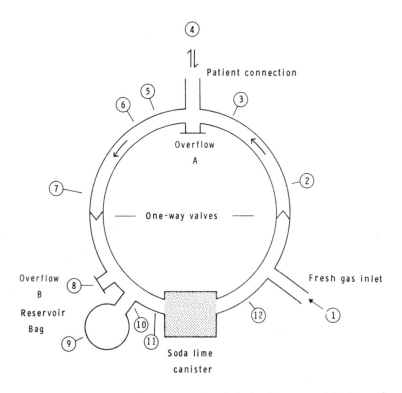

Fig. 2.7   Suggested arrangement of components in a circle absorber system. Numbers refer to alternative positions mentioned in the text. Overflow A is used with spontaneous respiration and overflow B with controlled respiration.

The arrangement recommended by Dorsch and Dorsch,[57] and by Schreiber,[58] as best meeting all requirements, and which corresponds with the 'second choice' of Eger and Ethans is shown in Figure 2.7. Jørgensen and Jørgensen[59] examined various arrangements of the Hafnia circuit (which uses an Ambu-E valve) and other circuits, for economy, and their suggested arrangement is similar to that shown in Figure 2.7 except that inspiratory and expiratory valves are combined upstream of the absorber.

The arrangement is logical in that fresh gas is included in the inspired gas stream, ensuring maximum inspired concentrations of oxygen and anaesthetic gas; expired gas is vented from the circuit upstream of the absorber and fresh gas inlet, conserving fresh gas and sodalime, and the lowest flow rate occurs in the region of the absorber between the overflow and fresh gas inlet, reducing respiratory resistance and allowing adequate time for absorption. With spontaneous respiration the overflow at position 4 is used, and the one at position 8 with controlled ventilation.

A recent clinical assessment of three circle systems confirmed the earlier predictions of Eger,[52] but found that the differences between the systems in terms of economy were somewhat smaller than had been suggested and were of only modest clinical significance.[60] More importantly, it was found that, when using halothane, the inflow rate need not exceed 3 litres/min after the first 10 minutes in order to sustain an inspired halothane concentration close to the delivered concentration.

Individual components[52,57,58]

Fresh gas inlet. The best compromise is obtained with the inlet at position 1 (Fig. 2.7). Increased humidity of inspired gases can be obtained by introducing fresh gas upstream of the absorber at position 11 but fresh gas may be lost through the overflow at the end of expiration. Anaesthetic absorption in sodalime will also be increased, especially with the drying effect of fresh gas on the sodalime.

Some systems have the fresh gas inlet downstream of the inspiratory valve at position 2, with the object of continuously flushing the inspiratory limb. However gas cannot now flow backwards into the reservoir bag during expiration as the inspiratory valve is closed, and will pass around the circuit to be lost through the overflow with expired gas. This will occur especially during spontaneous respiration with the overflow valve at position 4 or 5. A respirometer placed in the expiratory limb will over-read because of this continued fresh gas flow during expiration.

Location of the inlet upstream of the expiratory valve at position 7 is wasteful and will permit inhalation of a proportion of gas from the expiratory limb during inspiration, although the expiratory valve is closed. This gives rise to the unusual situation where rebreathing increases with increased fresh gas inflow, as the proportion of gas inhaled from the expiratory limb is increased.

Overflow. With spontaneous respiration overflow occurs in late expiration: the overflow is best sited at a position close to the patient at position 4 or 5 so that deadspace gas is conserved and alveolar gas ejected, as in the Magill circuit. With controlled ventilation using a pop-off valve, overflow occurs during inspiration. Fresh gas and expired gas cleared of CO_2 will be lost if the overflow is sited at the Y-piece or in the inspiratory limb at positions at 4, 2 or 12. An overflow valve at 2 or 3 will also allow exhalation into the inspiratory limb despite closure of the inspiratory valve with the production of CO_2 rebreathing. The best site is therefore between the expiratory valve and the absorber at positions 8 or 10, upstream of the reservoir bag. A pop-off valve can be conveniently replaced with a ducted spill valve by inserting the latter at position 10 before the reservoir bag, or at position 5 at the Y-piece junction.

As mentioned above, with inspiratory and expiratory valves at positions 3 and

5, the most economical arrangement is obtained with the overflow at position 6. A low-pressure relief valve which closes with high-pressure is best placed at position 4, as venting will occur at end-expiration with both spontaneous and controlled respiration. A modification of the system illustrated, incorporating a reservoir of 250 ml capacity upstream of the reservoir bag with low and high pressure relief valves, has been developed by workers at the University of Tottori, Japan,[61] (the Tottori circuit*) and is designed to increase efficiency by ejecting alveolar gas during spontaneous respiration with the overflow remote from the patient. The overflow closes during controlled respiration so that venting of excess gas still takes place during late expiration.

Reservoir bag. During spontaneous respiration, the bag can be placed in positions 9 or 12, according to whether reduced respiratory resistance is required during inspiration or expiration. Both positions allow retrograde filling of the bag by fresh gas during expiration. During controlled respiration, at position 12, compression causes retrograde flow of cleared gases through the absorber, again, to be vented. As previously mentioned, at positions 7 or 2 the bag becomes a reservoir for exhaled CO_2-containing gas which will be re-inhaled.

Sodalime absorber. The absorber body forms the hub of the circle system with other components mounted on it, and is usually attached to the anaesthetic machine, though there is no reason why it cannot be mounted on the head of the operating table if this is more convenient, or attached to a drip stand. A large canister allows increased absorption efficiency in the circle, compared with the to-and-fro system. Other advantages are increased transit time for gases allowing complete CO_2 removal, lower flow velocity with reduced resistance and less risk of dust formation, and longer intervals between changes. The divided canister permits complete exhaustion of one charge of sodalime before renewal.

Gas passes through the sodalime in one direction only and an internal or external bypass channel is provided. If the absorber unit is not assembled with a gas-tight seal then bypass of the sodalime will occur with profound hypercapnia; this fault is liable to occur with some earlier models.[62]

Lumley and Morgan measured temperatures reached in currently-available brands of sodalime with CO_2 flow of 200 ml/min and a fresh gas flow of 3 litres/min at tidal volumes of 500 ml at 20 times a minute.[63] With all brands, temperatures reached between 40°C and 50°C in 30 minutes at normal room temperature and then stabilised. Temperatures were higher in the centre of the canister than at the periphery, and the to-and-fro canister became approximately 5°C warmer than the circle canister. Lloyd reported that even with modern sodalime he had observed a temperature of 104°C with steam emerging when large volumes of CO_2 were being absorbed.[64] Although maximum decomposition of trichlorethylene occurs in the presence of alkali at temperatures over 60°C, small amounts of dichloracetylene are still formed at 15°C, and it is therefore still unsafe to use trichlorethylene even with modern sodalime in a jumbo canister. The patient next to use the circuit may be the one most at risk.

* Penlon Ltd., Radley Road, Abingdon, Berks.

Circle without absorber

Patients are customarily hyperventilated during anaesthesia when ventilation is controlled: this results from difficulty in calculating the precise level of alveolar ventilation required and therefore erring on the safe side, and from a desire to inhibit efforts at spontaneous respiration, enhance unconsciousness, ensure oxygenation and maintain full lung inflation. As arterial Pco_2 varies directly with alveolar ventilation, this practice often results in undesirably low levels of arterial CO_2 tension, especially during long operations. Marked hypocapnia results in peripheral and cerebral vasoconstriction, reduced cardiac output, leftward shift of the oxygen dissociation curve with reduced P50 and tissue oxygen extraction, and postoperative hypoventilation while body CO_2 stores are replaced.[20] As a result, there is a growing tendency to attempt to maintain $Paco_2$ at near-normal levels while retaining the advantages of large volume ventilation; this can be done by adding CO_2 to inspired gases, using a deadspace of appropriate volume, or allowing rebreathing of expired CO_2 to take place. With adequate total ventilation the amount of rebreathing is determined by the fresh gas inflow and this becomes the major determinant of the resulting $Paco_2$.

Mechanical ventilation with a circle absorber can be achieved in two ways. Usually, inspiratory pressure is produced by the ventilator acting as a mechanical bag squeezer; some ventilators can use circle absorber circuits, the mechanical valves of the ventilator acting as the inspiratory and expiratory valves, or a bag-in-bottle type of ventilator can be plugged into the circle in place of the bag. Venting of excess gas takes place during expiration. Alternatively, inspiratory pressure can be produced by a pulse of gas from a ventilator delivering air or oxygen or some respirable gas: mixing of circuit and driving gas during the inspiratory phase is prevented by interposing a deadspace of suitable volume between the circle and the ventilator outlet. Excess circuit gas mixes with driving gas and is ejected through the expiratory port of the ventilator. A minute volume dividing ventilator can be used in this way if a separate gas source is available to power it. A recent assessment of the method,[65] using a pressure-cycled flow generator as originally described by Voss,[66] showed that lengths of standard corrugated tubing could be used satisfactorily as buffer space, and related buffer space and fresh gas flow to tidal volumes obtainable without dilution of circuit gas. The author routinely used four one-metre lengths of tubing between ventilator and circle absorber.[65]

Several workers have investigated the use of the circle with the absorber removed for ventilating patients during anaesthesia. Both the total minute volume of ventilation and the fresh gas inflow were found to be important for carbon dioxide homeostasis by Benson and his colleagues.[67] In their studies a $Paco_2$ of 40 mmHg or below was produced by a combination of 50 ml/lb body weight/min fresh gas inflow with 100 ml/lb body weight/min total ventilation. Achievement of a steady state took forty minutes but the circuit volume of eight litres was large. Suwa and Yamamura,[68] by a theoretical analysis, proposed that, with some assumptions and sufficiently large total ventilation, alveolar CO_2 tension would be dependent on the relationship of CO_2 production to fresh gas inflow. They set the fresh gas inflow, in litres/min, at 0.02 times the minute CO_2 production (ml/min) calculated from the formulae of Kleiber,[69] and ventilated their patients with a tidal volume of 15 ml/kg body weight at a frequency of 16 per minute. Observed values of $Paco_2$ tended to be higher than those predicted, though for calculated values above 30 mmHg agreement was closer. Scholfield and Williams[70] assumed that, with adequate mixing, composition of alveolar and circuit gas would approximate, and that elimination of CO_2 from the overflow would be proportional to fresh gas flow; fresh gas flow could therefore be equated with effective alveolar ventilation. They used the Nunn blood gas predictor to calculate the alveolar ventilation necessary to achieve the chosen level of $Paco_2$, and set the fresh gas inflow at this value. Patients were hyperventilated with a minute volume twice to four times the fresh gas inflow. Their results showed a tendency for $Paco_2$ to be lower than predicted for high values, and higher than predicted for low values. Drummond suggested that siting of the overflow may have led to loss of fresh gas at higher fresh gas inflow rates, and that the influence of ventilation becomes more pronounced as fresh gas flow approaches minute ventilation.[71]

Harris et al confirmed the relation between fresh gas inflow and $Paco_2$ and the influence of minute volume.[72] They measured CO_2 production by measuring the volume and CO_2 content of the overflow, and found that this correlated better with $Paco_2$ than the predicted value.

Snowden and his colleagues varied fresh gas inflow, tidal volume and frequency in all combinations, using two types of circle according to the position of the fresh gas entry.[73] Results from a model lung and from patients demonstrated the importance of tidal volume. Large tidal volumes generally increased efficiency, assessed as effective utilisation of fresh gas. The system with fresh gas entry downstream of the inspiratory valve proved to be more efficient than the one with an upstream position. As venting occurred from the bag during expiration, the latter arrangement may have allowed some loss of fresh gas before it reached the patient. Efficiency did not depend on CO_2 production.

Patel and his colleagues[74] found an almost linear relation between $Paco_2$ and fresh gas flow at inflows between 60 and 120 ml/kg body weight/min, when using a circle system and a bellows-in-bottle ventilator. Fresh gas inlet and overflow were separated from the patient by the inspiratory and expiratory valves. $Paco_2$ at a fresh gas inflow of 60 ml/kg body weight/min was 38.4 mmHg with a standard deviation of 3.3 in 28 patients, and 31.3 mmHg with a standard deviation of 3.1 at an inflow of 100 ml/kg body weight/min.

The circle without absorber is a useful method of providing large volume ventilation without excessive CO_2 washout; though fresh gas inflow is the chief determinant of $Paco_2$ it seems important to provide a minute volume well in excess of the fresh gas flow. Frequency appears less important. With the variety of circle and ventilator arrangements possible, together with the inevitable limitations in predicting CO_2 output, the variation in results is not surprising and is probably no greater than the variation in $Paco_2$ seen with non-rebreathing systems. Suwa and Yamamura consider it important that venting of excess circuit gas should take place from the ventilator bellows.[68]

Methods based on complicated calculations are unlikely to achieve wide usage. The performance of a system should be checked by gas or blood gas analysis to ensure that adequate alveolar ventilation has been provided.

Use of basal or low flows

With the better availability of monitoring devices, attention has turned again to the use of the once-popular technique of basal or low flow anaesthesia with the circle absorber, primarily with the aim of greatly reducing the outflow of anaesthetic vapours and gases into the atmosphere. There is no doubt, however, that use of the circle absorber in the totally-closed mode or with minimal flows presents many practical problems.

In theory, once saturation of tissues with an appropriate anaesthetic tension has been achieved, uptake will cease and anaesthesia can be maintained indefinitely with a totally-closed circuit supplying only a basal flow of oxygen to match consumption. In reality such conditions take an impossibly long time to achieve, and variations in oxygen consumption and anaesthetic uptake and elimination, together with leaks, uptake into rubber and sodalime and continued nitrogen elimination, make higher than basal flows a necessity.

With high-flow non-rebreathing circuits, the gas flows set on the flowmeters represent the inspired concentrations. With a low-flow rebreathing circuit, inspired concentrations differ from delivered concentrations in ways which are difficult to predict and which change with time. Elimination of nitrogen will dilute inspired concentrations significantly for a considerable time unless gaseous nitrogen is first washed out from the lungs.

Many factors conspire to reduce inspired and alveolar concentrations.[52] The circuit itself contains a large volume which must first be washed out before inspired concentrations can rise. The time constant for washout is given by the ratio of circuit volume to inflow rate. The smaller the constant the more rapid the rise in inspired concentrations. This initial delay can be reduced by raising the delivered concentration, but hypoxia limits the extent of this manoeuvre with nitrous oxide.

Inflow rate, uptake and ventilation all affect the inspired concentration to a greater extent with a rebreathing circuit. Rebreathing dilutes fresh gas and thus decreases inspired concentrations, and the extent of rebreathing is determined by inflow rate and by alveolar ventilation. Rapid uptake will also reduce inspired concentrations. The rate at which alveolar concentrations approach inspired concentrations is affected by inflow rate and ventilation, both independently and in series: for instance, alveolar concentration cannot rise regardless of ventilation if inflow ceases and vice versa. Although an increase in ventilation accelerates uptake of more soluble agents, with a closed circuit this effect is offset by the limitation imposed by low inflow rates. A low inflow system does have the advantage of producing more stable alveolar levels in the face of changing alveolar ventilation, but concentrations will be affected by changes in cardiac output.

Low flows may not permit vaporisation of sufficient mass of volatile anaesthetic to meet the requirements of induction and maintenance, with the vaporiser in the fresh gas supply line, though the Fluotec Mark II was redesigned specifically to provide a rising characteristic to meet this problem. Although high-output calibrated vaporisers are available for halothane, and direct injection of measured doses of liquid anaesthetic directly into the circuit has been used, the more usual solution is to use an in-circuit vaporiser, whose responses are modified by factors quite different from those which control out-of-circuit vaporisers. The vaporising flow now consists of mixed fresh and expired gas. The latter, after the first breath, will already contain some vapour, and the output of the vaporiser will therefore be higher than its set value. The output concentration will rise as fresh gas inflow falls and expired gas forms a greater proportion of the vaporising flow. Similarly an increase in ventilation will increase vaporisation and lead to an increased output concentration, and this effect will also be more marked as fresh gas inflow is reduced. To a certain extent, with spontaneous respiration, anaesthetic levels will be self-regulating as respiratory depression associated with deepening anaesthesia will reduce the amount of anaesthetic vaporised. However, taken to its absurd conclusion, this means that vaporisation will cease only when total apnoea or death supervenes. Controlled or assisted ventilation with an in-circuit vaporiser will rapidly produce excessively high anaesthetic concentrations, especially if the vaporiser is positioned in the circle in such a way that the issuing concentration cannot be diluted by fresh gas entering the circuit: the vaporiser must first be turned off and the circuit flushed with fresh gas.

Many modern Rotameters do not allow the fine control of low flows required for closed circuit anaesthesia with nitrous oxide and oxygen.

The control of anaesthesia with a low-flow circle absorber must therefore be by inference rather than implication, and close observation of patient responses is required. Cullen, not unreasonably, thinks this not at all a bad thing, and has urged a return to closed circuit anaesthesia to discipline the clinical skills of anaesthetists which are being increasingly replaced by electronic monitors and the application of the MAC concept.[75]

Nitrogen elimination and nitrous oxide uptake

The most rapid changes in inspired concentrations occur with induction, when nitrogen is washed out from the lungs and replaced with nitrous oxide. The body of the average adult contains almost three litres of exchangeable nitrogen, of which about 1600 ml are in the functional residual capacity, the remainder being dissolved in blood, body tissues and fat. The gaseous nitrogen can be washed out quite rapidly, leaving about 900 ml which will evolve at varying, but much slower rates. If a patient is connected directly to a circle absorber with low fresh gas inflows, elimination of nitrogen will occur over a long period and interfere considerably with inspired concentrations of oxygen and anaesthetics. Holmes and Spear,[76] using a model consisting of a volume of 6 litres (representing a circuit volume of 4 litres and a functional residual capacity (FRC) of 2 litres) as a basis for a computer programme showed that the curve of nitrogen elimination followed an exponential form and demonstrated the extent of interference that could occur. Using a value of 225 ml/min for oxygen consumption and basing nitrous oxide uptake on the formula of Severinghaus (derived with an inspired concentration of 80 per cent), of $1000 \, t^{-0.5}$, (where $t =$ time since induction in minutes), with a fresh gas inflow of 500 ml/min they calculated that the concentration of nitrogen in the circuit would still be 40 per cent after about 30 minutes and that it would take about two hours to fall to 10 per cent. With fresh gas inflows of 7 litres/min, circuit nitrogen concentration would fall to less than 5 per cent in 5 minutes. No allowance was made for dissolved nitrogen in this study. Barton and Nunn found that almost all of the nitrogen of the FRC can be eliminated in five minutes breathing oxygen with high flows.[77] Forbes used flow rates of 6 litres/min until a reasonably steady state had been achieved, as demonstrated by identical repeated readings of inspired oxygen concentrations, and found that this usually took about 20 minutes.[78]

Uptake of nitrous oxide falls from its initially high level in a biphasic exponential manner. Smith found that the rate of uptake changes rapidly during the first 20–30 minutes of inhalation of a constant inspired tension, and that uptake continued for hours.[79] Average uptake (in his patients) was 75 ml/min after one hour and 20 ml/min after 170 minutes (keeping mixed expired oxygen concentration between 15 and 35 per cent), though there was considerable variation both within and between patients, and periods of excretion of nitrous oxide during maintenance were occasionally seen. This will occur of course if the inspired concentration of nitrous oxide is reduced during maintenance and will result in reduced inspired oxygen concentrations until a new steady state is achieved.

Virtue, using a closed circuit and keeping the inspired oxygen concentration at 35 per cent after a 15 minute high flow denitrogenation period, found a wide range of values for nitrous oxide uptake at 15 minutes post-induction (mean 406 ml/min, SD 232) but with time the uptake values became more consistent.[80] At 35 minutes uptake was less than 100 ml/min then slowly decreased to a mean of 73 ml/min (SD 24) at 60 minutes. A totally-closed circuit was also used by Barton and Nunn: maintaining an inspired oxygen concentration of 30 per cent, nitrous oxide was about 500 ml/min during the first two minutes, and 110–120 ml/min at one hour. The curve obtained from their results shows a short time constant of 25 minutes and a long time constant of about 500 minutes. The values include gas removed for sampling and not returned to the circuit.

Homes and Spears' computer study produced a graph of theoretical requirements of nitrous oxide inflow to maintain a constant inspired nitrous oxide concentration which has the expected bi-exponential shape.

There is therefore great practical advantage in allowing an initial period of breathing with high fresh gas inflows, for 5 minutes if denitrogenation and pre-oxygenation only are required, and for up to twenty minutes to allow for the maximum uptake of nitrous oxide at a time when inspired concentrations will be changing most rapidly. Bushman et al, however, using only oxygen and halothane in a circle absorber, deliberately omitted pre-oxygenation as a way of avoiding very high inspired oxygen concentrations, and suggested that retention of nitrogen might act as a scaffold to prevent peripheral lung collapse at low tidal volumes.[81] Inspired oxygen concentrations with pre-oxygenation settled at about 85 per cent and without pre-oxygenation at 50 per cent.

With a totally-closed circuit, nitrogen dissolved in tissues will gradually accumulate in the circuit over a period of time. Barton and Nunn found a mean concentration at one hour of 10 per cent. As the inspired oxygen concentration was kept constant, this resulted in a small dilution of inspired nitrous oxide.

Oxygen uptake

Oxygen consumption remains reasonably constant during anaesthesia. The difficulty lies in predicting the actual level for an individual patient. Smith found values of 125–230 ml/min, usually with a variation of less than 30 ml/min above and below, for long periods; in 3 patients, though, consumption fell, and in 6 rose markedly during the last half hour of the operation. As was the case with nitrous oxide, there was no reliable agreement between observed and predicted values at inflows below 1200 ml/min.

Forbes used varying inflow rates of nitrous oxide and oxygen and measured the inspiratory oxygen concentration when steady states had been achieved. With an inflow of 1 litre/min of nitrous oxide and 0.5 litre/min of oxygen, the mean inspired oxygen concentration was 27 per cent; with inflows of 0.5 litre/min of each, it was 40 per cent. The discrepancy between delivered and inspired concentrations predictably increased as fresh gas inflow was reduced.

Barton and Nunn found that oxygen consumption in their patients remained constant after two minutes stabilization, at a mean value of 227 ml/min, with a range of 180–260 ml/min. This figure included sampling gas. Holmes and Spears used their computer programme to calculate the effects upon inspired concentration of differing levels of oxygen consumption. With a steady state and an inflow of 700 ml/min of Entonox, inspired oxygen concentrations at consumption figures of 150, 225 and 300 ml/min would be about 45 per cent, about 33 per cent and about 17 per cent respectively. With an inflow of 1000 ml/min of nitrous oxide and 600 ml/min of oxygen, inspired concentrations for the same values of oxygen consumption would be 33 per cent, 28 per cent and 25 per cent respectively. This clearly demonstrates the significant effect which varying rates of uptake have on inspired concentrations at low inflow rates. It seems essential therefore to use an oxygen analyser to monitor inspired oxygen concentrations when using nitrous oxide in a circle absorber with very low flows. The advent of the compact, inexpensive fuel-cell meters now makes this a practical proposition.[82] They also have the advantage of being unaffected by the moisture content of gases, compared with the paramagnetic analysers, but it must be emphasised that this type of device has so slow a response time that it may give a false sense of security.

If an oxygen analyser is unavailable, what are the lowest flows of nitrous oxide and oxygen which can be used to provide a useful narcotic effect from nitrous oxide yet ensure that inspired oxygen concentrations remain at a safe level? Smith considered that variations in gas exchange made the use of an oxygen analyser mandatory with total inflows of less than 1200 ml/min. Forbes found that the mean inspired concentration of oxygen of 40 per cent, with an inflow of 500 ml/min of each gas, remained consistent after a steady state was achieved, usually after twenty minutes, though this seems a relatively short time. Inspired oxygen concentrations are likely to fall gradually as further saturation of body tissues with nitrous oxide occurs and its uptake falls.

With an inflow of 300 ml/min of oxygen and 200 ml/min of nitrous oxide, Virtue measured inspiratory oxygen concentrations of 30 per cent, with controlled ventilation, in patients weighing up to 80 kg, after one hour. At three hours, the lowest value found was 22 per cent. Increased inflows were needed with some patients weighing over 80 kg. With inflows of 500 ml/min of each gas, mean inspired oxygen concentrations at one, two and three hours were 37, 34 and 30 per cent respectively. Cullen suggests figures of 200 ml oxygen and 200–400 ml nitrous oxide per minute: from Virtue's results it would seem that slightly higher flows are needed.

Holmes and Spears' chosen regime as a result of their computer studies was 1000 ml/min nitrous oxide and 600 ml/min oxygen. Clinical trials using an oxygen analyser gave good agreement with their predicted values, resulting in inspired oxygen concentrations between 25–35 per cent over a range of values of oxygen consumption from 150–300 ml/min.

Care must be taken to avoid leaks in the circuit when using low inflows as inspired oxygen concentrations may fall rapidly to hypoxic levels. Barton and Nunn's patients were all intubated and the circuit was made leak-free to a pressure of 60 cm H_2O by using rubber sleeves over the connections. Bushman and his colleagues used oxygen and halothane only and employed a novel method of refilling the circuit with oxygen via a demand valve when pressure became sub-atmospheric. A face mask was used successfully in most cases, and leaks were overcome by using low-flow suction from the circuit. An air-entrainment valve was also included as an added safety feature, set at a higher pressure than the oxygen demand valve.

Inhalational agents

Any volatile anaesthetic with the exception of trichlorethylene can be used in the closed circuit, though if a non-flammable agent is required, choice is limited to halothane, methoxyflurane and enflurane. Most of the information on volatile agents in the closed circuit refers to halothane and this is the most widely used agent. Methoxyflurane has the disadvantages of low volatility and high rubber solubility.[54] Up to 50 per cent of the delivered concentration may be absorbed into rubber during the first ten minutes of administration, and absorption continues for hours; similarly methoxyflurane will continue to be released for considerable periods of time after the vaporiser is turned off. The rubber-gas partition coefficient of methoxyflurane is 630, compared with 120 for halothane, which means that 100 ml of rubber when equilibrated with 1 per cent vapour will absorb 630 ml of vapour. A single corrugated breathing tube could therefore absorb 3000 ml of vapour, the equivalent of 15 ml of liquid methoxyflurane. Absorption can be reduced by the use of polyethylene or polymethane tubes, but polyvinylchloride absorbs more anaesthetic than rubber. Trichlorethylene has an even higher rubber-gas partition coefficient than methoxyflurane (830) which would make it an unsuitable agent for use in the closed circuit even if it were not degraded by sodalime. The administration of methoxyflurane in the closed circuit is therefore beset by difficulties in achieving a suitable inspired concentration. A most valuable monograph has been prepared by Lowe on the subject.[54]

Little experience has yet been gained with enflurane. Although anaesthesia requires inspired concentrations approximately twice those of halothane, vaporisation is no problem and the rubber:gas partition coefficient is 74, half that of halothane. The circle absorber with low flows may prove to be a suitable method for its administration, not least on account of its cost.

Absorption of volatile agents by sodalime adds another hindrance to the development of an inspired concentration. Absorption of these agents is increased as the water content of sodalime falls. Circle absorbers which have been used with high flows may cause a delay in induction when used subsequently with low flows and may then release large amounts of vapour when the humidity increases. Dry sodalime may absorb 300–400 ml of halothane vapour during induction.

The principles which govern the concentrations of anaesthetics in closed circuits were clearly set out in a classic series of papers from Cardiff in 1960.[83–85] Most of the accurately-calibrated vaporisers used in the fresh gas supply line give an inadequate vapour output to meet the needs of induction and maintenance in the closed circle because of the diluting effect of rebreathing on low inflows. The simplest alternative is to place the vaporiser inside the circuit. Vaporisation then occurs both from the fresh gas inflow and the tidal circuit gas. Vaporisers for in-circuit use need to have a limited maximum output, a low resistance to gas flow, and should not have wicks on which exhaled water vapour will condense. Condensation will in any event occur on the surface of the liquid anaesthetic and may reduce vaporisation after a time. This can be minimised by placing the vaporiser in the inspiratory limb downstream of the fresh gas inlet.

The vaporisers originally designed for use with intermittent-flow dental gas machines such as the Goldman and McKesson fulfil the above requirements. The Goldman is the one most commonly used as an in-circuit vaporiser.[86] It is found in two versions: an earlier model (Mark II) made by A. C. King, with four arbitrary output settings, and the current model, made by BOC Medishield, which has three settings. Output from a vaporiser in circuit is unknown: not only is the vaporiser uncalibrated, but output depends on the vaporiser flow, itself dependent on fresh gas inflow and minute volume of ventilation, on uptake and on the vaporiser setting and characteristics which alter according to flow rate. With a totally-closed circuit and basal flows, halothane concentration in the circle will eventually rise to the saturation concentration, i.e., about 35 per cent, if there is no uptake, but Mushin and Galloon found that in practice, with continuous patient uptake of halothane, this does not occur, and the concentration stabilises after 10–12 minutes at a concentration dependent on the setting of the vaporiser, with no tendency to build up. The Goldman was designed to give a maximum output of no more than 3 per cent under all flow conditions; as a plenum vaporiser with a steady gas flow of 8 litres/min, output concentrations for the Mark II model at settings 1, 2, 3 and ON are 0.1, 1, 2.5 and 3 per cent respectively.[87] Considerably greater ranges of concentrations are found however when used as an in-circuit vaporiser with very low flows. A recent assessment[81] showed that with intermittent flows, when tidal volumes fall to less than 200 ml the output of the vaporiser starts to rise; thus the lower the tidal volume at high settings the higher the output, which is the opposite response to that ideally required. The vaporiser is also sensitive to movement, which can produce high peak outputs taking several breaths to settle. For example, at a tidal volume of 100 ml, peak output was 9 per cent after a shake, and 18 per cent at a tidal volume of 50 ml. Mounting of the vaporiser in the circle renders it particularly liable to movement; however, these extreme concentrations occurred at tidal volumes which would be unlikely to occur clinically without the vaporiser being turned off, and under usual conditions the vaporiser appears to function satisfactorily if output is limited by use of a lower setting. Inspired concentrations varying between 0.5 per cent and 1.2 per cent were obtained with a totally closed circuit by Barton and Nunn with the Goldman vaporiser at setting 1. Setting 2 was used briefly to deepen anaesthesia in two patients.

If ventilation needs to be controlled in a patient who has been breathing halothane spontaneously from a circle with an in-circuit vaporiser, high concentrations may be inhaled unless the circuit is first flushed, with consequent wastage of gas and the possibility of pollution. Bushman and colleagues,[81] as an alternative, incorporated a switched charcoal absorber into the circuit which produced rapid falls in the circuit halothane concentration. Within 5 breaths (thirty seconds), concentration of halothane fell from 1.8 per cent to 0.15 per cent, and to 0.03 per cent after three minutes.

The problems of using halothane and volatile anaesthetics in the closed circuit can be greatly reduced if inspired concentrations can be measured continuously. The Narkotest (Draeger Medical Ltd.) is a simple, fairly inexpensive monitor which depends on the relaxation of stretched silicone-rubber strips with absorption of anaesthetics, producing movement of a pointer on a scale.[88] It has the advantages of being able to respond to all inhalational anaesthetics (a correction is required if nitrous oxide is used) and of being compact and not requiring a power supply. Response time depends on rubber and oil/gas partition coefficients and is prolonged with more-soluble agents. Ninety-five per cent response time ranges from 7 seconds for nitrous oxide to 843 seconds for methoxyflurane. 1 per cent halothane requires approximately 100 seconds.[89]

An alternative to measuring the output of a vaporiser in circuit is to use measured doses of volatile agents calculated to produce an appropriate alveolar concentration, taking into account circuit volume, patient size and uptake into body tissues and circuit components. Such an approach requires apparatus and data which may not be readily available. Liquid anaesthetics may be injected directly into the closed circuit where the tidal volume is available for their vaporisation.[90] All agents produce almost the same amount of vapour per ml liquid volume (112 ml ± 20 ml); liquid agent is unaffected by fluctuations in circuit pressure, and temperature corrections are not required. Agents may also be mixed in proportion to provide equipotent anaesthesia. Lowe has used a motorised syringe pump controlled by a potentiometric curve follower tracking data from a programmed card.[54]

Titel and colleagues used a temperature-compensated automatic pressurised halothane vaporiser producing a constant 20 per cent halothane vapour in oxygen, with flows calculated to produce the required induction dose over a five-minute period into a closed circuit.[91] Patients were ventilated with an assistor/controller ventilator and maintenance of anaesthesia was by either following a pre-calculated programme with step-wise reduction in inspired concentration according to time, or by clinical judgement, producing depth of anaesthesia which allowed the patient to trigger the ventilator regularly.

There is no doubt that with careful technique use of the closed circuit can greatly reduce levels of atmospheric contamination. The highest halothane concentrations found in the theatre atmosphere by Barton and Nunn when using their totally-closed circuit method were 0.03 ppm, compared with control figures of 0.02 ppm. Nitrous oxide contamination was presumably reduced by an equivalent amount. The halothane levels are approximately 500 times less than those which have been reported with semi-closed methods of administration; however the meticulous technique required is certainly time-consuming and not easily adaptable to routine use with short operations.

FLEXIBLE PIPELINES FOR MEDICAL GASES

Safety rules and procedures for medical gas installations are required to ensure that an adequate, safe and reliable service is provided for patient care. The potential hazard to patients arises from terminal units of such installations being either incorrectly labelled or incorrectly assembled, cross-connection (transposition) of hoses, incorrect pressure settings or sudden disruption of supply without the knowledge or permission of the hospital staff.

Crossed oxygen and nitrous oxide supplies

The tragedy of the 'wrong cylinder' has been known for years. The classical situation is where a nitrous oxide cylinder is coupled to the oxygen yoke of an anaesthetic machine.[92] The 1946 thriller film *Green for Danger* highlighted the situation which existed before the days of pin-index valve fittings; several people died mysteriously during their operations—the explanation was that the murderer had substituted carbon dioxide for oxygen and painted the cylinders to circumvent the colour code!

The risk of the 'wrong cylinder' has been greatly reduced since the introduction of the pin-index flush valve fitting system for medical gases. The hole/pin locations are subject to international agreement by the countries using the pin-index system. Hole/pin positions are prescribed in Great Britain by BSS 1319:1955 and are the same as those of the International Standards Organisation ISO 407.[93] The pin-index system is not absolutely fool-proof as it is still possible, accidentally or deliberately, to connect the wrong cylinder. This can be done either by damaging or removing the index locating pins on the yoke of the anaesthetic machine, or by 'standing-off' the cylinder flush valve from the indexing pins by the use of several Bodok seals. The chance of the latter method being successful is minimised by the use of narrow fixed aperture yokes instead of those fitted with a hinged retaining bar of 'gate'. Pin-index valves attached to medical gas hoses supplied from overhead have been known to be connected incorrectly to the yokes of anaesthetic machines.[94] This follows from the use of the pin-indexing valve in the 'upside-down' position. Apart from the obvious absurdity, this situation does not occur with cylinders because the shoulder of the cylinder prevents the valve from entering the yoke to the required extent.

The introduction of piped medical gases has greatly reduced the risks of the oxygen supply running out during operations. However, instances have continued to be reported of accidental cross-connection of the nitrous oxide and oxygen pipelines. Cross-connection can occur during the installation or the modification or extension of piped medical gas systems. After the introduction of piped medical gases into Great Britain, it was possible to connect either the piped medical gas service or a cylinder containing the same medical gas to a single pin-index yoke on some anaesthetic machines. On some anaesthetic machines provision is sometimes made by means of a Schrader or other temporary fitting for quick dis-connection of the flexible medical gas supply lines (hoses) at the point where they enter the anaesthetic machine. This has been described to facilitate the use of 'take-up reels' for medical gas hoses.[101] The use of Schrader or other tem-porary couplings at this site is condemned by the Department of Health and Social Security.[102] The joints between the piped medical gas supply hoses and the anaesthetic machine should be permanent, i.e. the use of special tools are required; this should also be the case if a pin-index yoke is used. It is hoped that

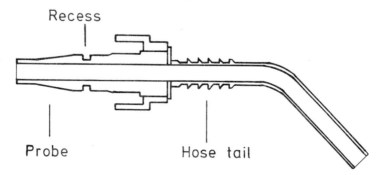

Fig. 2.8   Diagram of remote probe used in the Schrader form of temporary connexion for medical gas lines. The probe mates with the outlet socket (terminal unit) at the end of the run of metal distribution pipe. The flexible hose and remote probe form a permanent union; this is made by pushing the hose over the angled hose tail (which forms the spigot) until it is engaged by the serrations. A short metal tube or ferrule is then crimped over this part of the hose by using a special crimping tool to make a tight fastening. Non-inter-changeability of probes between the various medical gases and vacuum supplies is achieved by varying the diameter of the indexing collar. The hoses should be colour-coded.

the abolition of the Schrader or other temporary connections of flexible hoses to yokes on anaesthetic machines will prevent the type of accidents described recently where disruption followed by accidental cross-connection of the wrong hose has occurred. The new British Standard for medical gas pipeline systems specifies permanent joints being made between the anaesthetic machine and the flexible medical gas hose by the use of non-interchangeable screw thread (NIST) unions.[103]

Figure 2.8 shows the mode of connection of the flexible hose to the hollow spigot (which is the end piece of a connection fitting into a high pressure hose and which helps to anchor this connection to the hose) and the terminal probe. The probe mates with the female socket of the terminal unit or outlet of the medical gas supply. The spigot usually forms an integral part of the terminal probe.

The most recently reported case of accidental cross-connection of oxygen and nitrous oxide hoses in Great Britain occurred following accidental disconnection of both hoses from the spigots of Schrader valves fitted to an anaesthetic machine.[98,99] This tragic case has again drawn attention to the fact that it is not universally realised that internal and external diameters of hoses and sizes of spigots vary.[104] A safe design demands hoses and spigots of matching sizes and agreement amongst manufacturers to produce a British Standard for such hoses and spigots which prevents mismatch between equipment of different manu-facturers.

It is suggested that anaesthetists and those with responsibilities for hospital pipelines should test the joints by pulling vigorously on the hoses (the so-called 'tug test').[98] There should be no movement between the spigot and hose as a result of the applied stress. The test is recommended because the security of a crimped joint on a medical gas hose is not necessarily proved by a pressure test, even when this is combined with a leak test using a soapy solution as a bubble

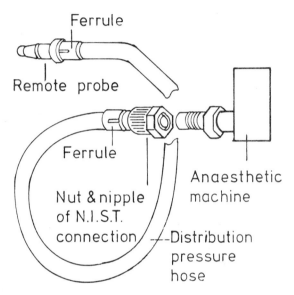

Fig. 2.9   Diagram of a complete hose assembly showing the remote probe fitted to one end of the hose and the permanent non-interchangeable screw threaded (NIST) connexion between the other end of the hose and the anaesthetic machine or lung ventilator.

detector. Unfortunately, the application of the tug-test to some Schrader valve unions may result in ejection of the male probe from its socket. This occurs because wear at the shoulder of the groove on the male probe allows the retaining clips of the socket to slip out of that groove. The use of harder metals in the manufacture of the probe should reduce the amount of wear.

The temporary connection between the medical gas hoses (permanently connected to the anaesthetic machine) and the appropriate medical gas supply should be made only by inserting the male terminal probe into the corresponding socket of the terminal unit. The hoses are to be colour coded for the appropriate medical gas (i.e. oxygen or nitrous oxide) and the whole hose assembly will be a 'declared item', i.e. a complete hose assembly is required should repair be indicated and on-site repairs are not to be made[105] (Fig. 2.9).

Testing anaesthetic machines

The single-hose or qualitative test mentioned in the recommendations of an inquiry has been adopted by many anaesthetic departments. However, the final conclusion that 'the machine is now ready for safe use' appears incompatible with the fact that the tests on the machine mean that it has been left completely disconnected from all sources of supply of oxygen and nitrous oxide. Furthermore, anaesthetic machines which incorporate a safety N_2O/O_2 interlock device (i.e. a mechanism which automatically shuts off the supply of N_2O when the supply of O_2 is interrupted) prohibit those tests which check whether N_2O from cylinders or pipeline can enter the flowmeters.

The following qualitative checking scheme for pipeline-supplied anaesthetic machines fitted with N_2O/O_2 interlock devices has been suggested to the authors by Dr Nicholas I Newton:

Before starting the tests, the machine must be disconnected from all piped medical gas supplies and with oxygen and nitrous oxide cylinders turned off.

Procedure

1. Check that full cylinders of oxygen and nitrous oxide are properly attached to their yokes on the anaesthetic machine and the cylinders are all turned off.
2. Open the O_2 and N_2O flowmeter valves from 2 to 3 full turns each (ensure all other flowmeter valves are closed). No flow should be registered at this stage.
3. Turn on O_2 cylinder and check that O_2 gauge for that cylinder registers adequate oxygen content. The O_2 flowmeter should now register a flow of gas. Check that the O_2 flowmeter valve can deliver the maximum flow indicated, and then accurately adjust the bobbin to register a suitable test flow (e.g. 4 litres/min). *If N_2O flowmeter registers any flow when O_2 cylinder alone is turned-on reject the machine.*
4. Turn on N_2O cylinder and check that N_2O flowmeter bobbin now also registers a flow of gas. *If O_2 flowmeter bobbin demonstrates any flow when the N_2O cylinder is turned on—reject the machine.*
5. Set the O_2 failure warning device in operation (where this is not automatic).
6. Turn off O_2 cylinder, and check that O_2 failure alarm functions correctly when bobbin of O_2 flowmeter falls. Check that this bobbin falls completely to the bottom of the flowmeter tube. *If O_2 flowmeter still registers any flow when only N_2O cylinder is turned on—reject the machine.*
7. Insert O_2 probe of hose leading from the anaesthetic machine into piped O_2 supply connection at wall (terminal unit). This must cancel the noise (and/or warning light) of the O_2 failure alarm. Apply 'tug-test' to this connection. Again check that O_2 flowmeter valve can deliver the maximum indicated flowrate, and then accurately reset the flowmeter bobbin to register the original test flow (4 litres/min).
8. Turn off N_2O cylinder, and note whether there is any change in O_2 flowmeter bobbin setting as the N_2O flowmeter bobbin falls. *If O_2 flowmeter bobbin demonstrates any fall when N_2O cylinder is turned off—reject the machine.*
9. Insert N_2O probe from anaesthetic machine into piped N_2O supply connection at wall (terminal unit). Apply 'tug-test' to this connection. Check that the N_2O flowmeter valve can deliver the maximum flow indicated, and note if there is any change in O_2 flowmeter bobbin-setting. *If O_2 flowmeter bobbin demonstrates any use when piped N_2O supply is connected, reject the machine.*

10. To complete the check test for leaks by occluding the outlet from the machine until the pressure-relief valve on the backbar is seen or heard to operate. The anaesthetic machine is now ready for use.

The back-pressure test should not be applied unless the anaesthetic machine is fitted with a pressure-relief valve as damage to the flowmeter tubes and their seatings can occur.[26] Leakage at such seatings or cracks in the carbon dioxide or cyclopropane flowmeter tubes may allow metered oxygen to escape and result in a hypoxic mixture being delivered to the patient.[106-108]

The tests outlined above assume, however, that the correct gases are being supplied to the respective terminal units. Even in a correctly-piped installation contamination of O_2 pipelines by N_2O can occur and has been reported following the introduction of early versions of O_2/N_2O blender devices. There has been one instance where a liquid oxygen vessel was filled with nitrogen.[109] The use of O_2 gas analysers appears obvious as a means of checking the purity of the oxygen supply but the user must be thoroughly familiar with them. Wright has recently suggested the use of an inexpensive and reliable whistle discrimination for O_2 and N_2O.[110] The velocity of sound in O_2 is 317 m/s and in N_2O it is 262 m/s. The pitch of a whistle is directly proportional to the velocity of sound in the gas so a change from O_2 to N_2O will cause the pitch to fall by about 17 per cent, i.e. equal to an interval of one and a half tones, the interval between the third and fourth notes of 'God Save the Queen' (in the U.S.A. 'My Country 'tis of Thee'). A closed pipe type of whistle of pitch C″ is suitable. The test would be carried out at the start of an operating session or at any other time as necessary. The whistle is connected to the outlet from the machine and O_2 passed at about 8 l/m. When the note becomes steady the O_2 is turned off and N_2O turned on at the same flow rate. After the residual O_2 is swept out the note drops $1\frac{1}{2}$ tones. The note rises again when the N_2O is turned off and O_2 substituted. The first note will be low should the gases have been interchanged but the fact that it rises (instead of falls) when the N_2O valve is turned on is said to be apparent to even those who claim to be tone deaf. Carbon dioxide provides almost exactly the same pitch as N_2O and cannot be distinguished from it.

Accidents due to the inadvertent administration of carbon dioxide during an anaesthetic may be reduced by adopting the same procedure as should always be used with cyclopropane, that is by removing the cylinder from the machine; the cylinder should only be attached by the anaesthetist himself when its use is intended.

'Permit to Work' system

The 'permit to work' system is a form of declaration in the form of a certificate in six parts for signature as appropriate.[111,112] It has been introduced in order to prevent maintenance or service engineering work commencing on systems for piped medical gases, medical compressed air and medical vacuum systems without the prior knowledge of hospital staff (doctors and nurses), pharmacists, administrators, engineering department staff or contractors' staff.

The certificate states the degree of hazard involved, defines all services to be worked on and the points where isolation of the affected sections are made. It also gives an indication of the work to be carried out. The system is particularly necessary when the actions of one group of people can directly or indirectly expose others to a hazard or create difficulty in operation.

The system is applicable to the security, repair, alteration and extension of existing installations within a hospital, or any action, such as the closure of an isolating valve, which restricts the supply. However, permits are not necessary for the routine replacement of cylinders on manifolds nor for the re-charging of liquid oxygen vessels, provided there is no danger of the supply being disrupted when these tasks are undertaken.

The 'Permit to Work' document defines the responsibilities of the people who are involved in the Permit, the principles and operational conductors, the scope and procedures to be followed. Three levels of hazard are identified, high, medium and low. High hazard work includes any work involved in cutting an in-service pipe-line and any work in which brazing is required. Such work introduces hazards of cross-connection or pollution or both. Medium hazard work includes work at any terminal unit, boom or pendant where there is a piped service of more than one medical gas or medical vacuum service, i.e. in operating theatres and anaesthetic rooms. Again, the hazard is one of cross-connection. Low hazard work includes work on terminal units only and on pipe-lines where there is a piped service of only one gas, or in addition to a piped service of medical vacuum (e.g. in wards).

The Permit to Work Certificate does not authorise the use of the installation for clinical purposes until the appropriate part of the form has been completed by the personnel as defined in the Supplement to HTM 22.

Acknowledgements

Figure 2.4 is reproduced by kind permission of the Editor of *Anaesthesia*. Dr Adams would also like to thank Professor W. E. Spoerel for his help in studies of spontaneous breathing with the Bain circuit (Fig. 2.5).

REFERENCES

1. Macintosh, R. R. & Mushin, W. W. (1945) Anaesthetics research in war-time. *Medical Times*, **73(2)**, 53.
2. Macintosh, R. R. & Pask, E. A. (1957) The testing of life jackets. *British Journal of Industrial Medicine*, **14**, 168.
3. Obituary: Professor E. A. Pask (1966) *Anaesthesia*, **21**, 437.
4. Macintosh, R. R. (1976) Personal communication.
5. Bain, J. A. & Spoerel, W. E. (1972) A streamlined anaesthetic system. *Canadian Anaesthetists' Society Journal*, **19**, 426.
6. Mapleson, W. W. (1954) The elimination of rebreathing in various semi-closed anaesthetic systems. *British Journal of Anaesthesia*, **26**, 323.
7. Spoerel, W. E., Bain, J. A. & Heinrich, G. R. (1974) A redesigned anaesthetic gas machine. *Canadian Anaesthetists' Society Journal*, **21**, 335.
8. Henville, J. D. & Adams, A. P. (1976) A co-axial breathing circuit and scavenging valve. *Anaesthesia*, **31**, 257.
9. McGaughey, W. (1977) An adaptor for coaxial circuits. *Anaesthesia*, **32**, 50.
10. Farrar, M. D. (1977) An alternative mount for the Bain coaxial circuit. *Anaesthesia*, **32**, 918.
11. Henville, J. D. & Adams, A. P. (1976) The Bain anaesthetic system. An assessment during controlled ventilation. *Anaesthesia*, **31**, 247.
12. Chu, Y. K., Rah, K. H. & Boyan, C. P. (1977) Is the Bain breathing circuit the future anesthesia system? An evaluation. *Anesthesia & Analgesia; Current Researches*, **56**, 84.

13. Weeks, D. B. (1976) Provision of endogenous and exogenous humidity for the Bain breathing circuit. *Canadian Anaesthetists' Society Journal*, **23**, 185.
14. Bain, J. A. & Reid, D. (1975) A simple way to ventilate babies utilizing a mark VII Bird ventilator and a modified Mapleson "D" breathing circuit. *Canadian Anaesthetists' Society Journal*, **22**, 202.
15. Adams, A. P. (1976) Anaesthetic ventilators and associated breathing circuits. *British Journal of Clinical Equipment*, **1**, 133.
16. Adams, A. P. & Henville, J. D. (1977) A new generation of anaesthetic ventilators. The Pneupac and the Penlon A-P. *Anaesthesi* 32, 34.
17. Spoerel, W. E. (1977) The Bird Mark VII as anaesthesia ventilator. *Indian Journal of Anaesthesia*, **25**, 113.
18. Adams, A. P. (1977) The Bain circuit. Prevention of anaesthetic mixture dilution when using mechanical ventilators delivering non-anaesthetic gases. *Anaesthesia*, **32**, 46.
19. Prys-Roberts, C., Kelman, G. R., Greenbaum, R. & Robinson, R. H. (1967) Circulatory influences of artificial ventilation during nitrous oxide anaesthesia in man II. Results: the relative influence of mean intrathroacic pressure and arterial carbon-dioxide tension. *British Journal of Anaesthesia*, **39**, 533.
20. Salvatore, A. J., Sullivan, S. F. & Papper, E. M. (1969) Post-operative hypoventilation and hypoxaemia in man after hyperventilation. *New England Journal of Medicine*, **280**, 467.
21. Adams, A. P. & Salt, R. H. (1976) The resistance of the Bain and Penlon co-axial circuits. *Anaesthesia*, **31**, 562.
22. Nott, M. R. (1977) Resistance of anti-pollution circuits. *Anaesthesia*, **32**, 917.
23. Hannallah, R. & Rosales, J. K. (1974) A hazard connected with use of Bain's circuit: a case report. *Canadian Anaesthetists' Society Journal*, **21**, 511.
24. Paterson, J. G. & Van Hooydonk, V. (1975) A hazard associated with improper connection of the Bain breathing circuit. *Canadian Anaesthetists' Society Journal*, **22**, 373.
25. Mansell, W. H. (1976) Bain circuit: 'The hazard of the hidden tube.' *Canadian Anaesthetists' Society Journal*, **23**, 227.
26. Newton, N. I. & Adams, A. P. (1978) Excessive airway pressure during anaesthesia. Hazards, effects and prevention. *Anaesthesia*, **33**, 689.
27. Pethick, S. L. (1975) Correspondence. *Canadian Anaesthetists' Society Journal*, **22**, 115.
28. Baraka, A. (1969) Pco_2 control by fresh gas flow during controlled ventilation with a semi-open circuit. *British Journal of Anaesthesia*, **41**, 527.
29. Bain, J. A. & Spoerel, W. G. (1973) Flow requirements for a modified Mapleson 'D' system during controlled ventilation. *Canadian Anaesthetists' Society Journal*, **20**, 629.
30. Bain, J. A. & Spoerel, W. E. (1975) Prediction of arterial carbon dioxide tension during controlled ventilation with a modified Mapleson 'D' system. *Canadian Anaesthetists' Society Journal*, **22**, 34.
31. Rayburn, R. L. & Graves, S. A. (1976) The use of the Bain circuit anesthetic system for children during controlled ventilation. *Abstracts of Scientific Papers, p. 9. American Society of Anesthesiologists Meeting 1976.*
32. Mansell, W. H. (1976) Spontaneous breathing with the Bain circuit at low flow rates: a case report. *Canadian Anaesthetists' Society Journal*, **23**, 432.
33. Eger, E. I. II (1974) *Anesthetic uptake and action, p. 209. Williams & Williams Co., Baltimore.*
34. Willis, B. A., Pender, J. W. & Mapleson, W. W. (1975) Rebreathing in a T-piece: volunteer and theoretical studies of the Jackson-Rees modification of Ayre's T-piece during spontaneous respiration. *British Journal of Anaesthesia*, **47**, 1239.
35. Conway, C. M., Seeley, H. F. & Barnes, P. K. (1977) Spontaneous ventilation with the Bain anaesthetic system. *British Journal of Anaesthesia*, **49**, 1245.
36. Spoerel, W. E., Aitken, R. R. & Bain, J. A. (1978) Spontaneous respiration with the Bain breathing circuit. *Canadian Anaesthetists' Society Journal*, **25**, 30.
37. Enright, A. C., Moore, R. L. & Parney, F. L. (1976) Contamination and resterilization of the Bain circuit. *Canadian Anaesthetists' Society Journal*, **23**, 545.
38. Lack, J. A. (1976) Theatre pollution control. *Anaesthesia*, **31**, 259.
39. Barnes, P. K., Seeley, H. F., Gothard, J. W. W. & Conway, C. M. (1976) The Lack anaesthetic system. An assessment during spontaneous ventilation. *Anaesthesia*, **31**, 1248.
40. Norman, J., Adams, A. P. & Sykes, M. K. (1968) Rebreathing with the Magill attachment. *Anaesthesia*, **23**, 75.
41. Kain, M. L. & Nunn, J. F. (1968) Fresh gas flows and rebreathing in the Magill anaesthetic circuit with spontaneous ventilation. *Proceedings of the Royal Society of Medicine*, **60**, 749.
42. Lack, J. A. (1976) Pollution control by co-axial circuits. *Anaesthesia*, **31**, 561.
43. Lack, J. A. & Davies, R. J. (1976) Theatre pollution control with the 'Lack' circuit. *Anaesthesia*, **31**, 951.

44. Lack, J. A. (1976) Addendum. *Anaesthesia*, **31**, 1253.
45. Nott, M., Walters, F. & Norman, J. (1977) A comparison of the Lack and Bain semi-closed circuits in spontaneous respiration. *British Journal of Anaesthesia*, **49**, 512.
46. Christensen, K. N., Thomsen, A., Hansen, O. & Jørgensen, S. (1978) Flow requirements in the Hafnia modifications of the Mapleson circuits during spontaneous respiration. *Acta Anaesthesiologica Scandinavica*, **22**, 27.
47. Jørgensen, S. (1974) The ejector flowmeter and its clinical application. *Acta Anaesthesiologica Scandinavica*, **18**, 29.
48. Jørgensen, S. & Thomsen, A. (1976) The dumping valve and its clinical application. *Acta Anaesthesiologica Scandinavica*, **20**, 409.
49. Thomsen, A. & Jørgensen, S. (1976) The Hafnia circuit. *Acta Anaesthesiologica Scandinavica*, **20**, 395.
50. Waters, R. M. (1924) Clinical scope and utility of carbon dioxide filtration in inhalation anesthesia. *Anesthesia and Analgesia ; Current Researches*, **3**, 20.
51. Sword, B. C. (1930) The closed circle method of administration of gas anesthesia. *Anesthesia and Analgesia ; Current Researches*, **9**, 198.
52. Eger, E. I. II (1974) *Anesthetic uptake and action. Baltimore : Williams and Wilkins Company.*
53. Jørgensen, B. & Jørgensen, S. (1977) The 600 gram CO_2 absorption canister: an experimental study. *Acta Anaesthesiologica Scandinavica*, **21**, 437.
54. Lowe, H. J. (1972) Dose-regulated penthrane anesthesia. *Abbot Laboratories, North Chicago.*
55. Eger, E. I. II & Ethans, C. T. (1968) The effects of inflow, overflow and valve placement on economy of the circle system. *Anesthesiology*, **29**, 93.
56. Brown, E. S., Seniff, A. M. & Elam, J. O. (1964) Carbon dioxide elimination in semi-closed systems. *Anesthesiology*, **25**, 31.
57. Dorsch, J. A. & Dorsch, S. E. (1975) Understanding anesthesia equipment. Construction, care and complications. *Baltimore. The Williams and Wilkins Company.*
58. Schreiber, P. (1972) Anaesthesia equipment. Performance, classification and safety. Berlin. *Springer-Verlag.*
59. Jørgensen, B., & Jørgensen, S. (1973) Carbon dioxide elimination from circle systems. *Acta Anaesthesiologica Scandinavica Supplement*, **53**, 86.
60. Harper, M. & Eger E. I. II (1976) A comparison of the efficiency of three anesthesia circle systems. *Anesthesia and Analgesia ; Current Researches*, **55**, 724.
61. Wakai, I & Sato, T. (1970) Experimental study on the efficiency of semi-closed circle absorption systems with a pressure equaliser valve and an expiratory trap. *Japanese Journal of Anesthesiology*, **19**, 1122.
62. Whitten, M. P. & Wise, C. C. (1972) Design faults in commonly used carbon dioxide absorbers. *British Journal of Anaesthesia*, **44**, 535.
63. Lumley, J. & Morgan, M. (1976) The temperature inside carbon dioxide absorbers. *Anaesthesia*, **31**, 63.
64. Lloyd, E. Ll. (1976) Correspondence. *Anaesthesia*, **31**, 950.
65. Jeal, D. E. (1977) A method of controlled ventilation with a circle absorber breathing system. *British Journal of Anaesthesia*, **49**, 273.
66. Voss, T. J. V. (1967) Adaptation of ventilator for anaesthesia with particular reference to paediatric anaesthesia. *South African Medical Journal*, **41**, 1079.
67. Benson, D. W., Graff, T. D., Hurt, H. H. & Lim, H. S. (1968) The circle semi-closed system control of $Paco_2$ by inflow rates of anesthetic gases and hyperventilation. *Anesthesiology*, **29**, 174.
68. Suwa, K. & Yamamura, H. (1970) The effect of gas inflow on the regulation of CO_2 levels with hyperventilation during anesthesia. *Anesthesiology*, **33**, 440.
69. Kleiber, M. (1947) Body size and metabolic rate. *Physiology Reviews*, **27**, 511.
70. Scholfield, E. J. & Williams, N. E. (1974) Prediction of arterial carbon dioxide tension using a circle system without carbon dioxide absorption. *British Journal of Anaesthesia*, **46**, 442.
71. Drummond, G. B. (1975) Prediction of $Paco_2$ in a circle system (correspondence). *British Journal of Anaesthesia*, **47**, 740.
72. Harris, P. H. P., Kerr, J. H. & Edmonds-Seal, J. (1975) Artificial ventilation using a circle circuit without an absorber. *Anaesthesia*, **30**, 269.
73. Snowdon, S. L., Powell, D. L., Fadl, E. T. & Utting, J. E. (1975) The circle system without absorber. Use with controlled ventilation. *Anaesthesia*, **30**, 323.
74. Patel, K., Bennett, E. J., Grundy, E. M. & Ignacio, A. (1976) Relation of $Paco_2$ to fresh gas flow in a circle system. *Anesthesia and Analgesia ; Current Researches*, **55**, 706.
75. Cullen, S. C. (1972) Who is watching the patient? *Anesthesiology*, **37**, 361.
76. Holmes, C. McK. & Spears, G. F. S. (1977) Very-nearly-closed-circuit anaesthesia. A computer analysis. *Anaesthesia*, **32**, 846.

77. Barton, F. & Nunn, J. F. (1975) Totally closed circuit nitrous oxide/oxygen anaesthesia. *British Journal of Anaesthesia*, **47**, 350.
78. Forbes, A. R. (1972) Inspired oxygen concentrations in semi-closed circle absorber circuits with low flows of nitrous oxide and oxygen. *British Journal of Anaesthesia*, **44**, 1081.
79. Smith, T. C. (1966) Nitrous oxide and low inflow circle systems. *Anesthesiology*, **27**, 266.
80. Virtue, R. W. (1974). Minimal-flow nitrous oxide anesthesia. *Anesthesiology*, **40**, 196.
81. Bushman, J. A., Enderby, D. H., Al-Abrak, M. H. & Askill, S. (1977) Closed circuit anaesthesia. A new approach. *British Journal of Anaesthesia*, **49**, 575.
82. Torda, T. A. & Grant, G. C. (1972) Test of a fuel cell oxygen analyser. *British Journal of Anaesthesia*, **44**, 1108.
83. Mapleson, W. W. (1960) The concentration of anaesthetics in closed circuits, with special reference to halothane. I: Theoretical study. *British Journal of Anaesthesia*, **32**, 298.
84. Galloon, S. (1960) The concentration of anaesthetics in closed circuits with special reference to halothane. II: Laboratory and theatre investigations. *British Journal of Anesthesia*, **32**, 310.
85. Mushin, W. W. & Galloon, S. (1960) The concentration of anaesthetics in closed circuits with special reference to halothane. III: Clinical aspects. *British Journal of Anaesthesia*, **32**, 324.
86. Gusterson, F. R. & Clark, J. M. (1960) The use of the Goldman halothane vaporiser in the closed circuit. *British Journal of Anaesthesia*, **32**, 388.
87. Goldman, V. (1962) The Goldman halothane vaporiser Mark II. *Anaesthesia*, **17**, 537.
88. Bennetts, F. E. (1976) Closed circuit halothane anaesthesia. Use of the Narkotest as an in-line monitor in a non-polluting technique. *Anaesthesia*, **31**, 644.
89. Velazquez, J. L., Feingold, A. & Walther, P. (1977) Response time of the Narkotest anesthetic gas monitor. *Anesthesia and Analgesia ; Current Researches*, **56**, 395.
90. Weingarten, M. & Lowe, H. J. (1973) A new circuit injection technic for syringe-measured administration of methoxyflurane: a new dimension in anesthesia. *Anesthesia and Analgesia ; Current Researches*, **52**, 634.
91. Titel, J. H., Lowe, H. J., Elam, J. O. & Groscholz, J. R. (1968) Quantitative closed-circuit halothane anesthesia. A clinical study employing a new pressurised temperature-compensated vaporizer. *Anesthesia and Analgesia ; Current Researches*, **47**, 560.
92. Macintosh, R. R. (1949) Deaths under anaesthetics. *British Journal of Anaesthesia*, 107.
93. Grant, W. J. (1978) Medical gases. Their properties and uses. *H.M. + M., Aylesbury, U.K.*, p. 6.
94. Rawston, R. E. & McNeil, T. D. (1962) Pin index system. *British Journal of Anaesthesia*, **34**, 591.
95. Mazze, R. I. (1972) Therapeutic misadventures with oxygen delivery systems: the need for continuous in-line oxygen monitors. *Anesthesia and Analgesia ; Current Researches*, **51**, 787.
96. Editorial (1974) Nitrous oxide asphyxia. *Lancet*, **i**, 848.
97. Feeley, T. W., Headley-Whyte, J. (1976) Bulk oxygen and nitrous oxide delivery systems: design and dangers. *Anesthesiology*, **44**, 301.
98. Abriged Report (1977) Committee of inquiry appointed by the Kensington and Chelsea and Westminster Area Health Authority (Teaching).
99. Editorial (1977) The Westminster inquiry. *Lancet*, **ii**, 175.
100. *Daily Telegraph* (1977) August 3rd, p. 15. '35 die' in laughing gas mix-up (Pa hospital).
101. Crawford, J. S. (1973) Two ancillary devices for use with a piped-gas system. *British Journal of Anaesthesia*, **45**, 763.
102. Department of Health & Social Security (1975) Anaesthetic equipment supplied from pipeline medical gas systems—hazard. *Health Equipment Information*, **61**, 38/75.
103. British Standards Institution (1978) British Standard specification for medical gas pipeline systems—terminal units, hose assemblies and connections to medical equipment. Document 77/64924.
104. Hunter, A. R. (1977) Pipe-line accident. *Anaesthesia*, 1977, **32**, 383.
105. Robinson, J. S. (1977) British Standard on pipeline connections. *Anaesthesia*, **32**, 809.
106. Eger, E. I. II & Epstein, R. M. (1964) Hazards of anesthetic equipment. *Anesthesiology*, **25**, 490.
107. Adams, A. P. (1969) Anaesthetic machines. *British Journal of Hospital Medicine*, April Supplement, 35.
108. Rendell-Baker, L. (1976) Some gas machine hazards and their elimination. *Anesthesia and Analgesia ; Current Researches*, **55**, 26.
109. Sprague, D. H. & Archer, G. W., jr. (1973) Intraoperative hypoxia from an erroneously filled liquid oxygen reservoir. *Anesthesiology*, **42**, 360.
110. Wright, B. M. (1977) Whistle discriminator for oxygen and nitrous oxide. *Lancet*, **ii**, 1008.
111. Health Technical Memorandum No. 22 (1977) Piped medical gases, medical compressed air and medical vacuum installations. *Department of Health & Social Security, London*.
112. Supplement to Hospital Technical Memorandum No. 22 (1977) Permit to work system. For medical gases, medical compressed air and medical vacuum installations. *Department of Health & Social Security, London*.

3. Techniques and complications in cardiac surgery

Alan Gilston

Advances in cardiac surgery in the past few years have chiefly affected cardiac surgical methods and the management of complications. Changes in anaesthetic and related techniques have been less dramatic, and are sometimes more related to personal taste or a desire for change than real patient benefit. The results of cardiac surgery continue to depend largely on the surgeon's ability and experience, though, of course, he cannot work without a skilled team. However, the anaesthetist plays a vital role in the management of difficult cases and serious postoperative complications. Some gravely ill patients with major circulatory or respiratory problems require resuscitation and intensive care even before the operation. The quality of care in these situations may critically influence the outcome in sick patients, however skilled the surgery. Lack of space alone does not permit a comprehensive review of current practice, and this chapter merely reflects some personal interests. It is particularly concerned with recent advances in intensive care and their impact on cardiac surgery. Overlap with several other contributions in this book is, therefore, inevitable, but most of the topics are sufficiently important to warrant the presentation of different viewpoints.

Fashion and conservatism complement each other in medicine. They change as their underlying dogmas and heresies change, or switch places. This review will examine some current concepts and problems, and indicate the limitations of our knowledge.

SURGICAL TECHNIQUES

The most important recent cardiac surgical advance has been the correction of ischaemic heart disease with saphenous vein grafts and endarterectomy. This operation has had a major and increasing impact on the surgical workload, forming approximately 30 per cent of the operations in the National Heart Hospital. In some North American centres other types of cardiac surgery have even been virtually eliminated. In this and other leading centres the mortality for this operation in uncomplicated cases is less than 1 per cent, and less than 3 per cent in grave cases, a very significant reduction in the natural mortality of the disease, even if treated with drugs. Resection of a ventricular aneurysm, repair of a ventricular septal defect, correction of mitral regurgitation from papillary muscle damage or the insertion of an artificial pacemaker may also be required. Preoperative coronary angiography is essential to demonstrate the blocked vessels and is often undertaken even in patients who require mechanical circulatory assistance for cardiogenic shock or intractable angina.

Whilst heart action may be seriously impaired by disease, in some cases aggravated by beta-adrenergic blockade, general anaesthesia need be no different from that used for other lesions, but merely requires the same precautions. There is little evidence that in skilled hands the choice of anaesthetic drugs influences the results in this or any other type of cardiac surgery, whatever its effect on a particular parameter. At the moment, morphine in high dosage is popular. Simplicity, using the minimum number of agents,[83] continues to have major advantages in a busy teaching centre.

A reduced cardiac output and even cardiogenic shock are common in the immediate postoperative period in high risk cases, and require appropriate therapy. Hypertension, due to excessive sympathetic activity, is also common after coronary vascular surgery and though we do not feel this is a major problem, it is undesirable since it increases heart work and may also rupture a vessel anastomosis. It usually responds to a vasodilator, or if this fails a beta-adrenergic blocker.

Various ingenious procedures have been designed for the more complex types of congenital heart disease. Whilst these are mainly of surgical interest, the revival of hypothermic techniques (below) has facilitated their execution in infants. The increasing volume of infant cardiac surgery, including neonates, has greatly increased the anaesthetist's involvement in the postoperative period, since many of these babies are gravely ill. Such work is best confined to specialised units which can also provide expert paediatric guidance.

Myocardial protection

Cardiac surgeons have now recognised, somewhat belatedly, what has long been established by physiologists and pathologists, namely the heart is readily and permanently damaged by ischaemia. Protracted ischaemia at normal temperature during cardiac surgery eventually leads to a grave and usually fatal condition, 'stone heart'.[53] Here, the heart is tense and oedematous, and contracts feebly if at all. Lesser degrees of ischaemia produce functional impairment varying from an intractable low cardiac output state to a brief requirement for inotropic support. Induced ventricular fibrillation, widely used to produce a quiet heart for the surgical procedure, can, like the use of some sympathomimetic agents, lead to subendocardial ischaemia and damage.[39,112,113] These and other insults may prove to be the *coup de grâce* for an already extensively diseased myocardium. The anaesthetist must, therefore, himself be scrupulously careful to avoid marked hypotension or hypoxaemia.

There are now a multiplicity of experimental and clinical methods for protecting the heart against damage.[118] Many are merely a disinterment of older techniques, such as cardioplegia with potassium chloride solution and cooling methods of varying complexity, reflecting the cyclical nature of surgical fashion. It is not yet clear which technique is best, and a combination of moderate hypothermia with the absolute minimum of myocardial ischaemia from interruption of coronary arterial flow at present seems as good as any other for the diseased heart. In the worst cases of ischaemic heart disease with aneurysm formation, extensive fibrosis, and gross impairment of cardiac function, even brief ischaemia may be disastrous.

Hypothermia

Surface cooling, used to produce moderate hypothermia for protection of the brain during circulatory arrest in the early days of cardiac surgery, has been revived by Japanese and subsequently other workers for deep hypothermia, alone or in combination with cardiopulmonary bypass.

The child is surrounded with ice, except for his extremities, and surface cooled until the nasopharyngeal temperature, the best index of brain temperature under these conditions, reaches 26–28°C, when it continues to fall from the 'afterdrop'. It is now further reduced with cardiopulmonary bypass to 16–20°C. At this point, the circulation is interrupted, the patient exsanguinated, and the perfusion cannulae removed. Circulatory arrest for up to an hour allows correction of the defect(s), after which the circulation is restored and the patient rewarmed either completely or partially with the heart-lung machine. This approach combines the advantages of surface cooling with those of cardiopulmonary bypass. It ensures an even fall in temperature, avoiding the danger of brain damage during circulatory arrest from uneven cooling, reduces the period of bypass, provides a relaxed heart in a bloodless field free from cannulae, facilitating the surgeon's task, and supports the circulation at critical stages. Moreover, should heart action suddenly fail during the thoracotomy after surface cooling, hypothermia will protect the brain and allow time for the careful introduction of cardiopulmonary bypass, the patient having already been heparinised. Some workers use surface cooling (to 20°C) and surface rewarming for the whole procedure.[239] The anaesthetic technique for this procedure varies from centre to centre, but there is no evidence that close adherence to any published method is required. As always, the nature of the lesion, the condition of the child, the skill of the surgeon and his choice of corrective procedure are the paramount factors determining the outcome.

The incidence of respiratory and other problems in the postoperative period is probably not influenced by this technique,[229] and largely depends on the nature of the lesion.[182] Intellectual function and development are not affected.[162]

ARTERIAL AND VENOUS PRESSURE MONITORING

Monitoring is fully discussed by Dr Clifford Franklin in Chapter 8 and only a few aspects will be examined here.

Arterial pressure

Percutaneous insertion of a plastic cannula or catheter into a peripheral artery is nowadays a simple and standard procedure and is advisable not only in cardiac surgery, whether 'open' or 'closed', but in all types of major surgery, especially in the very sick. Direct cannulation of the dissected vessel is rarely necessary except in infants. Where possible, it is best to cannulate the left radial artery since this will immediately reveal accidental insertion of the aortic perfusion cannula down the left subclavian artery during cardiopulmonary bypass (Fig. 3.1). It will also show if the aortic balloon catheter is inserted too far during counterpulsation therapy (p. 70), though here it is best to cannulate both left and right radial arteries, since for haemodynamic reasons the right side shows a different pressure wave to the left, and is the better guide to the effect of counterpulsation.

Percutaneous cannulation of the dorsalis pedis artery[217] is a simple and useful alternative to radial cannulation, whilst femoral cannulation[85] may be used when other routes fail, being most useful is shock and cardiac resuscitation.

An air bubble, oscillating in the pressure line, is a reliable and accurate monitor,[90] and requires no electronic equipment (Fig. 3.2). It demonstrates heart rate and heart rhythm, and if a sphygmomanometer cuff is inflated till the oscillation ceases, the systolic blood pressure even in profound hypotension. We routinely use this technique whilst transporting the patient to the Intensive Care Unit and on occasion when monitoring equipment fails.

Serious complications of radial arterial cannulation are rare in this centre. The Allen test is not a complete safeguard.[13] It is best to use the narrowest possible cannula,[14] size 20 F.G. in adults and older children, and size 22 F.G. in infants. We frequently leave the cannula in place for several days and even a week or more if necessary, removing it if there are trophic changes such as swelling or discolouration, which soon clear.

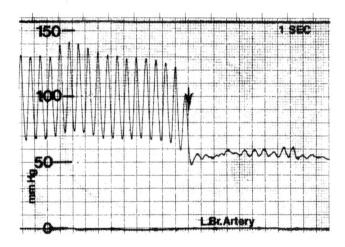

Fig. 3.1 Record of the left radial artery pulse wave during a cardiopulmonary bypass. The aortic cannula had been inserted too far, reaching the left subclavian artery, and the exaggerated pulse wave and high blood pressure returned to normal when the cannula was slightly withdrawn (arrow)

Central venous pressure

Cannulation of the right internal jugular vein for monitoring the central venous pressure and for long-term infusion is now a routine procedure in many centres. We prefer the 14 centimetre Bard Teflon Catheter* and the similar Deseret Angiocath† for adults and older children. These not only slide smoothly down their inner needle into the superior cava, but are much less likely to be misplaced than a longer catheter introduced through a short wide-bore needle, which is not only more traumatic, but narrows the size of the catheter, from which it cannot be separated.

These cannulae are also most useful in cannulating the femoral vessels when other routes fail or in an emergency.[90]

There are a variety of approaches to the internal jugular vein[57] but the operator

* C. R. Bard Inc., Murray Hill, New Jersey 07974, U.S.A.
† Deseret Pharmaceutical Co., Sandy, Utah 84070, U.S.A.

should be able to perform the technique even when the patient is in bed. This limits the 'head down' technique,[68] especially when the patient is conscious or breathless, and which may even be harmful in cardiac failure.[207] Like many 'blind' techniques, internal jugular cannulation has potential and even serious dangers,[40,52,54,57,248] but the 'high' approach is less likely to damage important intrathoracic structures than lower approaches or than subclavian vein cannulation, especially in inexperienced hands. A pneumothorax, for example, is a particularly undesirable complication in a sick cardiac patient. A suitable landmark is a point 3 to 4 centimetres above the apex of the triangle formed by the two heads of the sterno-mastoid, close to the angle of the jaw.

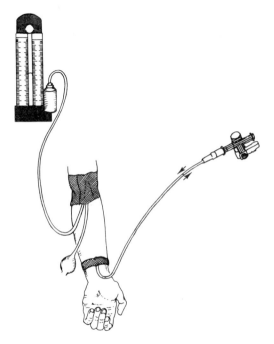

Fig. 3.2 An air bubble oscillating in the arterial pressure line is a valuable monitor of heart rate, heart rhythm and if the sphygmomanometer cuff is inflated till the oscillation ceases, systolic blood pressure

TEMPERATURE MONITORING

Skin blood flow falls when the cardiac output becomes unsatisfactory, leading eventually to the classical cold extremities of shock in advanced cases. Even a very slight, almost imperceptible degree of cooling in the nose, ears, fingers, knees or toes is a valuable sign, and is a most sensitive index of parallel deterioration in heart action, far more sensitive, for example, than changes in urine output, blood pressure or acid-base state.[206] This vital sign has recently become more precise with the introduction of sensitive electric thermometers, one sensor being placed on the pad of the great toe, the other in the oesophagus or rectum for the central 'core' temperature[117] (Fig. 3.3). Despite these accurate sensors, it is still essential to examine frequently and carefully the other extremities in sick patients, and monitor changes in the junction between warm and cold zones.[82] One or more fingers, for example, may cool before the toes, though most published work refers to the toe-core gradient. Normally the covered toe temperature is about 34–35°C, or one to two degrees lower than core temperature. There is a close relation between femoral blood flow and the cardiac output,[3] and if the toe temperature falls to less than 27°C it indicates a cardiac output of about half normal,[75,117] though presumably inotropic agents and vasodilators modify this relationship. At

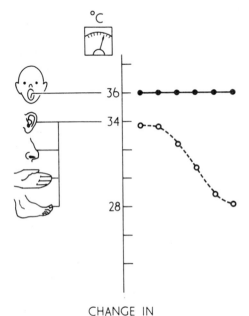

CHANGE IN
CENTRAL–PERIPHERAL
TEMPERATURE GRADIENT

Fig. 3.3 The central-peripheral temperature gradient is a sensitive guide to the cardiac output and circulatory state. Convergence or divergence of the readings has great significance

this temperature, the toes and fingers, though not always the nose and ears, are obviously cold. Asymmetrical cooling of the extremities, especially if marked, usually has a local vascular or neurological cause.

The extremities are often cold at the end of open-heart surgery, and may cool even more afterwards in the intensive care unit. This may reflect excessive sympathetic activity[115] triggered by various factors, including cardiopulmonary bypass, hypothermia, general or local heat loss, pain, or a fall in cardiac output. The toe-core gradient gradually diminishes over the next few hours, a change accelerated by vasodilator drugs and also by beta-adrenergic sympathomimetic agents, which increase not only skin flow directly but also the cardiac output. In general, patients with ischaemic heart disease take longer to rewarm completely than those with valve disease, often twenty-four hours or more, and this may be related to the raised catecholamine and plasma renin activity in these patients.[192] However, we have not been able to confirm that the rewarming period has any prognostic significance.[160] The cardiac output does not necessarily rise during the rewarming period, which is, therefore, less significant in this respect than cooling,[60] but a steady rise in peripheral temperature is an excellent sign of improvement in the treatment of a poor cardiac output, and often precedes other signs. The central temperature sometimes rises to high levels, 41°C or more when heart action is poor and the periphery cold. This rise in temperature has been attributed to increased heat formation as well as reduced heat loss.[242] If protracted, it has a bad prognosis, even if treated with cooling measures.

Poor heart action often requires treatment with adrenaline or other agents with an alpha and beta-sympathomimetic action. Here, cooling is often attributed to their vasoconstrictor effect on skin vessels. This explanation is rarely justified, even in part, since the peripheral temperature starts to rise, despite the alpha-sympathomimetic effect of the drug, once heart action improves. Moreover, some of these agents have no alpha effect in low dosage. The same argument applies to oliguria, which also improves as heart action improves, often despite considerable sympathomimetic support. The usual absence of sweating in cardiogenic shock immediately after cardiac surgery, the disproportionate fall in urine output in acute cardiac tamponade, and the marked sweating often seen in late tamponade suggest not only that the cholinergic and adrenergic activities of the sympathetic nervous system vary independently, but the response to endogenous catecholamines also varies after cardiac surgery. This may be linked to the ability of the adrenals to separately vary their production of adrenaline and noradrenaline.[115,181] Moreover, peripheral vasoconstriction and coldness after open heart surgery may not even be related to the levels of circulating adrenaline and noradrenaline, especially in patients who make satisfactory progress. The levels may not only be normal, but even if raised may show no fall and even a rise as the extremities become warmer.[237a]

Careful observation of changes in peripheral temperature is also invaluable when dealing with patients who may require or are receiving mechanical ventilation, and crucially affects decisions in this context.

POOR CARDIAC OUTPUT

Recent advances in our knowledge of the physiology and pharmacology of the failing heart have stimulated and assisted research into new drugs and new techniques for its management. But the evaluation and comparison of these advances are hindered by current methods of assessing cardiac function.[64] Concepts such as pre-load and after-load, left ventricular end-diastolic pressure or dp/dt (degree of acceleration of pressure during systole), for example, are invaluable but not infallible guides. In cardiac surgery, as in other fields, the ultimate test of a therapy is its benefit to the patient, but the difficulty of providing rigorously controlled trials in the very sick is well-recognised. The term 'low cardiac output' is often used loosely to mean any clinically obvious impairment in heart action, even in the ambulant patient with heart disease, though 'low cardiac output *state*' is generally used more precisely and synonymously with 'shock'. However, there is clearly a spectrum, varying from the normal cardiac output to the hardly measurable output of cardiac massage. From a practical viewpoint, it might be best to use 'poor cardiac output' as a general term, restricting the term 'low cardiac output state' to a situation where the absolute sign of tissue ischaemia is present, namely a metabolic acidosis which persistently recurs despite correction with alkali. This signifies a cardiac index of less than 1.8 litres,[75] or half to two-thirds of normal. Whilst the heart and liver in particular can metabolise lactic acid, eventually they can no longer accept the acid load and themselves join other tissues and organs in the formation and development of acidosis.[218] There is a close relationship between the degree of tissue hypoxia and blood lactate,[4,243] though a normal arterial oxygen tension antagonises its formation.[185] Persistent acidosis has a bad prognosis, whilst its absence or disappearance is a valuable sign of improved heart action and may precede clinical signs of improvement, except perhaps that of an increase in peripheral temperature.

A poor cardiac output after cardiac surgery is most often due to myocardial damage from preoperative and/or intraoperative factors. It also complicates uncorrected or intractable haemorrhage, postoperative myocardial infarction, therapy with myocardial depressants, in particular beta-adrenergic blockers, advanced respiratory distress, acute cardiac tamponade, septicaemia and very rarely acute adrenal insufficiency.[91]

Sympathomimetic drugs are a vital tool in treatment of this condition if it is due to poor heart action. Two of these, isoprenaline and adrenaline, have been used, often together, for many years. Noradrenaline has long been regarded as an undesirable agent because of its potent alpha-sympathetic properties, being used as a last and generally hopeless resort. However, it seems that like most sympathomimetic agents, it is most valuable and produces the best response when it is used early, and least effective when used late. We have used it with good effect when other sympathomimetic agents are unsuitable or unsatisfactory. It is specifically helpful in a heart poisoned by beta-adrenergic blockade when other agents fail to improve its action. The heart is also more sensitive to this drug when its endogenous stores have been depleted by chronic heart failure.[216] Noradrenaline is also invaluable in cardiac resuscitation where the peripheral resistance falls from intense tissue acidosis,[219] and it improves coronary and cerebral blood flow,[82] though here a massive dose (2–4 mg) is required. It can also occasionally be used with benefit during intraortic balloon pumping (see below), when the advantage of its raising of the diastolic blood pressure may outweigh the disadvantage of the accompanying increase in heart work from the rise in peripheral resistance. Some workers combine noradrenaline with an alpha-sympathetic blocker such as phentolamine[98] or phenoxybenzamine, though the alpha effect is anyway greatly reduced when the drug is highly diluted. It is uncertain whether, like adrenaline and isoprenaline, noradrenaline produces subendocardial ischaemia and necrosis,[104,151] one of the most important causes of cardiac dysfunction after open heart surgery. Other sympathomimetic agents are now available, each with claimed advantages and advocates. They include dopamine, dobutamine and salbutamol (Table 3.1). Some agents, for example, dopamine and isoprenaline,[170] have been compared with each other in the treatment of a low cardiac output state after cardiac surgery, but whilst there may be physiological benefits with this or that drug, none is ideal for all situations.[65,97,98] There is still no drug which in all dosages improves heart action without increasing its oxygen consumption or irritability, and specifically increases blood flow to vital organs and not skin or muscle. In one view, 'vascular changes in shock may simply represent the best possible balance between . . . priorities of pressure and flow under the particular circumstances. . . . We should concentrate on dealing with organ failure and with deficit where it exists, rather than tampering with a probably flawless homeostatic response'.[175]

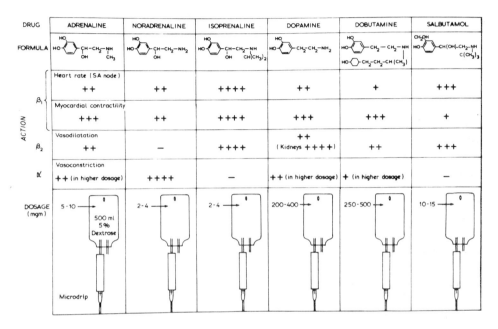

Table 3.1   Some sympathomimetic agents currently used in cardiac surgery. The 'microdrip' delivers 60 drops per ml of solution

The actions of sympathomimetic drugs are described in terms of alpha and beta (or more recently beta 1 and beta 2) sympathetic effects, but the limitations of this previously convenient classification are obvious when it is used to describe, for example, the qualitatively and quantitatively different beta effects of various drugs on the heart and specific vascular beds.

Ideally, the choice of drug, or drugs, should be based on continuous assessment of various physiological parameters, such as cardiac output, peripheral resistance, wedge pressure, stroke work and so on, and their response to therapy. In this centre, lacking the required investigative facilities, we judge the response largely on a clinical basis, and perhaps this is not really an inferior approach. We generally initiate therapy with isoprenaline and/or adrenaline, adding, or changing to, other agents if the response is unsatisfactory. The dose of sympathomimetic agent is often described in micrograms (μg) per kilogram body weight, an approach which has been criticised since the lean mass and not fat absorbs the drug.[232] We find it more convenient to make a standard solution and titrate the infusion rate according to the response, increasing the concentration if necessary (Table 3.1).

Dopamine[96,97,98]

This drug, like its immediate physiological derivative noradrenaline, has both alpha and beta sympathomimetic properties, but to a markedly different degree. It is said to act both directly on the adrenergic receptors and indirectly through the liberation of noradrenaline from body stores, and has several valuable actions which distinguish it from available sympathomimetic amines. One is improvement in cardiac contractility, and hence cardiac output, which is not accompanied by a significant rise in heart rate and hence myocardial oxygen consumption, a major disadvantage of isoprenaline[148] and an important cause of myocardial damage from subendocardial necrosis.[104] Dopamine, a vasodilator like isoprenaline and low concentrations of adrenaline, also specifically increases renal blood flow, an action attributed to hypothetical 'dopaminergic' receptors, though the term is merely an acknowledgement of our ignorance of how sympathomimetic drugs act. This increase in renal flow may produce a significant rise in urine output in a low cardiac output state when other agents have failed. But it is not known whether dopamine can prevent renal damage from shock. In high doses (more than 15–20 μg/kilogram body weight/minute), dopamine also has an alpha-adrenergic effect, though this can be abolished by vasodilators,[65,97] and may cause tachycardia and ventricular dysrhythmias. A combination of dopamine and adrenaline is superior to either drug alone in high dosage, producing a relatively greater increase in cardiac output than in heart rate or afterload.[77] Like isoprenaline[137] and other vasodilators such as phenoxybenzamine,[18] dopamine increases the physiological shunt in the lungs,[15,188] though the Pao_2 may not fall because of the simultaneous rise in cardiac output.[188] As with other powerful vasoconstrictors dopamine can produce extensive tissue necrosis if it escapes into the tissues or is infused into a peripheral vein.[224] Even infusion into a major central vein may not prevent digital gangrene from aggravation of the already grossly reduced peripheral blood flow in a protracted low cardiac output state. However, tissue loss may be slight if the patient finally recovers.

We generally use a solution containing 200–400 mg of dopamine in 500 ml 5 per cent dextrose solution.

Dobutamine[96,198]

This drug is a derivative of dopamine, but its action does not partly depend on the liberation of endogenous noradrenaline, nor does it have a specific effect on renal blood flow. It has both alpha and beta adrenergic properties, but is a less powerful vasodilator than isoprenaline, this being claimed an advantage as less blood is wastefully diverted to muscles. Its alpha effect, present in higher doses, is less than that of noradrenaline or dopamine. At the moment, it has no obvious place in the management of patients after open heart surgery.

Salbutamol

This valuable bronchodilator has been used in the treatment of bronchial asthma for many years and replaced isoprenaline for this purpose because of its minimal cardiac side effects in the usual dosage. In high doses, it also has a beta-sympathomimetic effect on the heart and is a powerful vasodilator. Some centres use it in the postoperative period after cardiac surgery,[32,255] in particular to reduce peripheral vascular resistance. We have found it has no advantage over isoprenaline in this context since doses required for a significant response produce obvious tachycardia.

Glucagon

We have found this non-sympathomimetic inotropic drug disappointing, despite its advantages of not being affected by beta-adrenergic blockers, increasing renal blood flow,[126] and the low risk of producing dysrhythmias. It rarely produces significant improvement in heart action when sympathomimetic drugs fail.

Steroid therapy

Despite encouraging experimental and clinical reports,[58] there is still no convincing evidence that massive doses of the potent glucocorticosteroid methylprednisolone, or any other drug of this type, are beneficial in cardiogenic shock or, indeed, any other major problem associated with open heart surgery;[5,178] nor is there certain evidence of its prophylactic value against shock or pulmonary damage, and such therapy may even be harmful.[46] If reduction in left ventricular afterload from vasodilatation is one real benefit, this can be more readily achieved with other agents. Few drugs in medicine have as wide a spectrum of claimed value as massive corticosteroid therapy, and this alone justifies a sceptical attitude.

Renal failure

Though primary renal failure is rare after open heart surgery, secondary renal failure from a low cardiac output is common. The treatment of a low cardiac output with vasoactive drugs does not increase the risk of kidney damage.[157] On the contrary, the improvement in cardiac output from their beta-adrenergic effect outweighs the alpha-adrenergic effect, though dopamine has the added advantage of specifically increasing renal blood flow. A poor urine output is, therefore, more likely to reflect a poor cardiac output in shock than vasoconstriction from the inotropic drugs. It is now recognised that sustained diuresis during the operation, and massive doses of diuretics before or during a low cardiac output state, do not prevent renal failure,[129,138] but a satisfactory urine output is later essential to correct the haemodilution of cardiopulmonary bypass.

METABOLIC ACIDOSIS AND ITS CORRECTION

Whilst severe metabolic acidosis is harmful, sodium bicarbonate therapy itself has serious disadvantages and for a number of reasons should be used with discretion, especially in patients with a major cardiac lesion. The popular belief that the aim in sick patients should always be 'normality' may not be justified with regard to acid-base therapy. Mild metabolic acidosis (standard bicarbonate $\geqslant 16$ mmol per litre) will soon be corrected spontaneously if heart action is satisfactory. Some workers do not even correct acidosis after deep hypothermia in infants because of this and to avoid the disadvantages of bicarbonate therapy.[222] The acidosis is due to a variety of factors,[20] and is also seen in normothermic cardiopulmonary bypass, pulsatile or non-pulsatile,[21] when it has been attributed to inadequate flow,[256] though it is lessened by vasodilators.[21] Sodium bicarbonate therapy can lead to a metabolic alkalosis since bicarbonate excretion is slower than lactate oxidation, normally a rapid process.[62,185] A metabolic alkalosis may develop in patients very sick for other reasons, including chronic potassium loss, and after massive blood transfusion. The ill effects of alkalosis include the Bohr effect on the oxyhaemoglobin dissociation curve, a fall in serum potassium and excessive loss of this ion in the urine.[48] Although severe metabolic acidosis can antagonise sympathomimetic amines, there is no evidence that a mild acidosis is harmful or depresses heart action. It may even be beneficial by assisting oxygen uptake in the tissues.

Sodium bicarbonate solution (8.4 per cent, 1 mmol/ml) contains about seven times as much sodium as physiological saline, and this can lead to considerable sodium loading with its danger of hyperosmolarity.[152,253] The dangers of this condition are now well-recognised and include cerebral damage and circulatory overload from the intravascular shift of fluid.[71,147,253]

For these and perhaps other reasons, the mortality in patients with severe alkalosis may be similar to those with severe acidosis.[246] Suitable formulae for the correction of severe acidosis have been described. Whilst the Astrup formula is widely used, it can lead to excessive doses, and a more suitable formula[142] is:

required dose of sodium bicarbonate in mmol

$$= \frac{K \text{ (weight of patient in kilograms)} \times D \text{ (base deficit in mmol)}}{5}$$

Correction should aim at a standard bicarbonate of not more than 20 mmol per litre.[185] In cardiac arrest, whilst the degree of acidosis remains unknown, the dose may be calculated[89] as

mmol of sodium bicarbonate required

$$= \frac{K \text{ (estimated wt of patient in kg)} \times M \text{ (duration of cardiac arrest in minutes)}}{10}$$

The immediate administration of 100–150 mmol of sodium bicarbonate in cardiac arrest, widely, even authoritatively recommended, has no justification and there is no evidence of its value. It represents an unnecessary sodium and bicarbonate load if cardiac arrest is too brief for the development of significant acidosis and is then followed by the return of satisfactory heart action. Severe depression of brain activity after cardiac arrest may be due to the swift passage of carbon dioxide liberated by alkali therapy across the blood-brain barrier,[17] as well as osmolar complications from excessive sodium bicarbonate.[152]

Bicarbonate therapy is not necessary in massive transfusion unless heart action is unsatisfactory[165] since the tissues can consume the extra lactate. Indeed, if renal excretion of the citrate preservative is impaired, a metabolic alkalosis may develop later.[150]

VASODILATOR THERAPY[49,167,172a]

The oxygen demand of the heart is related to a number of factors. They include the ventricular wall tension, the contractile state of the myocardium and the heart rate. The ventricular wall tension depends on the end-diastolic volume of the ventricle (pre-load, volume load), and the systemic vascular resistance (after-load, aortic impedance, pressure-load), both of which are often raised in heart failure.[49] A reduction in after-load allows the failing heart to devote more of its energy to expelling blood, than to generating pressure (Fig. 3.4), so increasing the cardiac output. At the same time, the reduction in venous return from peripheral pooling reduces the ventricular filling pressure and hence its end-diastolic volume. This fall in ventricular diameter allows the heart to beat more effectively, since in accordance with Laplace's Law it now has to generate less wall tension to produce the same pressure. These reductions in pre-load and after-load are the principle benefits of vasodilator therapy in heart failure. In contrast to other pharmacological methods of supporting the failing heart, in particular sympathomimetic amines,

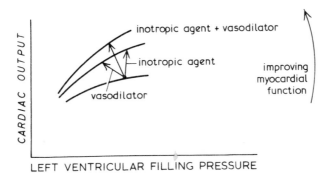

Fig. 3.4 The effect of inotropic agents and vasodilators on ventricular function curves in heart failure. (After Miller, R. R. et al (1977) *Circulation*, 55, 881)

vasodilator therapy decreases rather than increases oxygen demand, though unlike mechanical circulatory assistance devices, it does not also directly increase myocardial blood supply. On the other hand, a combination of vasodilator and inotropic drugs has a synergistic effect,[49,173] though the ideal combination for each clinical situation cannot be predicted.

Most of the evidence for the value of vasodilator therapy relates to the left side of the heart. Its effect on the right ventricle and pulmonary circulation is less clear, though it can reduce pulmonary vascular resistance,[49] and some workers have found it beneficial, especially in patients with pulmonary hypertensive mitral valve disease.[27] If heart function is normal or only slightly impaired, the combination of reduced venous return and vasodilatation can lead to a fall in cardiac output and hypotension.[49] In heart failure, the rise in cardiac output from the shift to an improved Frank–Starling curve outweighs the fall in peripheral vascular resistance so that hypotension, with its danger of myocardial ischaemia, does not occur unless there is hypovolaemia or the dose of vasodilator drug is excessive. However, vasodilator therapy must be used with great care, if at all, in a low cardiac output state since there may be a disastrous fall in blood pressure.

Several drugs are used for intravenous administration in vasodilator therapy.[49,167] They include phentolamine,[174] chlorpromazine, trimetaphan, and most recently sodium nitroprusside.[16,225,234]

CIRCULATORY ASSIST DEVICES

These devices have two major advantages in patients with severe heart failure, especially in patients with severe ischaemic heart disease. They decrease ventricular work, and hence myocardial oxygen consumption, and they increase coronary blood flow, and hence myocardial oxygen supply. No inotropic drugs, or combination of drugs have both these effects, which are of great benefit to the myocardial oxygen demand–oxygen supply ratio.

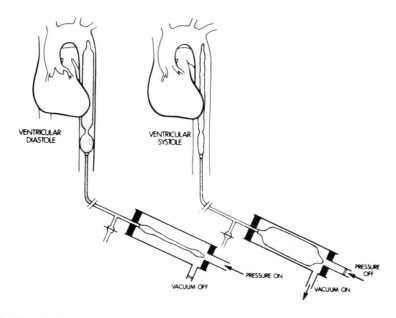

Fig. 3.5   The principle of circulatory assistance from intra-aortic balloon counterpulsation. The intra-aortic balloons are inflated during ventricular diastole by mechanically driven gas compression of the external balloon, and deflated by its inflation during ventricular systole. (Bregman, D. (1970) *Trans Am. Soc. Artif. Int. Organs*, **16,** 439.) (Reproduced by kind permission of the American Society for Artificial Internal Organs, Washington)

The most effective devices use internal (intra-aortic balloon catheter) counterpulsation,[37,169] a concept first described by Harken twenty years ago, but only recently introduced into clinical practice. External, non-invasive techniques are less satisfactory.[169] The principle of the internal device, commonly termed the 'balloon pump', is as follows. A long catheter with two balloons at its tip is introduced into the femoral artery and thence up the aorta to just below the origin of the left subclavian artery (Fig. 3.5). These balloons are now inflated and deflated together, with the aid of a pump, which alternately and in the opposite phase, deflates and inflates an external balloon joined to the internal pair. The aortic balloons inflate at the onset of ventricular diastole, just before the closure of the aortic valve. This prevents the 'run off' of blood into the descending aorta and increases the diastolic pressure (Fig. 3.6). Autoregulation of coronary blood flow is lost in ischaemic heart disease and coronary flow becomes pressure dependant. Since three-quarters of coronary flow occurs in diastole, this increase in diastolic pressure produces a significant rise in myocardial blood supply, which may even triple. The smaller, distal balloon is said to enhance this effect since it inflates slightly before the larger one, whose expansion, therefore, displaces its own volume of blood towards the heart. However, the balloons are generally not occlusive, and the displaced blood is also driven distally. The improvement in coronary arterial flow may also improve collateral vessel flow.[37] The balloons deflate at the onset of ventricular systole, reducing aortic tension and hence ventricular work (after-load), and increasing the stroke volume, with a fall in ventricular diastolic volume (pre-load). The cardiac output may rise by as much as one and a half litres.[169]

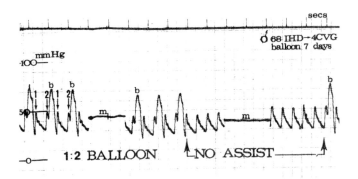

Fig. 3.6   Record of the radial artery pulse wave during intra-aortic balloon counterpulsation in a 68-year-old man who required this therapy for seven days after the insertion of four saphenous vein grafts for ischaemic heart disease. Note that although there is only a slight rise in mean blood pressure, the diastolic area of the curve is greatly increased. There is also a lower end-diastolic pressure with each assisted beat. (1 = pulse wave without circulatory assistance; 2 = pulse wave with circulatory assistance; b = effect of circulatory assistance; m = mean arterial blood pressure)

The balloon cycle can be linked either to the aortic ejection curve or more usually to the R wave of the electrocardiogram. Controls on at least one device permit great flexibility in the onset, pattern, and duration of balloon inflation to permit optimal assistance to the heart. Weaning from the device is facilitated by assisting every second or third heart beat.

Circulatory assistance is now widely used for some days or even weeks before cardiac surgery in patients with cardiogenic shock from acute myocardial infarction. It not only improves heart action, with its beneficial effects on other organs, but it can reduce the size of the infarct. In addition, it dramatically relieves anginal pain and abolishes grave dysrhythmias. It can also prevent infarction. Postoperatively the indications for using the device vary with the surgeon, some even using it electively in high risk cases with poor ventricular function. As with mechanical ventilation (page 75) earlier use inevitably produces better results since it includes patients who would have survived without it. However, it is often dramatically beneficial when severe heart failure after surgery for ischaemic heart disease responds poorly to liberal doses of inotropic drugs, though these may still be required during counterpulsation. The mortality rate for cardiogenic shock complicating acute myocardial infarction is over 95 per cent. The survival rate is improved to about 20 per cent with balloon pumping and to 30 to 40 per cent if this is combined with aortocoronary bypass surgery.[25] The results of circulatory assistance are less impressive when it is used for heart failure after other types of cardiac surgery. Balloon pumping can also be used during cardiac resuscitation.[37]

The main disadvantage of this technique is the cost of the machine and the balloon catheters, and the need for skilled supervision. Mechanical ventilation may be discontinued before the device is removed if the patient's condition, including his circulatory state, is stable and satisfactory. Serious complications are rare, though it is best to remove the catheter under general anaesthesia, exploring the femoral artery with a Fogarty catheter before repairing it, to remove clot. Thrombocytopaenia has also been reported and is probably a reflection of blood damage from the balloon.

RESPIRATORY PROBLEMS

(Note: the reader is referred to Chapter 7 for a full examination of the subject of mechanical ventilation.)

Lung function is depressed for several days after open heart surgery, as in other types of trauma, and this has been attributed to various factors, some special to cardiopulmonary bypass and its consequences. They include water retention, reduction in oncotic pressure, atelectasis, airway closure and perhaps reduction in surfactant, though this is now a less fashionable culprit. Continued ventilation during bypass is also deleterious.[220] Postoperative oxygen therapy usually ensures adequate oxygenation, but mechanical ventilation is generally continued for some hours, chiefly because of its many practical advantages, since its prophylactic value against pulmonary complications, and particularly the respiratory distress syndrome, is still uncertain. These practical advantages include ensured and adequate gas exchange, unrestricted use of narcotic analgesics, airway protection, immediately effective ventilation in cardiac arrest, and a rapid switch to general anaesthesia if countershock or thoracotomy is required. However, some centres allow infants to breathe spontaneously with positive end expiratory pressure immediately after surgery, if their cardiovascular state is satisfactory.[222] The decision to attempt discontinuation of mechanical ventilation is easy to make in most cases, and can be made by the trained nurse, using ordinary clinical criteria. It does not require blood gas analysis or any other test, though some centres use a whole range of these.[110,184] Neither in the immediate postoperative period nor in the treatment of long-term patients do we accept that 'the question of how one assesses the ability of a patient to come off the ventilator is a complex one'.[111] Essentially, the patient's respiratory, cardiovascular and neurological state should all be clinically satisfactory, and remain so during spontaneous respiration.[82] Typically, a suitable patient shows an active alert interest in his surroundings and his feet are completely warm. This unorthodox approach has proved safe and reliable for many years. Potentially difficult patients, in particular infants, and those with complex congenital heart disease or severe pulmonary hypertensive mitral valve disease, are disconnected from the ventilator only under medical supervision, though using identical criteria. The patient is reconnected if there is any clinical deterioration,[82] blood gas analysis being performed exceptionally and only in the most difficult cases, or as a baseline measurement if continued ventilation is judged necessary.

Respiratory distress requiring continued mechanical ventilation may be obvious shortly after the patient is allowed to breathe spontaneously, or it may develop some hours or even days later. Unless the problem has an obvious cause, such as pulmonary oedema or massive atelectasis, it can be regarded as a manifestation of the adult respiratory distress syndrome (ARDS), an inappropriate term since the condition also occurs in children, although it also has at least twenty-seven other labels.[24] Its cause has not been clearly established, though evidence suggests it is

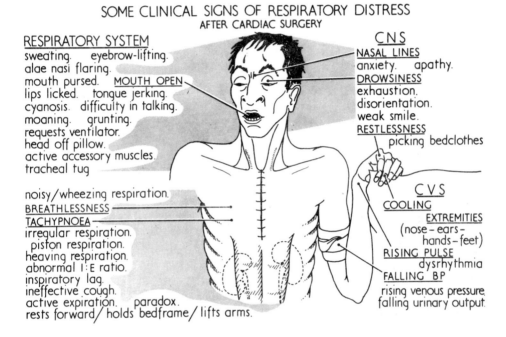

SOME CLINICAL SIGNS OF RESPIRATORY DISTRESS
AFTER CARDIAC SURGERY

RESPIRATORY SYSTEM
sweating.   eyebrow-lifting.
alae nasi flaring.
mouth pursed.   MOUTH OPEN
lips licked.   tongue jerking.
cyanosis. difficulty in talking.
moaning.   grunting.
requests ventilator.
head off pillow.
active accessory muscles.
tracheal tug

noisy/wheezing respiration.
BREATHLESSNESS
TACHYPNOEA
irregular respiration.
piston respiration.
heaving respiration.
abnormal I : E ratio.
inspiratory lag.
ineffective cough.
active expiration.   paradox.
rests forward/ holds bedframe/ lifts arms.

CNS
NASAL LINES
anxiety.   apathy.
DROWSINESS
exhaustion.
disorientation.
weak smile.
RESTLESSNESS
        picking bedclothes

CVS
COOLING
        EXTREMITIES
(nose – ears –
        hands – feet)
RISING PULSE
        dysrhythmia
FALLING BP
rising venous pressure.
falling urinary output.

Fig. 3.7   The clinical signs of respiratory distress after cardiac surgery can be classified under three systems, respiratory, cardiovascular and central nervous. A scoring system based on nine selected common signs (underlined) is a reliable guide to mechanical ventilation[87]

at first a mainly pulmonary vascular lesion.[23,200,247] The value of measures for its prevention such as microfilters during massive transfusion (see below), and massive corticosteroid therapy[7,46,205,245] remains uncertain. Its incidence is unrelated to colloid osmotic pressure.[51,235]

Patients with even obvious impairment of lung function before cardiac surgery do not seem to be more likely to require protracted ventilation afterwards, but certain conditions do greatly increase the risk, in particular advanced mitral valve disease associated with certain signs. These signs are breathlessness at rest, and this may be almost imperceptible even on talking, cachexia, a cold periphery, gross hepatomegaly, severe pulmonary hypertension (pulmonary artery pressure ⩾60 mm mercury), and a large heart (cardiothoracic ratio ⩾0.6) with a giant left atrium. Double or triple valve replacement in these patients with mechanical prostheses is very often followed by severe respiratory distress, and finally death from heart failure, despite mechanical ventilation. Massive blood transfusion, often required because of bleeding adhesions from previous surgery and prolonged myocardial ischaemia may be contributory factors.

The clinical features of ARDS after open heart surgery (Fig. 3.7) reflect the underlying changes in lung function and particularly lung structure, and their ill-effects[86] (Fig. 3.8). The most common of the important clinical signs, apart

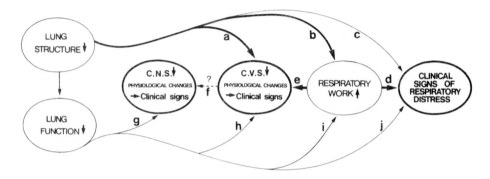

THE PATHWAY FOR CLINICAL SIGNS IN ARDS

Fig. 3.8   Mechanisms leading to the development of the clinical signs of respiratory distress after cardiac surgery. The thick arrows indicate the main pathways. (a) pulmonary hypertension, from deterioration in lung structure and pulmonary vasoconstriction, together with excessive respiratory work (e) leads to the clinical signs of heart failure, such as hypotension, tachycardia and peripheral cooling. (b) fall in lung compliance leads to signs of increased respiratory work (d), such as breathlessness, tachypnoea and an open mouth, as well as to heart failure (e). (c) deterioration in lung structure produces such signs as intercostal recession, and wheezing and other auscultatory abnormalities. (f) severe neurological deterioration is probably chiefly due to exhaustion and heart failure, but the cause of terminal coma is not clear, and is only occasionally attributable to profound hypoxia or respiratory acidosis (g) in the ventilated patient. Early neurological deterioration, with anxiety and restlessness is probably due to excessive respiratory work, and precedes marked blood gas derangement. (h) profound hypoxia and respiratory acidosis may finally depress heart action. (i) the loss of functioning lung tissue requires an increase in ventilation of the remaining lung. (j) sweating is usually due to excessive work, not respiratory acidosis, whose classical signs are rarely seen in cardiac patients. The need for increased ventilation may be obvious from the respiratory pattern

from increasing breathlessness, are a rising respiratory rate, a cooling periphery and drowsiness.[86,92] These reflect, in order, respiratory, cardiovascular and neurological deterioration. Death is usually due to heart failure, though there is often accompanying deterioration of other organ function. The heart failure is chiefly due to two factors, excessive respiratory work from the fall in lung compliance, and pulmonary hypertension, which is one consequence of the lesion.[93,108,257] The oxygen cost of breathing may rise to more than half the total intake, with a third of the cardiac output going to the respiratory muscles. The situation is aggravated when lung dysfunction, pulmonary hypertension and heart failure[41] are already present, as just described in mitral valve disease.

There are also important changes in the blood gas state, reflecting simultaneous deterioration in lung function. The $Paco_2$ initially falls because of hyperventilation, and this may be associated with increasing respiratory distress and an increasing need for mechanical assistance, though finally it rises from exhaustion and progressive deterioration in lung function. The arterial oxygen tension (Pao_2) falls and the alveolar-arterial tension difference ($AaDo_2$) rises, a consequence of the increase in venous admixture.

A scoring system based solely on selected but common and significant clinical signs indicates the appropriate moment for initiating mechanical ventilation,[87] whose chief advantage is the abolition of respiratory work, though a fall in pulmonary vascular resistance and improvement in lung structure and function also assist the heart. Most workers believe blood-gas analysis and sometimes other tests of lung function are crucially important in determining the need for mechanical ventilation;[24,247] but there is no evidence that these are essential, that the proposed critical, though arbitrary values, are optimal values, or that this approach produces the best results. Indeed, the mortality of ARDS is high in most reported series, differences perhaps depending not only on the indications for initiating mechanical ventilation but on the type of material and on the criteria for diagnosis. Earlier mechanical ventilation can improve results simply by including patients who would anyway survive without it, as much as by its therapeutic effect. There is little relationship between the clinical picture and the blood gas state,[92] and this is not surprising since the first is closely linked to *respiratory work* and cardiac function (whose deterioration finally kills the patient, ventilated or not), the second to *respiratory function*, whose impairment, however gross, rarely threatens life except in the terminal stages (Fig. 3.9). At most, a group of patients judged to require mechanical ventilation after open heart surgery purely on clinical grounds have a mean $Paco_2$ somewhat lower than a group with milder respiratory distress who all survive without it, but there is a wide and overlapping range of $Paco_2$ values between an acceptable level and hypoxia in each group.[92] There is no difference between mean $Paco_2$ values which are normal, though here, too, there is a wide range. An unsatisfactory blood gas state, therefore, does not necessarily indicate the need for mechanical ventilation, nor does an acceptable one rule it out.

A combination of sedation, muscle paralysis and mild hypothermia (34°C) to reduce metabolic rate and hence oxygen requirements appeared to increase the survival rate in one small series.[74] The pulmonary vascular resistance in ARDS is not fixed but is inversely related to the cardiac output,[257] and this is also the case in normal lungs.[244] For this reason, we now introduce a slow infusion of an inotropic agent such as isoprenaline in difficult cases. Dangerous complications of prolonged endotracheal intubation are rare, whilst those of tracheostomy are not. Sick patients are easily infected even with bacteria of low virulence, in particular *Ps. pyocyaneus*, and a tracheostomy, however carefully managed, swiftly exposes the lungs to this problem. We, therefore, prefer the risk of laryngeal damage to the risks of tracheostomy.

Mechanical ventilation is continued until the previously described criteria are satisfied, weaning being based solely on clinical signs in most cases.[82] These indicate the patient's ability to work, and his cardiac response to this work and to the rise in venous return and pulmonary vascular resistance. As in the immediate postoperative period, most centres regard blood gas analysis and perhaps other tests of lung function as crucial throughout the weaning period,[70,212] but they are guides neither to respiratory work nor to heart function, and occasionally are dangerously misleading.

The circulatory state is the best guide to the prognosis. As long as it is satisfactory, the outlook is hopeful, but once the peripheral circulation, as judged by the warmth of the extremities, starts to deteriorate, survival is unlikely.

A recently described technique, intermittent mandatory ventilation (IMV) is now widely used.[59] We have found it offers little advantage over our present methods, and its value has yet to be clearly demonstrated. Most accounts are anecdotal and there is little evidence that it shortens the necessary period of

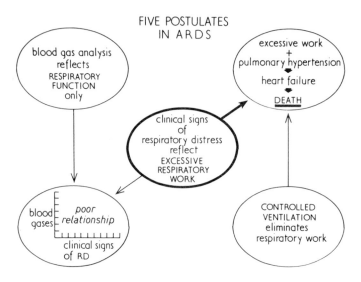

Fig. 3.9   Five postulates in ARDS after cardiac surgery. The main value of mechanical ventilation is the abolition of respiratory work

mechanical ventilation or accelerates removal of the tracheal tube. Patients with stiff lungs may not be suitable,[70] and one favourable report did not bear critical examination.[176]

The survival rate of patients requiring immediate and uninterrupted mechanical ventilation after open heart surgery seems to be higher than in those who require it much later. If this difference is established, it may be due to various factors, and it has been reported in other conditions, when sepsis was a vital element in the difference.[108,240] Amongst its many ill-effects, sepsis intensifies the rise in pulmonary vascular resistance, possibly by release of vasoactive agents[51] which aggravate capillary damage, encouraging fluid leakage into the tissues and compression of the vascular bed. A persistently high $AaDO_2$ in ARDS also has a bad prognosis, especially if it has a rapid onset, whereas a return to normal within forty-eight hours without relapse has the best outlook.[12] A swift and marked improvement in the $AaDO_2$ with positive end expiratory pressure (PEEP) is another favourable sign,[69] especially if it is due to a fall in physiological shunt rather than a rise in cardiac output.[215] Lung function is at most only slightly depressed after recovery from ARDS,[125,132,194] probably reflecting the reversible nature of the histological lesion in those who survive and the absence of fibrosis.[69]

Clearly, there are still many uncertainties about the adult respiratory distress syndrome after cardiac surgery and other conditions. Is mechanical ventilation merely supportive or is it also curative? How can we conclusively determine when to initiate it and when to discontinue it? Is there an optimum point for its use and a critical point for its delay, and does even 'safe' delay nevertheless postpone recovery? What are the indices for these points? How are they related to pulmonary anatomical changes, physiological disturbances and clinical signs, and how are these factors linked to each other? Why is the mortality still so high, at least 50 per cent in most centres? Most important, how can we prevent the condition?

POSITIVE END EXPIRATORY PRESSURE (PEEP)

This technique was first described over forty years ago, but it has only recently been combined with mechanical ventilation ($PEEP_{mech}$). Its main advantages are improvement in arterial oxygenation, allowing a lower inspired oxygen fraction (Fio_2), a reduction in small airways resistance, and in some patients with severe right heart failure, a rise in cardiac output because of the fall in venous return and hence right ventricular filling pressure.[84,236]

PEEP is now widely used in the treatment of ARDS, including patients after open heart surgery. It is generally indicated if the Pao_2 is unsatisfactory despite oxygen therapy ($Pao_2 \leqslant 75$–80 mm mercury, $Fio_2 \geqslant 0.6$). Its effect on the Pao_2 depends on many factors and is unpredictable in the very sick. Two factors in particular influence it. These are the cardiac output and hence the mixed venous oxygen tension ($P\bar{v}o_2$), the 'quality' of the shunt, and the shunt fraction (Q_s/Q_t), the 'quantity' of the shunt[88] (Figs 3.10a and 3.10b). The Pao_2 may rise or fall to a variable degree, or even remain unaffected, depending on the balance between these two factors.

Despite its popularity, there is no evidence that PEEP has a significant effect on the mortality or morbidity of ARDS, and it can produce serious problems such as hypotension and barotrauma. Favourable reports are mostly retrospective or uncontrolled studies, and one comparative trial suggested it had no effect on mortality.[221] However, it may have a prophylactic effect, reducing the likelihood of ARDS developing in susceptible patients,[10,201] or the need for mechanical ventilation in those who develop it,[101] though here the evidence is less impressive. For these reasons, we now use $PEEP_{mech}$ 5–10 cm water after open heart surgery for 36–48 hours in the type of patients with mitral valve disease we have previously described, even if their condition is satisfactory. Whilst 'high PEEP'[124] ($PEEP_{mech} > 20$ cm water) is occasionally required, we have not found it beneficial, since on the whole the greater the level of PEEP needed, the worse the degree of lung damage, and the worse the prognosis.

PEEP with spontaneous ventilation ($PEEP_{spont}$, CPAP, CRAP) is now widely used after cardiac surgery in infants and small children. In some centres, it is used almost routinely after discontinuation of mechanical ventilation and gradually reduced to a prescribed pattern according to the Pao_2.[223] There is no evidence that such routine use is beneficial. Very sick infants with major circulatory and ventilatory problems are best mechanically ventilated, and $PEEP_{spont}$ should be used only where the circulatory state remains satisfactory, despite a respiratory problem, and the child is obviously content to breathe on his own without increasing distress. Its greatest value is in infants with stiff lungs, increased airway resistance and a high venous admixture. Here $PEEP_{spont}$ may be of

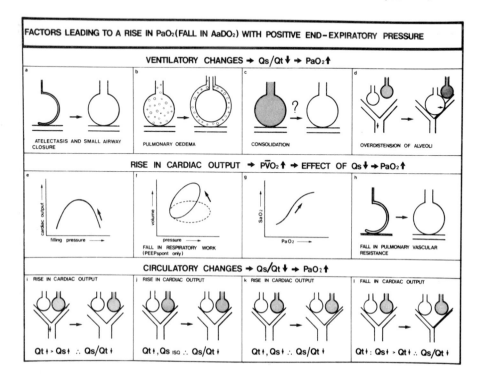

Fig. 3.10a   Factors leading to a rise in arterial oxygen tension (Pao_2) and fall in alveolar-arterial oxygen tension difference ($Aado_2$) with positive end-expiratory pressure. (Reproduced with kind permission of Springer-Verlag, Heidelberg.)

assistance, since the improved alveolar ventilation leads to a more acceptable respiratory pattern because of the significant fall in respiratory work, as well as a rise in Pao_2.[47,107] The effects of PEEP on the injured brain are discussed below.

BRAIN DAMAGE

This once common and feared complication of open-heart surgery is now relatively rare. The single most important factor in this change is almost certainly the careful prevention of embolism, particularly air embolism,[83] during and immediately after cardiopulmonary bypass, and the use of arterial filters.[33] Nevertheless, cardiopulmonary bypass remains a brain insult. The greatly reduced need for anaesthesia during perfusion[83] and the often delayed recovery of consciousness or even brain damage after a protracted bypass are evidence of this, though it is probably not the only factor. Pulsatile perfusion improves cerebral blood flow and function during cardiopulmonary bypass.[251]

Cerebral function often suddenly, but usually transiently, deteriorates at the moment of starting bypass, though the commonly associated clinical signs such as pupil dilatation, facial and other movements, and breathing are often attributed to the patient's 'waking up', an unlikely event because of the swiftness of their

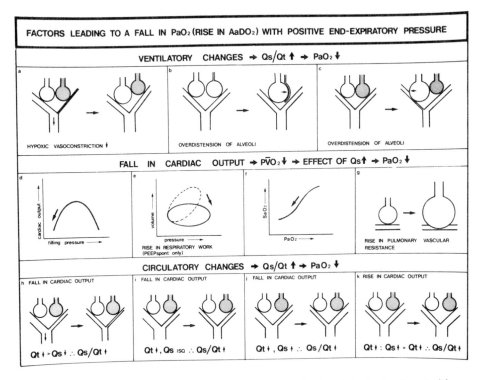

FACTORS LEADING TO A FALL IN PaO₂ (RISE IN AaDO₂) WITH POSITIVE END-EXPIRATORY PRESSURE

VENTILATORY   CHANGES   → Qs/Qt ↑   → PaO₂ ↓

a   b   c

HYPOXIC VASOCONSTRICTION ↑   OVERDISTENSION OF ALVEOLI   OVERDISTENSION OF ALVEOLI

FALL   IN   CARDIAC   OUTPUT   → PⱽO₂ ↓   → EFFECT OF Qs↑   → PaO₂ ↓

d   e   f   g

cardiac output / filling pressure   volume / pressure — RISE IN RESPIRATORY WORK (PEEPspont only)   SaO₂ / PaO₂ —   RISE IN PULMONARY VASCULAR RESISTANCE

CIRCULATORY   CHANGES   → Qs/Qt ↑   → PaO₂ ↓

h FALL IN CARDIAC OUTPUT   i FALL IN CARDIAC OUTPUT   j FALL IN CARDIAC OUTPUT   k RISE IN CARDIAC OUTPUT

Qt ↓ > Qs ↓ ∴ Qs/Qt ↑   Qt ↓, Qs iso ∴ Qs/Qt ↑   Qt ↓, Qs ↑ ∴ Qs/Qt ↑   Qt ↑ : Qs ↑ > Qt ↑ ∴ Qs/Qt ↑

Fig. 3.10b   Factors leading to a fall in arterial oxygen tension (PaO₂) and rise in alveolar-arterial oxygen tension difference (AaDO₂) with positive end expiratory pressure. (Gilston, A. (1977) *Intensive Care Medicine*, **3**, 267.) (Reproduced with kind permission of Springer-Verlag, Heidelberg)

appearance. There is an associated transient but marked deterioration in the electroencephalogram.[31]

Autoregulation persists during cardiopulmonary bypass,[109] but it does not immediately respond to sudden changes in perfusion pressure,[155] being largely a chemical mechanism. The sudden fall in mean blood pressure at the onset of bypass, due in part at least to the reduction in blood viscosity with haemodilution,[99] is therefore, one possible cause of this cerebral ischaemia,[30] though it does improve cerebral blood flow once the perfusion pressure rises.[195] The change from pulsatile to non-pulsatile flow is another possibility since pulsatile flow is physiologically superior.[251] Additional factors may be the abrupt perfusion of the brain with a cold perfusate which has a reduced oxygen carrying capacity, and the release of gas bubbles as the fluid warms to body temperature and responds to other complex physical changes.[19] Occasionally, the aortic cannula is accidentally inserted into the left subclavian artery (Fig. 3.1) but this is an easily corrected cause of cerebral ischaemia. The degree of gaseous and particulate embolism is related to the duration of bypass,[1,35] and together with hypotension it is one of the most likely factors in brain dysfunction after prolonged bypass. Some centres use a device which records the overall electrical activity of the brain very slowly,* facilitating the detection of neurological abnormalities during and after open heart surgery.[33,202] A recent device† monitors gaseous emboli in the perfusion line. The degree of gaseous embolism is also closely related to the Pao_2 during bypass,[143] and this is often unnecessarily high. A mean perfusion pressure

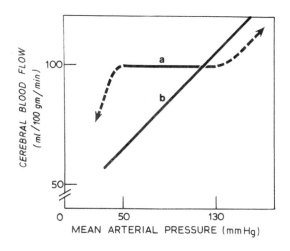

Fig. 3.11   The normal relationship between perfusion pressure and cerebral blood flow (a) and the effect of loss of autoregulation (b)

below 50–60 mmHg at normothermia greatly increases the incidence of electro-encephalographic abnormalities.[120] This pressure corresponds with the lower limit of autoregulation in normotensives. Whilst ischaemic depression of brain function is not synonymous with brain damage,[136] there is a risk of such damage,[226,237,249] and it therefore seems best to avoid prolonged hypotension during normothermia, especially in older patients, and during prolonged bypass. The critical level may be higher in hypertension, where the autoregulation curve (Fig. 3.11) is shifted to the right. A mean perfusion pressure over 100–120 mmHg, approaching the upper limit of autoregulation, is also undesirable, and should be treated with a vasodilator if it does not respond to a narcotic. Some workers have detected lactic acidosis in the cerebrospinal fluid during bypass,[78] as well as a gradual fall in oxygen tension,[106] and these are possibly related to brain damage.[106] However, there is no relationship between the pHa or $Paco_2$ and the electro-encephalogram during bypass.[119]

Hypoglycaemia is a well-recognised complication in children undergoing major

---

* Devices Cerebral Function Monitor (Devices Ltd., Welwyn Garden City, Herts.).
† TMB Microbubble Activity Monitor (Technique Laboratories Ltd., High Street, Hartley Wintney, Hampshire).

surgery,[241] and it also occurs in cardiac surgery.[145] To protect the brain, it is wise to administer appropriate amounts of glucose during and after the operation in this age group, such as 0.2 gram/kilogram body weight/hour as an infusion.[211]

If brain damage does occur, its degree varies from merely delayed return of consciousness or slight restlessness to profound areflexic coma and early death. Some workers believe careful examination reveals a high incidence of neurological abnormalities.[139] Psychiatric complications seem to be more common in North America,[61,139] than in this country, though depression is very common in the first postoperative week. The psychoses are probably organic, but lesser psychiatric complications may also be related to intensive care and social problems. Apart from overt brain damage, various cranial and peripheral nerve lesions have been reported. They include visual damage of varied types,[103,230] deafness,[9,252] and facial palsy.[61] A curious peripheral neuropathy, mononeuritis multiplex, is a common but only recently described entity after bypass,[123] with motor and sensory changes in cranial and peripheral nerves. The lesions in our experience often affect the upper limbs, with weakness and irregular scattered patches of numbness, paraesthesiae and even pain. They often show an irregular glove distribution on the hands, and do not correspond with any nerve area or dermatome. The cause is not known, but it may be due to embolism, and the condition clears after some weeks.

Investigation of brain damage after cardiac surgery

It is best to use an anaesthetic technique for cardiac surgery which allows the patient to regain consciousness swiftly afterwards.[83] This facilitates the early detection and interpretation of neurological problems. Profound but unexplained brain dysfunction requires the most careful investigation, though it is fortunately rare. Measurement of the serum osmolality is essential as well as estimation of the blood sugar, especially in diabetics who may be in hyperosmolar coma.[36,168] The advent of coronary artery surgery has made diabetes a common postoperative problem. Computerised axial tomography, 'brain scanning', a major advance in neuroradiology,[155] may prove to be an increasingly important diagnostic aid in patients with brain damage after cardiac surgery. Though not infallible,[158] it is exceedingly reliable in intracranial haemorrhage,[8] a recognised complication of open heart surgery[114,131] (Fig. 3.12). It can even reveal the precise degree of cerebral oedema.[133] Unfortunately, few centres possess this costly equipment and if the patient's circulatory state is also poor, as is often the case, he may be unfit for the necessary journey at a critical stage.

Management

Whilst heart failure, respiratory failure, renal failure and even liver failure can be attacked with powerful drugs and equipment, our management of brain damage still lacks specific techniques of proven value. Much continues to be learned from experimental work. However, at the moment, the temporal and quantitative relationships between such factors as the degree of brain insult, the degree and distribution of damage and depression of brain function, lactic acidosis, impairment of autoregulation, cerebral oedema, changes in intracranial and intracerebral pressure and alterations in cerebral blood flow after cerebral hypoxia or ischaemia are largely unknown. The influence of current therapy on these and other patho-physiological changes is equally uncertain. Heart failure itself may modify the various changes, for example, the response to a rise in intracranial pressure. What little we know about treatment largely relates to head injury, and we still cannot say whether the different forms of brain damage, traumatic, embolic, ischaemic and hypoxic require different or similar specialised management. Whilst they can produce histologically very similar lesions,[38] apart from the gross damage of trauma, their distribution and pathophysiology is very different.[127] If an effective

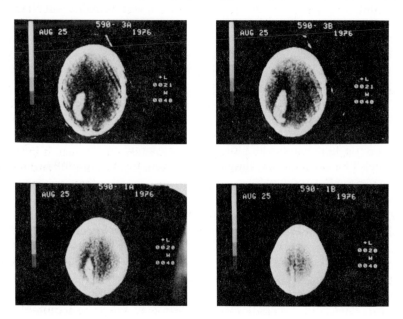

Fig. 3.12   Part of a 'brain scan' showing a cerebral haemorrhage in the posterior horn of the left ventricle. The patient was a young man who had undergone aortic valve replacement. He had major fits and remained comatose for several weeks, finally leaving hospital with a residual right hemiparesis

therapy is developed, perhaps it should always be applied prophylactically even in mild cases since even transient neurological abnormalities are associated with permanent damage.[22]

The specialised techniques for treating brain damage can be considered under three main, though overlapping, headings: neurological, respiratory and circulatory.

Neurological

There are a variety of special neurological measures, none of certain value. They include osmotic dehydration, steroids, hypothermia, the control of fits, and most recently barbiturate therapy. It is generally assumed that vasogenic cerebral oedema inevitably follows ischaemic or hypoxic brain injury, but this is not necessarily so;[122,214] nor is later deterioration of brain function inevitably due to increasing oedema.[102,122] Osmotic dehydration acts by dehydrating normal brain tissue,[187] but the agent can leak into damaged tissues, which may be widespread after a global insult such as hypoxia or ischaemia. If oedema does develop, it may take several days to reach its peak,[214] though the period is very variable.[95] It is not clear if the immediate administration of an osmotic diuretic, the usual practice, can prevent or reduce oedema formation, and the sudden expansion of the circulating volume can be hazardous in a patient already in heart failure. For these reasons, and to avoid any risk of osmolar complications,[214] we rarely use this therapy. Whilst steroids, in particular dexamethasone, can be dramatically beneficial in the type of cerebral oedema associated with brain tumours, their value in global ischaemic and hypoxic brain damage remains uncertain,[153,190] and they may even be harmful.[208] However, recent work suggests that massive dosage in head injury can prevent a rise in intracranial pressure.[94] The drug is used for six to nine days in combination with a gastric antacid to prevent ulceration, starting with 48 mg immediately, then 96 mg the first day, in divided doses, and gradually reducing this to 24 mg per day. Unfortunately, such massive dosage would probably delay healing and inhibit the response to infection after cardiac surgery. Hypothermia, also, is disappointing, despite its experimental promise, and whilst this may be because it is usually induced too slowly and too late, we use it only for treating hyperpyrexia. Cerebral metabolism is increased by fits (even if the motor activity is suppressed by muscle relaxants)[180] and by pain[135] and anxiety.[44] Adequate analgesia and sedation are, therefore, essential in brain damage after cardiac surgery.

Some workers[26,171] found a massive dose of thiopentone, 30 mg/kg body weight, given after severe brain ischaemia in monkeys, greatly reduces the degree of damage, though it does not eliminate it. Whilst the experimental model is very different from the clinical situation,[172] a combination of this treatment and circulatory support is under clinical trial.[34,197] The inverse relation between body weight and cerebral metabolic rate[210] suggests that a lesser, and, therefore, safer dose of thiopentone from a cardiovascular viewpoint, might be acceptable in man.

Respiratory
The importance of a clear airway and adequate ventilation and oxygenation in brain damage are widely appreciated, but more recently mechanical ventilation or hyperventilation initially seemed to offer major advantages, despite its special requirements.[155] The concept had a plausible theoretical basis. Lactic acidosis, with its ill-effects on cerebrovascular responses and dynamics, and other consequences, is now a well established complication of brain injury. Since it cannot be corrected by sodium bicarbonate therapy as this drug does not cross the blood-brain barrier, respiratory alkalosis seems a logical alternative, and it has important, though not entirely beneficial effects on vasoactivity.[50,155] Mechanical ventilation also reduces intracranial pressure, though only by reducing blood flow in vasoactive areas of the brain, and in addition, it ensures optimal ventilation and oxygenation. Unfortunately, despite widespread use, there have been few acceptable trials and its value in the various types of brain damage remains uncertain. It may at best increase the survival rate in patients with residual and permanent brain damage,[100] and even this may be due to improved care rather than specific benefit. At worst, the survival rate may fall.[128] Despite this uncertainty, mechanical ventilation with mild respiratory alkalosis

($Paco_2$ 30–35 mmHg) seems best continued in patients with brain damage after cardiac surgery, at least until the respiratory and cardiovascular status is satisfactory.

There are several ways in which PEEP may affect the injured brain. They include its mechanical effects on the cardiac output and on central (and hence cerebral) venous pressure, both being influenced by the physical state of the lungs,[88] as well as its effect on the Pao_2. A change in cerebral venous pressure may influence intracranial pressure, net perfusion pressure and transcapillary pressure. However, intracranial pressure may not change,[2] even if PEEP is suddenly terminated.[76] A rise is most likely when the compressibility of the brain is reduced by disease.[76,202a] The effect of such a rise on cerebral blood flow probably depends on a number of factors, including the physical and physiological state of the brain and its vascular bed. Sitting the patient up is not necessarily beneficial since it reduces cerebral perfusion pressure as well as cerebral venous pressure. Clearly, the effects of PEEP on the damaged brain depend on the net result of the interplay of many cardiovascular, pulmonary and neurological factors. At the moment, without special facilities it is virtually impossible to assess the cerebral consequences of PEEP in a patient who also has brain damage after cardiac surgery, though a fall in cardiac output or mean blood pressure is undesirable, especially when autoregulation is disturbed, and it may not be an acceptable price for a rise in Pao_2. Grave ill-effects, including irreversible neurological deterioration, have been reported with the use of PEEP after head injury.[202a]

Routine turning of the comatose patient may also have grave consequences for brain function,[183a] possibly from its disturbance of blood flow through the paralysed cerebrovascular bed and from the fall in Pao_2 if lung function too is impaired.

Circulatory

The need for an adequate circulation to protect the brain from hypoxic insult, and to improve and accelerate its recovery after severe ischaemia, has long been established,[82] but its clinical importance has only recently been recognised. The apparent extreme vulnerability of the brain to ischaemia is in large measure due to secondary neuronal damage from the circulatory failure which often follows it, for example after cardiac arrest. Experimentally, the safe period of cerebral ischaemia can be greatly prolonged by restoring an adequate cerebral circulation immediately afterwards. The explanation for this probably lies in the loss of autoregulation in intracerebral acidosis and its important consequences. Cerebral blood flow, instead of being an active physiological process, nicely responsive to changes in mean blood pressure and local metabolic needs, now becomes a purely passive hydrostatic response in the damaged areas, and critically dependant on mean blood pressure (Fig. 3.11). This abnormal situation is especially important after cardiac surgery where circulatory support is often required. If there is brain damage the mean blood pressure should be kept at 80–100 mmHg. Hypertension is also undesirable as it encourages the leakage of oedema fluid from damaged vessels if cerebral oedema does develop.[134] If lung function is also gravely impaired, hypoxia will aggravate the cerebral ill-effects of a poor circulation.[209]

Haemodilution increases cerebral blood flow after ischaemia. It may act by reducing the viscosity of the blood,[231] and even a slight change in haematcrit has a marked effect on this factor,[144] whose optimal level is about 30 per cent.[163] A combination of haemodilution, heparin, carotid flushing and noradrenaline has a markedly beneficial and protective effect on the brain after experimental ischaemia.[196] Since heparin alone has slight value,[228] and the 'no reflow' phenomenon is of little importance in primates,[105,141] these results were probably due to improved cerebral blood flow from circulatory support and haemodilution.

In summary, at the moment the most important measures in the treatment of ischaemic and hypoxic brain damage after cardiac surgery are the maintenance of a satisfactory circulation and blood pressure, and adequate ventilation and oxygenation, if necessary, with the aid of mechanical ventilation and guarded use of PEEP. Adequate analgesia and sedation are also important. Haemodilution, mild hypothermia and thiobarbiturate therapy are additional possible measures. Corticosteroids at the moment seem to have least value, but high dosage may alter this view.

HAEMORRHAGE AND TRANSFUSION

Normal clotting has three main components, vascular integrity, platelet function and the coagulation cascade.[67] Deficiencies in one or more of these mechanisms can lead to intractable and even fatal haemorrhage, one of the commonest causes of death after open-heart surgery. There may be abnormalities even before surgery, for example, from anticoagulant therapy, cyanotic heart disease,[66] Marfan's syndrome and haemoglobinopathies.[56] In the postoperative period it is often exceedingly difficult to decide whether excessive bleeding is due to 'surgical' factors, such as inadequate haemostasis, often aggravated by adhesions from previous surgery, or from 'medical' factors. Such 'medical' factors include inadequate heparin reversal or heparin 'rebound', a condition related to the swifter metabolism of protamine,[79,193] the damaging effects of cardiopulmonary bypass,[11] though membrane oxygenators reduce this,[156] and massive transfusion with stored blood.[164] Disseminated intravascular coagulation (DIC) though reported after cardiac surgery,[29] is rare and few would have the temerity to use heparin, especially since its value in the established condition is at best uncertain.[67,203]

Full laboratory investigation[67] only occasionally indicates the precise cause of the problem and its treatment, such as the presence of free heparin or platelet deficiency, though mild abnormalities or 'low normal' results of tests are common. In most cases, the only effective solution is continued infusion with clotting elements, namely fresh blood, fresh frozen plasma, and platelets. Calcium chloride, extra doses of protamine, vitamin K, and epsilonaminocaproic acid (EACA) are also commonly used on an empirical basis and later regarded as beneficial if bleeding ceases. It is unwise to use EACA prophylactically, except perhaps in cyanotic heart disease[154] since it inhibits the conversion of plasmin into plasminogen, which in turn, activates the degradation of fibrin, a constant natural process which prevents intravascular coagulation and also lyses clot. In the worst cases, re-exploration of the chest is imperative. No bleeding point may be found, but the bleeding may abruptly improve. This effect has been attributed to the removal of clot and the associated reduction in the amount of circulating fibrinolysins and their breakdown products which have an anticoagulant effect.[193] In the worst cases, bleeding continues despite all measures and the patient dies with a steadily deteriorating circulatory state. This is not uncommon in Marfan's syndrome, grave cyanotic heart disease and after protracted cardiopulmonary bypass.

Massive transfusion has other ill-effects apart from depletion of clotting factors. One is 2,3 diphosphoglycerate (2,3 DPG) deficiency. But despite its role in the release of oxygen in the tissues, there is little clinical evidence its deficiency is harmful,[28] though a poor circulatory state might enhance its importance. Particulate embolism seems a more important problem, since experimental and clinical studies show wide precapillary obstruction in the lungs after massive transfusion, from microaggregates.[55,189] It is one of the postulated causes of the adult respiratory distress syndrome, and some workers have claimed a reduction in the incidence of this condition with the use of fine pore filters.[189] These filters, which are highly efficient,[116] have pores about one-quarter of the conventional size.[42] However, the matter is not settled since other reports suggest that micro-aggregates do not have a clinically important effect on lung function.[77a,79,238] As most available microfilters hinder rapid transfusion, this factor alone indicates the need for convincing evidence of their importance, apart from the extra cost.

Some centres store blood taken from the patient himself before and during the operation, reinfusing it after cardiopulmonary bypass. We remove and store 400–500 ml of blood in adults during the thoracotomy. Whilst it is not certain whether this reduces bleeding,[121,179] we feel it is nevertheless an advantage to use the patient's own fresh heparinised and uncooled blood at this critical period. Jehovah's Witnesses accept open-heart surgery with cardiopulmonary bypass, whilst refusing the administration of any blood, including their own if it is stored. Cardiac surgery is only possible in these patients when the lesion is simple and unlikely to have bleeding complications. Despite the inevitable anaemia, like other centres,[199] we have had good results, an indication perhaps of an excessive use of blood in other patients. I, personally, would not hesitate to use blood in such patients if the situation was critical.

Autotransfusion, the collection and transfusion of blood which is normally discarded during and after surgery, reduces the need for stored donor blood, with its associated disadvantages and dangers.[186] The equipment is simple and easily constructed and it is most useful in closed cardiac surgery, though some centres also use it for open heart surgery. A recent device,* in principle a centrifuge, allows the separation of red cells from fluid left in the heart-lung machine after cardiopulmonary bypass. The salvaged cells can then be reinfused without overloading the patient with fluid.

* Haemonetics Cell Saver, Haemonetics Corporation, Natick, Massachusetts, 01760, U.S.A.

REFERENCES

1. Aberg, T. & Kihlgren, M. (1977) Cerebral protection during open heart surgery. *Thorax*, **52**, 525.

2. Aidinis, S. J., Lafferty, J. & Shapiro, H. M. (1976) Intracranial pressure response to PEEP. *Anesthesiology*, **45**, 275.

3. Aksnes, E. G., Cappelen, C. & Hall, K. V. (1966) Cardiac output and regional femoral blood flow in the early postoperative period after heart surgery. *Acta Chir. Scand.* suppl., **357**, 299.

4. Alpert, N. R. (1970) Regulation of lactate metabolism. *Helv. Med. Acta*, **35**, 335.

5. Altura, B. M. & Altura, B. J. (1974) Effects of local anaesthetics, antihistamines and glucocorticoids on peripheral blood flow and vascular smooth muscle. *Anesthesiology*, **41**, 197.

6. Apuzzo, M. J. J., Weiss, M. H. et al (1977) Effect of positive end expiratory pressure ventilation on intracranial pressure in man. *J. Neurosurg.*, **46**, 227.

7. Anderson, R., Sibbald, W. J. et al (1977) Increased pulmonary capillary permeability in human sepsis. *Intens. Care Med.*, **3**, 110, Abst. 24.

8. Abrams, H. L. & McNeil, B. J. (1978) Medical implications of computed tomography (first of two parts). *New Engl. J. Med.*, **298**, 255.

9. Arenberg, I. K., Allen, G. W. & Boer, A. D. (1972) Sudden deafness immediately following cardiopulmonary bypass. *J. Lar. Otol.*, **86**, 73.

10. Askanzi, J., Neville, J. F. et al (1975) Prevention of pulmonary insufficiency by prophylactic use of PEEP and rapid respiratory rates. *Surg. Forum*, **26**, 198.

11. Barrer, M. J. & Ellison, N. (1977) Platelet function. *Anesthesiology*, **46**, 202.

12. Bartlett, R. H., Drinker, P. A. et al (1976) Indications for extracorporeal membrane oxygen support: quantitating pulmonary insufficiency. In *Artificial Lungs for Acute Respiratory Failure*, ed. Zapol, W. M. & Qvist, J. (Academic Press, New York, San Francisco and London), p. 373.

13. Bedford, R. F. & Wollman, H. (1973) Complications of percutaneous radial artery cannulation. *Anesthesiology*, **38**, 228.

14. Bedford, R. F. (1977) Radial arterial function following percutaneous cannulation with 18 and 20 gauge catheters. *Anesthesiology*, **47**, 37.

15. Berk, J. L., Haagen, J. F. et al (1977) The use of dopamine to correct the reduced cardiac output resulting from positive end-expiratory pressure. *Crit. Care Med.*, **5**, 269.

16. Benzing, G. & Helmsworth, J. A. (1976) Nitroprusside after open heart surgery. *Circulation*, **54**, 467.

17. Berenti, K. J., Wolk, M. & Killip, T. (1975) Cerebrospinal fluid acidosis complicating therapy of experimental cardiopulmonary arrest. *Circulation*, **52**, 319.

18. Berk, J. L. (1975) Use of vasoactive drugs in the treatment of shock. *Surg. Clin. N. America*, **55**, 721.

19. Bethune, D. W. (1976) Organ damage after open heart surgery. *Lancet*, **2**, 1410 (Letter).

20. Black, P. B., Devanter, S. V. & Cohn, L. H. (1976) Current research review: effects of hypothermia on systemic and organ system metabolism and function. *J. Surg. Res.*, **20**, 49.

21. Black, A. M. S. (1976) Bicarbonate requirements during hypothermic cardiopulmonary bypass: the relative effects of pulsatile flow. *Anaes. Intens. Care*, **4**, 232.

22. Blagbrough, A. E., Brierly, J. B. & Nicholson, A. N. (1973) Behavioural and neurological disturbances associated with hypoxic brain damage. *J. Neurol. Sci.*, **18**, 475.

23. Blaisdell, F. W. (1974) Pathophysiology of the respiratory distress syndrome. *Arch. Surg.*, **108**, 44.

24. Blaisdell, F. W. & Schlobohm, R. M. (173) The respiratory distress syndrome: a review. *Surgery*, **74**, 251.

25. Bleifeld, W. (1977) Myocardial infarction: present knowledge and future prospects. *Triangle*, **16**, 69.

26. Bleyaert, A. L., Nemoto, E. M. et al (1976) Thiopental therapy after 16 minutes of global brain ischaemia in monkeys. *Crit. Care Med.*, **4**, 130 (Abst.).

27. Borman, J. B., Merin, G. et al (1971) The beneficial effects of chlorpromazine on pulmonary hemodynamics after cardiopulmonary bypass. *Ann. Thorac. Surg.*, **11**, 570.

28. Bowen, J. C. & Fleming, W. H. (1974) Increased oxyhemoglobin affinity after transfusion of stored blood. *Ann. Surg.*, **180**, 760.

29. Boyd, A. F., Engelman, R. M. et al (1973) Disseminated intravascular coagulation following extracorporeal circulation. *J. Thorac. Cardiovasc. Surg.*, **64**, 685.

30. Branthwaite, M. A. (1974) Cerebral blood flow and metabolism during open heart surgery. *Thorax*, **29**, 633.

31. Branthwaite, M. A. (1973) Detection of neurological damage during open heart surgery. *Thorax*, **28**, 464.

32. Branthwaite, M. A. (1977) *Anaesthesia for Cardiac Surgery*. Blackwell Scientific Publications, Oxford.

33. Branthwaite, M. A. (1975) Prevention of neurological damage during open heart surgery. *Thorax*, **30**, 258.

34. Breivik, H. (1977) Feasibility of barbiturate loading of patients for brain resuscitation after cardiopulmonary arrest. *Int. Care Med.*, **3**, 165, Abst. 233.

35. Brennan, R. W., Patterson, R. H. & Kessler, J. (1971) Cerebral blood flow and metabolism during cardiopulmonary bypass: evidence of microembolic encephalopathy. *Neurology*, **21**, 665.
36. Brenner, W. I., Lansky, Z. et al (1973) Hyperosmolar coma in surgical patients. *Ann. Surg.*, **178**, 651.
37. Bregman, D. (1976) Mechanical support of the failing heart. *Curr. Problems in Surg.*, **13** (12).
38. Brierly, J. B., Meldrum, B. S. & Brown, A. W. (1973) The threshold and neuropathology of cerebral 'anoxic-ischemic' cell change. *Arch. Neurol.*, **29**, 367.
39. Buckberger, G. D. & Hottenrott, C. E. (1975) Ventricular fibrillation: its effect on myocardial flow distribution and performance. *Ann. Thorac. Surg.*, **20**, 76.
40. Butsch, J. L., Butsch, W. L. & Da Rosa, J. F. T. (1976) Bilateral vocal cord paralysis: a complication of percutaneous cannulation of the internal jugular veins. *Arch. Surg.*, **111**, 828.
41. Buhlmann, A. A. & Frick, P. (1977) Acute respiratory distress consequent to cardiac surgery in relation to preoperative hemodynamics and pulmonary function patterns. *Physiopath. Resp.*, **13**, 32P.
42. Buley, R. & Lumley, J. (1975) Some observations on blood microfilters. *Ann. Royal Coll. Surg.*, **57**, 262.
43. Bynny, R. L. (1976) Withdrawal from glucocorticoid therapy. *New Engl. J. Med.*, **295**, 30.
44. Carlsson, C., Hagerdal, M. & Siesjo, B. K. (1975) Increase in cerebral oxygen uptake and blood flow in immobile stress. *Acta Physiol. Scan.*, **95**, 206.
45. Clowes, G. H. A., Hirsch, E. et al (1975) Septic lung and shock lung in man. *Ann. Surg.*, **181**, 681.
46. Coffin, L. H., Shinozaki, T. et al (1975) Ineffectiveness of methylprednisolone in the treatment of pulmonary dysfunction after cardiopulmonary bypass. *Am. J. Surg.*, 1975, **130**, 555.
47. Cogswell, J. J., Hatch, D. J. et al (1975) Effects of continuous positive airway pressure on lung mechanics of babies after operation for congenital heart disease. *Arch. Dis. Childh.*, **50**, 799.
48. Cohen, R. D. & Simpson, R. (1975) Lactate metabolism. *Anesthesiology*, **43**, 661.
49. Cohn, J. N. & Franciosa, J. A. (1977) Vasodilator therapy of cardiac failure: (second of two parts). *New Engl. J. Med.*, **297**, 254.
50. Cold, G. E., Jensen, F. T. & Malmros, R. (1977) The effects of Paco$_2$ reduction on regional cerebral blood flow in the acute phase of brain injury. *Acta Anaesth. Scand.*, **21**, 359.
51. Collins, J. A. (1977) The acute respiratory distress syndrome. *Advances in Surg.*, **11**, 171.
52. Cook, T. L. & Dueker, C. W. (1976) Tension pneumothorax following internal jugular vein cannulation and general anesthesia. *Anesthesiology*, **45**, 554.
53. Cooley, D. A., Reul, G. J. & Wukasch, D. C. (1972) Ischemic contracture of the heart: 'stone heart'. *Am. J. Cardiol.*, **29**, 575.
54. Dane, T. E. B. & King, E. G. (1975) Fatal cardiac tamponade and other mechanical complications of central venous catheters. *Brit. J. Surg.*, **62**, 6.
55. Davidson, I., Barret, J. A. et al (1975) Pulmonary microembolism associated with massive transfusion. *Ann. Surg.*, **181**, 51.
56. de Laval, M. R., Taswell, H. F. et al (1974) Open heart surgery in patients with inherited haemoglobinopathies, red cell dyscrasias and coagulopathies. *Arch. Surg.*, **109**, 618.
57. Defalque, R. J. (1974) Percutaneous catheterization of the internal jugular vein. *Anesth. Analg. Curr. Res.*, **53**, 116.
58. Dietzmann, R. H., Castaneda, A. R. et al (1970) Corticosteroids as effective vasodilators in the treatment of low output syndrome. *Chest*, **57**, 440.
59. Downs, J. B., Perkins, H. M. & Modell, J. H. (1974) Intermittent mandatory ventilation. *Arch. Surg.*, **109**, 519.
60. Eberhart, R. C. & Trelek, G. J. (1973) Central and peripheral rewarming patterns in postoperative cardiac patients. *Crit. Care Med.*, **1**, 239.
61. Ebido, B., Weinreich, A. & Lipton, B. (1973) Anesthetic agents and neuropsychiatric complications following extracorporeal circulation. *Bull. N.Y. Acad. Med.*, **48**, 545.
62. Editorial (1970) Lactic acidosis. *Br. Med. J.*, **4**, 258.
63. Editorial (1972) Intra-aortic balloon pumping. *Lancet*, **2**, 1238.
64. Editorial (1977) Pump failure. *Br. Med. J.*, **1**, 1430.
65. Editorial (1977) Intravenous dopamine. *Lancet*, **2**, 231.
66. Eernisse, J. G., Brand, A. et al (1977) Prevention of bleeding tendency after open heart surgery for tetralogy of Fallot. *Scand. J. Cardiov. Surg.*, **11**, 105.
67. Ellison, N. (1977) Diagnosis and management of bleeding disorders. *Anesthesiology*, **47**, 171.
68. English, I., Frew, R. M. et al (1969) Percutaneous catheterization of the internal jugular vein. *Anaesthesia*, **24**, 521.
69. Fallat, R. J., Lamy, M. et al (1976) Use of physiologic and pathologic correlations in evaluating adult respiratory distress syndrome. In *Artificial Lungs for Acute Respiratory Failure*, ed. Zapol, W. M. & Qvist, J. Academic Press, San Francisco, New York and London, p. 391.

70. Feeley, T. W. & Hedley-Whyte, J. (1975) Weaning from intermittent positive pressure ventilation. *New Engl. J. Med.*, **292,** 903.
71. Feig, P. U. & McCurdy, D. J. (1977) The hypertonic state. *New Engl. J. Med.*, **297,** 1444.
72. Feuer, H. (1975) Early management of pediatric head injury: physiologic aspects. *Ped. Clin. N. Amer.*, **22,** 425.
73. Fischer, E. G. (1973) Impaired perfusion following cerebrovascular stasis. *Arch. Neurol.*, **29,** 361.
74. Flachs, J., Bookallil, M. & Clarke, B. (1977) Extracorporeal oxygenation or hypothermia in respiratory failure. *Lancet*, 1977, **1,** 489. Letter.
75. Forrester, J. S., Diamond, G. et al (1976) Medical therapy of acute myocardial infarction by application of hemodynamic subsets (first of two parts). *New Engl. J. Med.*, **295,** 1356.
76. Frost, E. A. M. (1977) Effects of positive end expiratory pressure on intracranial pressure and compliance in brain injured patients. *J. Neurosurg.*, **47,** 195.
77. Gattiker, R. & Schmid, E. (1978) Haemodynamic effects of dopamine, epinephrine and orciprenaline (Alupent) after cardiac surgery. *Int. Care Med.*, 1978, **4,** 55.
77a. Geelhoed, G. W. & Bennett, S. H. (1975) 'Shock Lung' resulting from perfusion of canine lungs with stored bank blood. *Am. Surg.*, **41,** 671.
78. Geha, A. S., Malt, S. H. et al (1971) Effect of cardiopulmonary bypass on cerebral metabolism. *J. Thorac. Cardiovasc. Surg.*, **61,** 200.
79. Gervin, A. S. (1975) Complications of heparin therapy. *Surg. Gynec. Obstet.*, **140,** 789.
80. Gervin, A. S., Mason, K. & Wright, C. B. (1975) The filtration limitations of ultrapore filters. *Surgery*, 77, 186.
81. Ghani, M. F., Parker, B. M. & Smith, J. R. (1974) Recognition of myocardial infarction after cardiac surgery and its relation to cardiopulmonary bypass. *Am. Heart J.*, **88,** 18.
82. Gilston, A. & Resnekov, L. (1971) *Cardio-Respiratory Resuscitation.* Heinemann Medical Books, London.
83. Gilston, A. (1971) Anaesthesia for cardiac surgery. *Br. J. Anaesth.*, **43,** 217.
84. Gilston, A. (1976) Venous hypertension after mechanical ventilation. *Anaesthesia*, 1976, **31,** 513.
85. Gilston, A. (1976) Cannulation of the femoral vessels. *Br. J. Anaesth.*, **48,** 500. Letter.
86. Gilston, A. (1976) Facial signs of respiratory distress after cardiac surgery. *Anaesthesia*, **31,** 385.
87. Gilston, A. (1976) A clinical scoring system for adult respiratory distress. *Anaesthesia*, **31,** 448.
88. Gilston, A. (1977) The effects of PEEP on arterial oxygenation. An examination of some possible mechanisms. *Intens. Care Med.*, **3,** 267.
89. Gilston, A. (1965) Clinical aspects of cardiac resuscitation. *Lancet*, **2,** 1039.
90. Gilston, A. (1972) A simple method of monitoring the arterial blood pressure. *Brit. J. Anaesthesia*, **44,** 1334. Letter.
91. Gilston, A. (1962) Adrenal haemorrhage after open heart surgery. *Br. Med. J.*, **2,** 451.
92. Gilston, A. (1978) Further report on a clinical scoring system for respiratory distress after cardiac surgery. (*Submitted for publication.*)
93. Ginestal, R. J., Paylos, J. & Lovano, F. (1977) Pulmonary vascular pressures and resistance in adult respiratory distress syndrome. *Intens. Care Med.*, **3,** 106, Abst. 5.
94. Gobiet, W., Grote, W. & Bock, W. J. (1975) The relation between intracranial pressure, mean arterial pressure and cerebral blood flow in patients with severe head injury. *Acta. Neurochir.*, **32,** 13.
95. Gobiet, W. (1977) Monitoring of intracranial pressure in patients with severe head injury. *Neurochir.*, **20,** 35.
96. Goldberg, L. I. (1977) Recent advances in the pharmacology of catecholamines. *Intens. Care Med.*, **3,** 233.
97. Goldberg, L. I. (1974) Dopamine: clinical uses of an endogenous catecholamine. *New Engl. J. Med.*, **291,** 707.
98. Goldberg, L. I. (1972) Cardiovascular and renal actions of dopamine: potential clinical applications. *Pharmac. Rev.*, **24,** 1.
99. Gordon, R. J., Ravin, M. et al (1975) Changes in arterial pressure, viscosity and resistance during cardiopulmonary bypass. *J. Thorac. Cardiovasc. Surg.*, **69,** 552.
100. Gordon, E. (1971) The effect of controlled ventilation on the clinical course of patients with severe traumatic brain injury. In *Brain and Blood Flow*, ed. Russell, R. W. R. Pitman, London, p. 365.
101. Greenbaum, D. M., Millen, J. E. et al (1976) Continuous positive airway pressure without tracheal intubation in spontaneously breathing patients. *Chest*, **69,** 615.
102. Gurvitch, A. M. & Mutuskina, E. A. (1977) Experimental model of delayed postresuscitation encephalopathy. *Intens. Care Med.*, **3,** 165, Abst. 235.
103. Guttman, F. A. & Zegarra, H. (1971) Ocular complications of cardiac surgery. *Surg. Clin. N. Amer.*, **51,** 1095.
104. Haft, J. I. (1974) Cardiovascular injury induced by sympathetic amines. *Prog. Cardiovasc. Dis.*, **17,** 73.

105. Harrison, M. J. G., Sedal, L. et al (1975) No reflow phenomenon in the cerebral circulation of the gerbil. *J. Neurol. Neurosurg. Psychiat.*, **38**, 1190.
106. Hasbrook, J. D. & Rigor, B. M. (1969) The oxygen tension of cerebrospinal fluid during cardiopulmonary bypass. *J. Thorac. Cardiovasc. Surg.*, **58**, 754.
107. Hatch, D. J., Cogswell, J. J. et al (1973) Continuous positive airway pressure after open heart operations in infancy. *Lancet*, **2**, 469.
108. Hedley-Whyte, J., Burgess, G. E. et al (1976) *Applied Physiology of Respiratory Care*. Little Brown and Co., Boston.
109. Held, K., Gottstein, V. & Neidermayer, E. R. (1969) C.B.F. in non-pulsatile perfusion. In *Cerebral Blood Flow*, ed. Brock, M., Fieschi, I. C. et al. Springer-Verlag, Berlin, p. 94.
110. Hilbermann, M., Kamm, B. et al (1976) An analysis of potential physiological predictors of respiratory inadequacy following cardiac surgery. *J. Thorac. Cardiovasc. Surg.*, **71**, 711.
111. Hilbermann, M. & Osborn, J. J. (1976) Monitoring of the patient in shock. In *Shock. Clinical and Experimental Aspects*, ed. Ledingham, I. McA. Excerpta Medica, p. 111.
112. Hoffman, J. I. E. (1975) Pathophysiology of subendocardial ischaemia. *Brit. Med. J.*, **1**, 76.
113. Hottenrott, C. E., Towers, B. et al (1973) The hazard of ventricular fibrillation in hypertrophied ventricles during cardiopulmonary bypass. *J. Thorac. Cardiovasc. Surg.*, **66**, 742.
114. Humphreys, R. P., Hoffman, H. J. et al (1975) Cerebral haemorrhage following heart surgery. *J. Neurosurg.*, **43**, 671.
115. Jaatela, A., Alho, A. et al (1975) Plasma catecholamines in severely injured patients: a prospective study in 45 patients with multiple injuries. *Br. J. Surg.*, **62**, 177.
116. James, O. (1977) The use of blood microfilters. *Br. J. Clin. Equipment*, **2**, 199.
117. Joly, H. R. & Weil, M. H. (1969) Temperature of the great toe as an indication of the severity of shock. *Circulation*, **39**, 131.
118. Thorac, J. (1975) *Cardiovasc. Surg.*, **70** (6).
119. Juneja, I., Flynn, R. E. & Berger, R. L. (1972) The arterial pH, P_{CO_2} and the electroencephalogram during open heart surgery. *Acta Neurol. Scand.*, **48**, 169.
120. Juneja, I., Flynn, R. E. & Berger, R. L. (1972) The arterial and venous pressures and the electroencephalogram during open heart surgery. *Acta Neurol. Scand.*, **48**, 163.
121. Kaplan, J. A., Cannarella, C. et al (1977) Autologous blood transfusion during cardiac surgery. *J. Thorac. Cardiovasc. Surg.*, **74**, 4.
122. Katzman, R. & Pappius, H. M. (1973) Cerebral edema-intracranial pressure. In *Brain Electrolytes and Fluid Metabolism*, ed. Katzman, R. & Pappius, H. Williams and Wilkins Co., Baltimore, p. 366.
123. Keates, J. R. W., Innocenti, D. M. & Ross, D. N. (1975) Mononeuritis multiplex: a complication of open heart surgery. *J. Thorac Cardiovasc. Surg.*, **69**, 816.
124. Kirby, R. R., Downs, J. B. et al (1975) High level positive and expiratory pressure (PEEP) in acute respiratory insufficiency. *Chest*, **67**, 156.
125. Klein, J. J., Haeringen, J. R. V. et al. Pulmonary function after recovery from the adult respiratory distress syndrome. *Chest*, **69**, 350.
126. Kones, R. J. & Phillips, J. H. (1971) Glucagon: recent studies in cardiovascular disease. *Clin. Pharmac. Therap.*, **12**, 427.
127. Kovach, A. G. B. & Sandor, P. (1976) Cerebral blood flow and brain function during hypotension and shock. *Ann. Rev. Physiol.*, **38**, 571.
128. Krenn, J., Steinbereithner, P. et al (1975) The value of routine respirator treatment in severe brain trauma. In *Advances in Neurosurgery*. Springer-Verlag, Berlin, Heidelberg and New York, p. 134.
129. Krian, A. (1976) Incidence, prevention and treatment of acute renal failure following cardiopulmonary bypass. *Intern. Anesth. Clinics*, **14**, 87.
130. Kritikou, P. E. & Branthwaite, M. A. (1977) Significance of changes in cerebral electrical activity at onset of cardiopulmonary bypass. *Thorax*, **32**, 534.
131. Krous, H. F., Tenckhoff, L. et al (1975) Subdural hematoma following open heart surgery. *Ann. Thorac. Surg.*, **19**, 269.
132. Lakshminarayan, S., Stanford, R. E. & Petty, T. L. (1976) Progress recovery from adult respiratory distress syndrome. *Am. Rev. Resp. Dis.*, 1976, **113**, 7.
133. Lanksch, W., Oettinger, W. & Baethmann, A. (1977) Diagnosis of brain edema using C.T. In *Computer Assisted Tomography*, ed. Kuhler, W. J. Excerpta Medica, Amsterdam and Oxford, p. 13.
134. Lassen, N. A. & Agnoli, A. (1972) The upper limit of autoregulation of cerebral blood flow: on the pathogenesis of hypertensive encephalopathy. *Scan. J. Clin. Lab. Invest.*, **30**, 113.
135. Lassen, N. A. & Christinsen, M. S. (1976) Physiology of cerebral blood flow. *Br. J. Anaesth.*, **48**, 719.
136. Lassen, N. A. (1977) Cerebral ischemia. *Int. Care Med.*, **3**, 251.

137. Laver, M. B., Hallowell, P. & Goldblatt, A. (1970) Pulmonary function secondary to heart disease: aspects relevant to anaesthesia and surgery. *Anesthesiology*, **33**, 161.
138. Lee, H. A. (1977) The management of acute renal failure following trauma. *Br. J. Anaesth.*, **49**, 697.
139. Lee, W. H., Brady, M. P. et al (1971) Effects of extracorporeal circulation upon behaviour, personality, and brain function. *Ann. Surg.*, **173**, 1013.
140. Lefkowitz, R. J. (1976) Beta-adrenergic receptors: recognition and regulation. *New Engl. J. Med.*, **295**, 323.
141. Levy, D. E., Brierly, J. B. & Plum, F. (1975) Ischemic brain damage in the gerbil in the absence of 'no-reflow'. *J. Neurol. Neurosurg. Pschiat.*, **38**, 1197.
142. Li, W. K. & Holder, B. S. (1969) Sodium bicarbonate for correction of metabolic acidosis in open-heart surgery. *Anesth. Analg. Curr. Res.*, **48**, 381.
143. Licht, I. L., Simmons, E. M. & Almond, C. A. (1972) Detection of microembolism during cardiopulmonary bypass. *Surg. Gynec. Obstet.*, **134**, 977.
144. Litwin, M. S. (1976) Blood viscosity changes after trauma. *Crit. Care Med.*, **4**, 67.
145. Lockey, E. Personal communication.
146. Lindquist, O., Rammer, L. & Saldeen, T. (1972) Pulmonary insufficiency, microembolism and fibrinolysis inhibition in post-traumatic autopsy material. *Acta Chir. Scand.*, **138**, 545.
147. Loeb, J. N. (1974) The hyperosmolar state. *New Engl. J. Med.*, **290**, 1184.
148. Lowenstein, E. (1976) Anesthetic considerations in coronary artery disease. *Am. Soc. Anesth. Refresher Course in Anesth.*, **4**, 51.
149. Lundberg, N., Kjallquist, A. et al (1974) Non-operative management of intracranial hypertension. In *Advances in Neurosurgery*, **1**, ed. Krayen-Buhl, H. et al. Springer-Verlag, Vienna and New York, p. 3.
150. Lyons, J. H. & Moore, F. D. (1966) Post-traumatic alkalosis: incidence and pathophysiology of alkalosis in surgery. *Surgery*, **60**, 93.
151. Malcolm, A. D., Coltart, D. J. et al (1977) Computer assisted evaluation of hemodynamic effects of isoprenaline and noradrenaline after open heart surgery with aortic flow monitoring. *Int. Care Med.*, **3**, 202, Abst. 380.
152. Mattar, J. A., Weil, M. H. & Shubin, H. (1973) A study of the hyperosmolal state in critically ill patients. *Crit. Care Med.*, **1**, 293.
153. Maxwell, R. E., Long, D. M. & French, L. A. (1972) The clinical effects of a synthetic glucocorticoid used for brain edema in the practice of neurosurgery. In *Steroids and Brain Edema*, ed. Reulen, H. J. & Schormann, K. Springer-Verlag, Berlin, Heidelberg and New York, p. 219.
154. McClure, P. D. & Izsak, J. (1974) The use of epsilonaminocaproic acid to reduce bleeding during cardiac bypass in children with congenital heart disease. *Anesthesiology*, **40**, 604.
155. McDowall, D. G. (1976) Neurosurgical anaesthesia and intensive care. In *Recent Advances in Anaesthesia and Analgesia*, ed. Hewer, C. L. & Atkinson, R. S. Churchill Livingstone, London, p. 16.
156. McKenzie, F. N., Heimbecker, R. O. et al (1975) The blood sparing effect of an atraumatic circuit and membrane oxygenator. *Circulation*, **52**, 4, Supplement 2.
157. McLeish, K. R., Luft, F. C. & Kleit, S. A. (1977) Factors affecting prognosis in acute renal failure following cardiac operations. *Surg. Gynec. Obstet.*, **145**, 28.
158. Messina, A. V. (1977) Cranial computerized tomography. *Arch. Neurol.*, **34**, 602.
159. Matsumoto, T., Wolfer, C. C. & Perlman, M. H. (1971) Effects of pulsatile and non-pulsatile perfusion upon cerebral and conjunctival microcirculation in dogs. *Am. Surg.*, **37**, 61.
160. Matthews, H. R., Meade, J. B. & Evans, C. C. (1974) Significance of prolonged peripheral vasoconstriction after open heart surgery. *Thorax*, **29**, 343.
161. Mattar, J. A., Weil, M. H. et al (1974) Cardiac arrest in the critically ill: II. Hyperosmolal states following cardiac arrest. *Am. J. Med.*, **56**, 162.
162. Messmer, B. J., Schallberger, U. et al (1976) Psychomotor and intellectual development after deep hypothermia and circulatory arrest in early infancy. *J. Thorac. Cardiovasc. Surg.*, **72**, 495.
163. Messmer, K. (1975) Hemodilution. *Surg. Clin. N. Amer.*, **55**, 659.
164. Miller, R. D. (1973) Complications of massive blood transfusions. *Anesthesiology*, **39**, 82.
165. Miller, R. D., Tong, M. J. et al (1971) Effect of massive transfusion of blood on acid-base state. *J. Am. Med. Assoc.*, **216**, 1762.
166. Miller, J. D. & Leech, P. (1975) Effects of mannitol and steroid therapy on intracranial volume-pressure relationships in patients. *J. Neurosurg.*, **42**, 274.
167. Miller, R. R., Vismara, L. A. et al (1977) The concept of afterload reduction in congestive heart failure: clinical application and spectrum of peripheral vasodilator drugs. In *Advances in Heart Disease*, ed. Mason, D. J. Grune and Stratton, New York, San Francisco and London, p. 25.
168. Mills, N. L., Beaudet, R. L. et al (1973) Hyperglycemia during cardiopulmonary bypass. *Ann. Surg.*, **177**, 203.

169. Mueller, H. (1977) Efficacy of intra-aortic balloon pumping and external counterpulsation in the treatment of cardiogenic shock. In *Recent Advances in Intensive Care*, ed. Ledingham, I. McA. Churchill Livingstone, Edinburgh, London and New York, p. 191.

170. Mueller, H. J. & Ayres, S. M. (1977) Dopamine in the treatment of low cardiac output state: comparison with l-norepinephrine and isoprotenerol. *Int. Care Med.*, **3**, 137, Abst. 126.

171. Nemoto, E. M., Bleyaert, A. L. et al (1977) Thiopental amelioration of brain damage after global brain ischemia. *Int. Care Med.*, **3**, Abst. 232.

172. Nemoto, E. M., Bleyaert, A. L. et al (1977) Global brain ischemia. A reproducible monkey model. *Stroke*, **8**, 558.

173. Parmley, W. W. & Chatterjee, K. (1977) Combined vasodilator and inotropic therapy: a new approach in the treatment of heart failure. In *Advances in Heart Disease*, ed. Mason, T. D. Grune and Stratton, New York, San Francisco and London, p. 44.

174. Perret, C., Poli, S. & Enrico, J. F. (1971) Phentolamine for vasodilator treatment of severe heart falure. *Lancet*, 1971, **2**, 978.

175. Perey, B. J. (1971) Vasoactive drugs in shock: the great disillusion. *Can. J. Surg.*, **14**, 295.

176. Petty, T. L. (1975) IMV versus IMC. *Chest*, **67**, 630.

177. Philips, P. A., Marty, A. T. & Miyamoto, A. M. (1975) A clinical method for detecting subendocardial ischemia after cardiopulmonary bypass. *J. Thorac. Cardiovasc. Surg.*, **69**, 30.

178. Piepenbrock, S., Hempelmann, G. & Westermann, C. (1977) Massive doses of methylprednisolone (30 mgm./kg) in man: immediate hemodynamic effects in 'low output state'. *Int. Care Med.*, **3**, 69.

179. Pliam, M., McGoon, D. C. & Tarhan, S. (1975) Failure of transfusion of autologous whole blood to reduce banked blood requirements in open heart surgical patients. *J. Thorac. Cardiocasc. Surg.*, **70**, 338.

180. Plum, F. I., Howse, D. C. & Duffy, T. E. (1974) Metabolic effect of seizures. In *Brain Dysfunction in Metabolic Disorders*, ed. Plum, F. Raven Press, New York, p. 141.

181. Pohorecky, L. A. & Wurtmann, R. J. (1971) Adrenocortical control of epinephrine synthesis. *Pharmac. Rev.*, **23**, 1.

182. Pooley, R. W., Hayes, C. J. et al (1976) Open heart experience in infants using normothermia and deep hypothermia. *Ann. Thorac. Surg.*, **22**, 415.

183. Powell, W. J. (1977) The physiology of mechanical pressure assist devices. In *Clinical Cardiology*, ed. Willerson, J. T. & Sanders, C. A. Grune and Stratton, New York, San Francisco and London, p. 509.

183a. Prior, P. F., Brigden, W. et al (1978) Nursing procedures and cardiovascular status. *Lancet*, **1**, 938. Letter.

184. Prakash, O. & Meij, S. (1977) Use of mass spectrometer and infrared CO_2 analyser for bedside measurement of cardiopulmonary function during anesthesia and intensive care. *Crit. Care Med.*, **5**, 180.

185. Rackwitz, R., Jahrmarker, H. & Haider, M. (1976) Sodium bicarbonate in cardiac arrest. *Lancet*, **2**, 474.

186. Raines, J., Buth, J. et al (1976) Intraoperative autotransfusion: equipment, protocols and guidelines. *J. Trauma*, **16**, 616.

187. Ransomoff, J. (1971) The effect of steroids on brain edema in man. In *Steroids and Brain Edema*, ed. Reulen, H. J. & Schurmann, K. Springer-Verlag, Berlin, Heidelberg and New York, p. 211.

188. Rapin, M., Lemaire, F. et al (1977) Increase of intrapulmonary shunting produced by dopamine. *Proc. Royal Soc. Med.*, **70**, 71.

189. Reul, G. J., Beall, A. C. & Greenberg, S. D. (1974) Protection of the pulmonary microvasculature by fine screen blood filtration. *Chest*, **66**, 4.

190. Reulen, H. J. (1976) Vasogenic brain edema. *Brit. J. Anaesth.*, **48**, 741.

191. Rittenhouse, E. A., Mohri, H. et al (1974) Deep hypothermia in cardiovascular surgery: current view. *Ann. Thorac. Surg.*, **17**, 65.

192. Roberts, A. J., Niarchos, A. P. et al (1977) Systemic hypertension associated with coronary artery bypass surgery. *J. Thorac. Cardiovasc. Surg.*, **74**, 846.

193. Rossi-Ferrini, P. (1976) Coagulation problems related to open heart surgery. *International Anesth. Clin.*, **14**, 103.

194. Rotmann, H. H., Lavelle, T. F. (1977) Long term physiologic consequences of the adult respiratory distress syndrome. *Chest*, **72**, 190.

195. Rudy, L. W., Heymann, M. A. & Edmunds, L. H. (1973) Distribution of systemic blood flow during cardiopulmonary bypass. *J. Appl. Physiol.*, **34**, 194.

196. Safar, P., Stezoski, I. W. & Nemoto, E. M. (1975) Amelioration of brain damage after cardiac arrest. *Crit. Care Med.*, **3**, 38, Abstract.

197. Safar, P., Myers, D. et al (1977) Clinical trial protocols for brain resuscitation. *Intens. Care Med.*, **3**, 165, Abstr. 234.

198. Sakamoto, T. & Yamada, T. (1977) Hemodynamic effects of dobutamine in patients following open heart surgery. *Circulation*, **55**, 525.

199. Sandiford, F. M., Chiariello, L. et al (1974) Aorto-coronary bypass in Jehovah's witnesses. *J. Thorac. Cardiovasc. Surg.*, **68**, 1.

200. Schlag, G., Voist, W. H. et al (1977) Ultrastructure of the human lung in shock. *Intens. Care Med.*, **3**, 113, Abstr. 34.

201. Schmidt, G. B., O'Neill, W. W. et al (1976) Continuous positive pressure in the prophylaxis of the adult respiratory distress syndrome. *Surg. Gynec. Obstet.*, **143**, 613.

202. Schwartz, M. S., Colvin, M. P. et al (1973) The cerebral function monitor. *Anaesthesia*, **28**, 615.

202a. Shapiro, H. M. & Marshall, L. F. (1978) Intracranial pressure responses to PEEP in head-injured patients. *J. Trauma*, **18**, 254.

203. Sharp, A. H. (1977) Diagnosis and management of disseminated intravascular coagulation. *Brit. Med. Bull.*, **33**, 265.

204. Shoemaker, W. C. (1974) Pattern of pulmonary hemodynamic and functional changes in shock. *Crit. Care Med.*, **2**, 200.

205. Shoemaker, W. C. & Brown, R. S. (1971) The dilemma of vasopressors and vasodilators in the therapy of shock. *Surg. Gynec. Obstet.*, **132**, 51.

206. Shubin, H. & Weil, M. H. (1970) Practical considerations in the management of shock complicating acute myocardial infarction. *Am. J. Cardiol.*, **26**, 603.

207. Sibbald, W. J., Paterson, N. A. M. et al (1977) Effect of Trendelenberg position on hemodynamics in the critically ill. *Int. Care Med.* **3**, 106, Abstr. 8.

208. Siegel, B. A., Studer, R. K. & Potchen, E. J. (1972) Effect of dexamethasone on triethylin induced brain edema and early edema in cerebral ischemia. In *Steroids and Brain Edema*, ed. Reulen, H. J. & Schurmann, K. Springer-Verlag, Berlin, Heidelberg and New York, p. 113.

209. Siesjo, B. K. (1977) The influence of respiratory disturbances on acid-base and energy metabolism of the brain. *Intens. Care Med.*, **3**, 245.

210. Siesjo, B. K., Carlsson, C. et al (1976) Brain metabolism in the critically ill. *Crit. Care Med.*, **4**, 283.

211. Simpson, J. C. (1976) Hypoglycaemia in children and undergoing operations. *Br. Med. J.*, **2**, 758. Letter.

212. Skillam, J. T., Malhotra, I. V. et al (1971) Determinants of weaning from controlled ventilation. *Surg. Forum*, **22**, 198.

213. Skinhoj, E. & Stransgaard, S. (1973) Pathogenesis of hypertensive encephalopathy. *Lancet*, **1**, 461.

214. Stern, W. E. (1972) The cerebral oedemas. In *Scientific Foundations of Neurology*, ed. Critchley, M. et al. Heinemann Medical Books, London, p. 289.

215. Sladen, A., Sweatman, A. & Klain, M. (1977) Computerized physiologic profiles of cardiorespiratory responses to PEEP challenge as an index of prognosis. *Intens. Care Med.*, **3**, 117, Abstr. 52.

216. Spann, J. F. & Braunwald, E. (1970) The sympathetic nervous system and cardiac catecholamines in congestive cardiac failure. In *Pre and Postoperative Management of the Cardiorespiratory Patient*, ed. Oaks, W. W. & Moyer, J. H. Grune and Stratton, New York and London, p. 207.

217. Spoerel, W. E. & Aitken, R. (1975) Direct arterial pressure monitoring from the dorsalis pedis artery. *Can. Anaesth. Soc. J.*, **22**, 91.

218. Sriussadaporn, S. & Cohn, J. N. (1968) Regional lactate metabolism in clinical and experimental shock. *Circulation*, **37**, Supplement VI, 187, Abstract.

219. Stalker, A. L. (1970) The microcirculation in shock. *J. Clin. Path.*, **23**, Supplement 4, 10.

220. Stanley, J. H., Liu, W. S. et al (1976) The influence of IPPB, CPAP and IPPB with CPAP during cardiopulmonary bypass on postbypass and postoperative pulmonary function. *Ann. Thorac. Surg.*, **22**, 182.

221. Steven, P. M. (1976) The effect of continuous positive pressure breathing on survival of patients with refractory hypoxemia. *Bull. Europ. Physiopath. Resp.*, **12**, 125P.

222. Steward, D. J., Sloan, I. A. & Johnston, A. E. (1974) Anaesthetic management of infants undergoing profound hypothermia for surgical correction of congenital heart defects. *Can. Anaesth. Soc. J.*, **21**, 15.

223. Stewart, S., Edmunds, L. H. et al (1973) Spontaneous breathing with continuous positive airway pressure after open intracardiac operations in infants. *J. Thorac. Cardiovasc. Surg.*, **65**, 37.

224. Stetson, J. B. & Reading, G. P. (1977) Avoidance of vascular complications associated with the use of dopamine. *Can. Anaesth. Soc. J.*, **24**, 727.

225. Stinson, E. B., Holloway, E. L. et al (1977) Control of myocardial performance early after open heart operations by vasodilator treatment. *J. Thorac. Cardiovasc. Surg.*, **73**, 523.

226. Stockard, J. J., Bickford, R. G. & Schauble, J. F. (1973) Pressure dependent cerebral ischemia during cardiopulmonary bypass. *Neurology*, **23**, 521.

227. Stone, H. H., Nusbaum, M. et al (1967) Lactate and pyruvate differences across the brain during cardiopulmonary bypass. *Circulation*, **36**, Supplement 11, 244, Abstract.

228. Stullken, E. H. & Sokoll, M. D. (1976) The effects of heparin on recovery from ischemic brain injuries in cats. *Anesth. Analg. Curr. Res.*, **55**, 683.

229. Sugimura, S. & Starr, A. (1977) Cardiopulmonary bypass under four months of age. *J. Thorac. Cardiovasc. Surg.*, **73**, 894.

230. Taugher, P. J. (1976) Visual loss after cardiopulmonary bypass. *Am. J. Opthal.*, **81**, 280.

231. Thomas, D. J., du Boulay, G. H. et al (1977) Effect of haematocrit on cerebral blood flow in man. *Lancet*, **2**, 943.

232. Thompson, W. L. (1977) Discussion; Dopamine in open heart surgery for congenital heart disease. *Proc. Royal Soc. Med.*, Supplement 2, 48.

233. Tinker, J. H., Tarhans, S. et al (1976) Dobutamine for inotropic support during emergence from cardiopulmonary bypass. *Anesthesiology*, **44**, 281.

234. Tinker, J. H. & Michenfelder, J. D. (1976) Sodium nitroprusside, pharmacology, toxicology and therapeutics. *Anesthesiology*, **45**, 340.

235. Tonnesen, A. S., Gabel, J. C. & McLeavey, C. A. (1977) Relation between lowered colloid osmotic pressure, respiratory failure and death. *Crit. Care Med.*, **5**, 239.

236. Trichet, B., Falke, K. et al (1975) The effect of pre-existing pulmonary vascular disease on the responses to mechanical ventilation with PEEP following open heart surgery. *Anesthesiology*, **42**, 56.

237. Tufo, H. M., Ostfeld, A. M. & Shekelle, R. (1970) Central nervous system function after open heart surgery. *J. Am. Med. Ass.*, **212**, 1333.

237a. Turton, M. B. & Matthews, H. R. (1974) Catecholamines and vasoconstriction after open heart surgery. *Clin. Chim. Acta*, **50**, 419.

238. Virgilio, R. W., Smith, D. E. et al (1977) To filter or not to filter. *Intens. Care Med.*, **3**, 144, Abstr. 151.

239. Wakusawa, R., Shibata, S. & Okada, K. (1977) Simple deep hypothermia for open heart surgery in infancy. *Can. Anaesth. Soc. J.*, **24**, 491.

240. Walker, L. & Eisemann, B. (1975) The changing pattern of post-traumatic respiratory distress syndrome. *Ann. Surg.*, **181**, 693.

241. Ware, S. & Osborne, J. P. (1976) Postoperative hypoglycaemia in small children. *Br. Med. J.*, **2**, 499.

242. Wedley, J. R., Lunn, H. F. & Vale, R. J. (1975) Studies of temperature balance after open heart surgery. *Crit. Care Med.*, **3**, 134.

243. Weil, M. H. & Henning, R. J. (1977) Acute circulatory failure (shock) associated with cardiogenic pulmonary edema. *Crit. Care Med.*, **5**, 215.

244. West, J. B. (1974) *Respiratory Physiology: The Essentials.* Blackwell, Oxford.

245. Wilson, J. W. (1971) Pulmonary morphologic changes due to extracorporeal circulation: a model for the 'shock lung' at cellular levels in humans. In *Shock in Low and High Flow States*, ed. Forscher, B. K. et al. Excerpta Medica, Amsterdam, p. 160.

246. Wilson, R. F., Gibson, D. et al (1972) Severe alkalosis in critically ill surgical patients. *Arch. Surg.*, **105**, 197.

247. Wilson, R. F. & Sibbald, W. J. (1976) Acute respiratory failure. *Crit. Care Med.*, **4**, 79.

248. Wisheart, J. D., Hassan, M. A. & Jackson, J. W. (1972) A complication of percutaneous cannulation of the internal jugular vein. *Thorax*, **27**, 496.

249. Witoszka, M. M., Tamura, H. et al (1973) Electroencephalographic changes and cerebral complications in open heart surgery. *J. Thorac Cardiovasc. Surg.*, **66**, 855.

250. Wright, G. (1972) Ultrastructural changes in dog brains immediately following non-pulsatile extracorporeal circulation and prolonged anaesthesia. *Br. J. Exp. Pathol.*, **53**, 501.

251. Wright, G., Sanderson, J. M. & Furness, A. (1978) Pulsatile flow for open heart surgery. *Lancet*, **1**, 217. Letter.

252. Wright, J. L. W. & Saunders, S. H. (1975) Sudden deafness following cardiopulmonary bypass surgery. *J. Laryngol. Otol.*, **89**, 757.

253. Worthley, L. I. G. (1976) Sodium bicarbonate in cardiac arrest. *Lancet*, **2**, 903.

254. Wukasch, D. C., Reul, G. J. et al (1972) The 'stone heart' syndrome. *Surgery*, **72**, 1071.

255. Wyse, S. D., Gibson, D. G. & Branthwaite, M. (1974) Haemodynamic effects of salbutamol in patients needing circulatory support after open heart surgery. *Br. Med. J.*, **3**, 502.

256. Yates, A. K. (1976) Maintenance of adequate hemodynamics during open heart procedures in the postoperative period. *Intern. Anesth. Clin.*, **14**, 1.

257. Zapol, W. M. & Snider, M. T. (1977) Pulmonary hypertension in severe acute respiratory failure. *New Engl. J. Med.*, **296**, 476.

4. Obstetric anaesthesia and analgesia

Donald D. Moir

The management of labour and delivery has been transformed within the last decade. More than 97 per cent of British babies were born in hospital in 1976. Labour hardly ever lasts for as long as 24 hours and accelerated labour is sometimes less painful labour. Labour is induced in 20 to 30 per cent of cases in many centres and epidural analgesia is now widely accepted as the most effective method of pain relief in labour.

Fetal growth and placental function are measured antenatally. Fetal lung maturity can be estimated and the respiratory distress syndrome avoided. Intrapartum monitoring of the fetal heart rate and scalp blood pH allow the detection of hypoxia. Chromosomal abnormalities and open neural tube defects can be diagnosed in time to allow termination of the pregnancy.

PERINATAL AND MATERNAL MORTALITY

By 1976 the perinatal mortality rate had fallen to 18 per 1000 births, but the rate varies from region to region and with social class. The contribution of anaesthesia and analgesia is unknown.

In 1970–72 in England and Wales 37 maternal deaths (10.4 per cent of true maternal deaths) were caused by anaesthesia.[1] All of these mothers had received general anaesthesia and 28 deaths were classed as avoidable. 14 women died of Mendelson's syndrome and 18 had a hypoxic cardiac arrest. General anaesthesia was the largest cause of death at Caesarean section, accounting for 17.2 per cent of deaths. The position in Scotland is comparable. Between 1972 and 1975 anaesthesia caused 14 per cent of maternal deaths[2] and Mendelson's syndrome and hypoxic cardiac arrest were prominent causes.

Deaths from Mendelson's syndrome are largely preventable because a single dose of 15 ml of magnesium trisilicate will raise the gastric pH above 2.5 in over 90 per cent of mothers.[3] Failed or difficult intubation of the trachea was an outstanding factor which lead to death from hypoxia or from Mendelson's syndrome in Scotland and was recorded in 5 cases in England and Wales. Persistent, unsuccessful attempts at intubation may lead only to hypoxia or to regurgitation. A failed intubation drill should be taught and practised. It will sometimes be safer to maintain anaesthesia with spontaneous ventilation by face mask, using a powerful volatile or gaseous agent as suggested by Tunstall. Regional analgesia will often be safer than general anaesthesia.

PHYSIOLOGICAL ADAPTATIONS IN PREGNANCY

Pregnancy is a unique physiological state in which most of the normal values of the non-pregnant condition are inapplicable. Many of the adaptations are important to the anaesthetist and some are outlined below.

Cardiovascular changes

Blood volume

By the final weeks of pregnancy the plasma volume has increased by over a litre. The increase in red cell mass is disproportionately less. The fall in plasma volume which was recorded after the 34th week was an artefact due to caval occlusion and is not seen in the lateral position.[4]

Cardiac output

By the 12th week cardiac output has increased by 30 to 60 per cent and remains at this level until term. Caval occlusion in the supine position reduces cardiac output by up to 50 per cent if accompanied by bradycardia[5] and blood flow to vital organs, including the placenta, may be impaired.

Venous pressure

Venous pressure in the lower limbs is elevated. The epidural veins are engorged and dilated so that solutions spread more extensively within the epidural space and a bloody tap is more likely. The pressure within the epidural space is increased.

Pulmonary function

Although tidal volume and inspiratory reserve volume are increased in pregnancy the expiratory reserve volume and functional residual capacity (FRC) are decreased with the net result that vital capacity and total lung capacity are unchanged. FRC falls by about 18 per cent.[6] Closing volume often exceeds the FRC and airway closure occurs within the tidal volume range in about 50 per cent of mothers.[7,8,9]

Hyperventilation is present from the 12th week, is due to an increase in tidal volume without alteration in rate and is a progesterone effect. The Pa_{CO_2} falls to 4 kPa (30 or 32 mmHg) and this may be nature's way of facilitating the transplacental elimination of fetal carbon dioxide.

Maternal and fetal oxygenation

Oxygen requirements increase by about 20 per cent in pregnancy. The diminished oxygen diffusing capacity is compensated for by hyperventilation. Earlier workers recorded Pa_{O_2} values below normal in late pregnancy and this phenomenon has been attributed to airway closure. However if measurements are made in the lateral position Pa_{O_2} is normal[10] and caval occlusion may be the cause of the mild hypoxaemia sometimes observed.

During apnoea the Pa_{O_2} falls more rapidly in pregnancy,[11] a finding which is due to the reduced FRC and which emphasises the importance of preoxygenation before anaesthesia. The hyperventilation associated with painful labour increases maternal Pa_{O_2}.[12]

The value for the fetus of maternal oxygen therapy has been disputed. Recently direct measurements on monkey fetuses have demonstrated that increasing the maternal FIO_2 consistently increases fetal PO_2 after an interval of about 50 seconds and that reducing placental blood flow reduces fetal PO_2.[13]

Coagulation and fibrinolysis

In pregnancy there is a shift in the balance between the haemostatic and fibrinolytic systems towards increased coagulability. Plasma fibrinogen concentration is almost doubled, averaging 0.4 to 0.6 g/100 ml and the concentration of factors VII, VIII and X is substantially increased. The concentration of plasminogen activator is decreased. These changes allow rapid haemostasis and fibrin deposition at placental separation but predispose to intravascular coagulation. In pre-eclampsia coagulability is even greater and in severe cases thrombocytopenia and fibrin degradation products in the serum are evidence of intravascular coagulation.

Disseminated intravascular coagulation (DIC). This may occur in the following states in pregnancy:

Abruptio placentae	Retained dead fetus
Amniotic fluid embolism	Sepsis
Severe pre-eclampsia	Hydatidiform mole
Missed abortion	Shock from any cause.

Abruptio placentae. This is the commonest cause of coagulation failure. The large retroplacental clot may produce a consumption coagulopathy and fibrinogen and other factors may be deficient. The entry of procoagulant substances into the circulation may produce DIC. Fresh whole blood or fresh frozen plasma will supply fibrinogen and other clotting factors.

Amniotic fluid embolism (AFE). This is a rare condition, but is a relatively important cause of maternal death because the mortality rate is as high as 80 per cent. Liquor amnii and fetal debris enter the pulmonary circulation causing intravascular coagulation. Cyanosis, dyspnoea, pulmonary oedema, profound shock, uterine haemorrhage and coagulation failure ensue. AFE is the probable explanation for sudden collapse and haemorrhage shortly after delivery. Treatment is based upon blood transfusion, heparin and IPPV.

Gastro-intestinal function

Gastric emptying time. This is prolonged from the 34th week[14] and is further delayed by analgesics given in labour. Although metoclopramide can accelerate gastric emptying in mothers who have not received analgesics, the inhibitory effect of analgesics is not reversed by metoclopramide.[15] Transit times in the small intestine are prolonged and drug absorption delayed.[16]

Intragastric pressure. At term intragastric pressure averages 13.6 to 17.2 cm H_2O and is substantially higher than in non-pregnant women.[17,18] Fortunately the high intragastric pressure is usually accompanied by an increase in the tone of the cardiac sphincter[18] and the risk of regurgitation is not increased. In women with heartburn the sphincter tone is not increased and there is a high risk of regurgitation. Heartburn is a warning symptom to the anaesthetist.

Fluid and electrolyte balance
There is a physiological retention of 3 to 4 litres of water in the intravascular and interstitial spaces in pregnancy. Sodium is retained with the water. The total body potassium increase is small and so the water retention results in a lowering of the potassium concentration. Renal plasma flow and glomerular filtration rate increase by 30 and 50 per cent respectively from the 12th week onwards.

Fat and carbohydrate metabolism
The pregnant woman shows accelerated adaptation to starvation. When nourishment is withheld in labour, or before surgery there is early activation of fat metabolism. Fatty acids are utilised and glucose is spared for the fetus. When nourishment is ingested there is accelerated deposition in energy depots.[19]

Blood sugar concentrations tend to be low in pregnancy due to decreased gluconeogenesis. Hypoglycaemia is associated with a large increase in ketone body formation. Maternal hypoglycaemia produces fetal hypoglycaemia, which in turn causes the fetus to call upon its own stores of glycogen.[19] These important consequences of maternal starvation do not justify a return to oral feeding in labour, but are arguments for the intravenous administration of sugar-containing solutions in all but the shortest of labours.

DRUGS ACTING ON THE UTERUS

Most drugs which influence uterine contractility have cardiovascular and other side-effects of concern to the anaesthetist.

β–adrenergic agents
Orciprenaline, ritodrine and salbutamol are used for the supression of premature labour. They have been recently used for the inhibition of uterine contractions while preparing for Caesarean section in cases of fetal distress in labour. The anaesthetist may have to anaesthetise a patient who has recently received an intravenous injection of a β–adrenergic drug, and who has hypotension and extreme tachycardia. These effects can be reversed by propranolol, but the β–blocker should if possible be withheld until after delivery of the fetus because it may cause neonatal bradycardia.[20]

Prostaglandins
Prostaglandins (PG's) cause uterine and other smooth muscle to contract. PGE_2 and $PGF_2\alpha$ are used in obstetrics and may be given orally, intravenously or by extra-amniotic injection to induce or to accelerate labour and for the termination of pregnancy. PGE_2 may cause tachycardia, hypertension and flushing when given intravenously and an intravenous injection of 0.5 g of $PGF_2\alpha$ causes slight hypertension. Cardiovascular effects are absent when PG's are given by mouth or by extra amniotic injection.

PGE$_2$ is a bronchodilator, whereas PGF$_2\alpha$ causes bronchoconstriction and should not be given to asthmatics. PG's may cause diarrhoea or vomiting when given orally.

Oxytocin

Continuous intravenous infusions of synthetic oxytocin are devoid of cardio-vascular side-effects. Bolus intravenous injections cause widespread vasodilation which lasts for 3 to 5 minutes. Quite severe, if transient hypotension can occur under general anaesthesia[21] but hypotension is mainly postural and is absent or minimal in the lithotomy, or in the laterally tilted position.[22,23] Central venous pressure changes are those which occur when no oxytocic drug is given.[24] Vomiting does not occur and blood loss at delivery is not increased when oxytocin is substituted for ergometrine.[23,25]

Ergometrine

Ergometrine causes powerful and prolonged spasm of arteries and veins through-out the body.[22,24,26] Arterial and central venous pressures rise[24] and the pressor response may last for several hours. Cerebral oedema, pulmonary oedema, convulsions and cerebro-vascular accident may occur.[22,27] Ergometrine is most dangerous for women with pre-eclampsia and with heart disease, who should receive oxytocin instead of ergometrine. Intravenous ergometrine causes vomiting in from 12 to 46 per cent of patients.[23,25]

ANALGESICS AND TRANQUILLISERS

There has been a welcome reduction in the prescribing of large and repeated doses of narcotic analgesics in labour, thanks to an awareness of the ineffective-ness of these drugs, [28,29] shorter labours,[30] the increasing availability of epidural analgesia and the recognition of the persistent depressant action of analgesics in the newborn infant.[31,32] Phenothiazines and other tranquillisers are less often used and happily the barbiturates have been abandoned.

The efficacy of systemic analgesics

Intramuscular injections of narcotic analgesics frequently fail to relieve or even alleviate pain in labour. In one study 40 per cent of mothers had unsatisfactory relief despite very large doses of various narcotic analgesics[28] while in another series 73 per cent got no relief, or inadequate relief from pethidine.[29] Labour was naturally painless in only 2 per cent.[29] While often failing to relieve pain, pethidine frequently produces unwelcome drowsiness, loss of self-control and nausea. Pentazocine is much less likely to cause nausea in equi-analgesic doses.[33]

When epidural analgesia is unavailable there is a need to increase the effective-ness of pethidine. Cardiff experiences with patient-controlled, intermittent intravenous injections have been encouraging.[34] Analgesia is better than that which is obtained by intramuscular injections, although it is rarely complete. Placental transfer is likely to be substantial.

Analgesics and the Fetus

The Apgar score. This evaluates clinical signs of hypoxia in the newborn but cannot quantify the subtle and long-lasting depressant effects of drugs upon the neonatal nervous system. A simple measure of the extent of drug-induced respiratory depression is the time to sustained respiration (TSR), which is prolonged by pethidine and other drugs.

Neurobehavioural assessment. This is a sensitive indicator of the effect of drugs on the newborn. Response to stimuli such as touch, light and sound and the sucking reflex are recorded. Pethidine consistently depresses many reflex responses, impairs the establishment of feeding for up to 48 hours after birth[31,32] and may influence the establishment of the bond between mother and child.

Pethidine analgesia. Pethidine analgesia is associated with a slight, progressive fall in the pH of the fetal scalp blood in the first stage of labour[36] and the neonatal $Paco_2$ is elevated for up to five hours after birth.[37] Although the newborn can excrete pethidine and its metabolite norpethidine in the urine, the elimination process requires two or three days for completion.[38] This observation is consistent with the known neurobehavioural effects of pethidine in the neonate.

Narcotic antagonists

Naloxone is now the narcotic antagonist of choice for administration to the newborn[39] and is available as a neonatal solution of 0.04 mg/ml. Naloxone has no depressant action and therefore the need for an accurate guess as to the role of analgesic drugs in a given situation is reduced. Naloxone is also moderately effective against pentazocine. An intravenous injection of 0.04 mg nalaxone increases alveolar ventilation for 30 minutes in the newborn whose mother has received pethidine. An intramuscular injection of 0.2 mg stimulates ventilation and also improves feeding and reflex responses for up to 48 hours after birth.[32]

Mixtures of narcotic analgesic and antagonist cannot be recommended. Pethilorfan does not reduce respiratory depression[40] and the analgesic effect is probably diminished. A pethidine and naloxone mixture lessens the analgesic action of pethidine and does not reduce the incidence of side effects.[41]

Diazepam and chlormethiazole

Diazepam is not a very effective tranquilliser in normal labour,[42] but is an excellent anticonvulsant in severe pre-eclampsia, when the effects on the neonate become acceptable. If more than 30 mg is given to the mother within 15 hours of delivery the infant may develop hypotonia, secondary apnoea, hypothermia, poor sucking and may aspirate feeds into the lungs. All these may result from loss of muscle tone and similar effects have been attributed to long-term therapy with diazepam and nitrazepam in pregnancy.[43] Neonatal jaundice has been attributed to the solvent in which diazepam is dissolved. Normal beat-to-beat variations in the fetal heart rate may be lost during labour.[44]

Continuous infusions of 0.8 per cent chlormethiazole solutions are also used to prevent convulsions in severe pre-eclampsia and are usually combined with anti-hypertensive and analgesic drugs, or epidural analgesia.[45,46] Plasma volume expanders, such as salt-poor albumin, may be used to correct hypovolaemia. Such treatment is a major advance over basal narcosis with bromethol or morphine. Chlormethiazole is not a hypotensive agent[47] and attempts to lower blood pressure by administering excessive doses are condemned. An infusion rate of 10 to 20 drops/minute is usually sufficient and the mother should be fully rousable.

Fetal effects of drugs in pregnancy

Many drugs may harm the fetus and should not normally be given in pregnancy. Tetracycline may discolour the developing teeth, dicoumarol may cause fetal bleeding and death, cancer chemotherapeutic agents may cause fetal abnormality or death, antithyroid drugs suppress fetal thyroid and oral hypoglycaemic agents cause fetal hypoglycaemia and may be teratogenic. Phenothiazines do not cause spontaneous abortion if taken as antimetics.[48] Psychotropic drugs are not associated with fetal abnormality.[49]

A fetal alcohol syndrome is recognised in the offspring of alcoholic mothers and includes microcephaly, micrognathia, micropthalmia, heart lesions and growth retardation.[50] Impaired growth is well recognized in the infants of mothers who smoke during pregnancy and is due to maternal and fetal carboxyhaemoglobinaemia and to a vasoconstrictor action of nicotine on the placental circulation.

Withdrawal symptoms occur in the newborn of narcotic-addicted mothers. Animal experiments indicate that morphine, diamorphine (heroin), pethidine and pentazocine can cause abnormalities of the fetal nervous system when given at the time of organogenesis.[51]

GENERAL ANAESTHESIA

The role of anaesthesia in the causation of maternal death has been considered early in this Chapter. A principal cause of death is Mendelson's syndrome, which accounted for 14 of 37 deaths in three years in England and Wales.[1]

Mendelson's syndrome

In 1946 Mendelson observed that the acid-aspiration syndrome which now bears his name was due to the pulmonary aspiration of gastic juice with a pH of less than 2.5 and this observation has been confirmed by others.[52,53]

Preventive measures include oral antacid therapy, the use of cricoid pressure and attempts to empty the stomach by tube, by intravenous apomorphine[54] and by metoclopramide.[15] There is no certain method of emptying the stomach. Metoclopramide may also reduce the risk of regurgitation by raising the tone of the cardiac sphincter.[55] The substitution of regional analgesia for general anaesthesia offers the most effective prevention.

Oral antacids

From 43 to 55 per cent of women in labour have a gastric pH below 2.5. A 15 ml dose of magnesium trisilicate keeps the gastric pH above this critical level for up to 2 hours in from 89 to 96 per cent of women, thereby substantially reducing the potential risk of death from Mendelson's syndrome.[3,56,57,58,65,66] A single dose of antacid may cause rebound acid secretion after three or four hours. It is vitally important that all women in labour should receive 15 ml magnesium trisilicate every two hours. The volume of gastric juice is not increased by antacids[58] and gastric pH is not clearly related to the volume of juice.[3] A secondary benefit of antacid therapy is an increase in the tone of the cardiac sphincter reducing the possibility of regurgitation.[59]

Magnesium trisilicate mixture BPC, with its content of sodium bicarbonate is the preferred antacid for rapid and sustained alkalinisation. Aluminium hydroxide gel is less effective[56] and a mother has died of Mendelson's syndrome after receiving a proprietory preparation containing magnesium and aluminium hydroxide.[2] 0.3 molar sodium citrate was effective in a single dose in 22 patients[60] but awaits fuller evaluation. A single dose of 30 ml magnesium trisilicate is recommended for all patients who are about to receive a general anaesthetic. The H_2-receptor blocker cimetidine merits evaluation for the inhibition of gastric secretion in labour, but cannot neutralise existing gastric acid.

Treatment of Mendelson's syndrome

The immediate management of suspected or known pulmonary aspiration of even a small volume of gastric juice may determine whether the patient lives or dies. Tracheobronchial suction and oxygenation should be followed by an intravenous injection of at least 300 mg hydrocortisone or 5 mg dexamethasone. The injection must not be delayed until signs of Mendelson's syndrome appear. Tracheobronchial lavage and intratracheal steroid injections are not recommended. A sample of gastric juice will give information of prognostic value when its pH is estimated.

If signs of Mendelson's syndrome develop then an intensive therapy regimen must be initiated and may be required for several weeks. Hypoxia and metabolic acidosis are usually severe, although the Pa_{CO_2} may be only slightly elevated, suggesting a severe ventilation/perfusion defect, a right to left shunt, or both.[52] Hydrocortisone 300 mg should be given at six hourly intervals. Dexamethasone 5 mg may be substituted and causes less sodium retention.[61] The effectiveness of steroid therapy is questioned, although it may relieve bronchospasm and reduce inflammation. Animal experiments suggest that steroids may increase survival rates when the aspirated liquid has a pH between 1.36 and 2.1 and that death is almost inevitable if the pH is below 1.36.[53,56]

The role of newer agents in obstetric anaesthesia

Intravenous induction agents

Ketamine. Ketamine is used in North America and Europe as the sole agent for outlet forceps delivery. The safety of this technique is questionable, neonatal depression is dose-related and the method is 'less than ideal'.[62] Ketamine increases uterine contractility and uterine artery blood flow is increased along with blood pressure and cardiac output.[63] This explains the relatively minor extent of fetal acidosis associated with ketamine, but this advantage is counterbalanced by a lower Apgar score and a prolonged TSR which result from the central depressant action of the drug.[64]

Propanidid and Althesin. These have the attraction of rapid biodegradation and short-lived central depression. Unfortunately fetal acidosis is greater with both these agents than with thiopentone,[65,66] suggesting that maternal cardiac output and placental blood flow are more severely depressed by propanidid and Althesin.

Methohexitone. Methohexitone seems not to cause fetal acidosis and Apgar scores are satisfactory with a dose of 1 mg/kg, although larger doses are associated with low scores. Thiopentone, like methohexitone does not reduce cardiac output in moderate doses[67] and placental blood flow is usually well maintained. On the available evidence the well tried agents thiopentone and methohexitone in low dosage seem best for fetal welfare and may have other advantages in avoiding awareness and adverse reactions. Thiopentone and ketamine have been shown to depress neurobehavioural responses for many hours after the birth of the infant[68] and it is likely that other agents would have comparable effects.

Etomidate. Etomidate awaits evaluation in obstetric anaesthesia.

Muscle relaxants
The placental transfer of fazadinium is clinically insignificant. This, together with the absence of fasciculations and cardiovascular stability, resulted in the suggestion that fazadinium might be suitable for obstetric anaesthesia.[69,70] Unfortunately conditions for intubation are too often unsatisfactory[71,72] and suxamethonium remains the agent of choice for emergency use. Although plasma cholinesterase levels are reduced in pregnancy, the action of suxamethonium is not prolonged.[73]

Newer inhalational agents
Fluroxene. Fluroxene has analgesic properties, induction and recovery are rapid, blood pressure and cardiac output are well maintained and it has been hailed as a non-explosive cyclopropane. Placental transfer is rapid and fluroxene is deposited in fetal tissues.[74] Uterine relaxation is dose-dependent and occurs before serious cardiovascular depression. Fluroxene is suitable for brief inhalational anaesthesia of the type much used in the U.S.A. for forceps delivery and is perhaps the agent of choice on the rare occasions when it is necessary to relax the uterus.

Enflurane. Enflurane relaxes the uterus in a manner comparable to halothane.[75] Light anaesthesia is associated with cardiovascular stability and minimal uterine relaxation and 0.6 per cent enflurane has been used to supplement nitrous oxide and relaxant anaesthesia for Caesarean section. The cerebral excitation sometimes produced by enflurane precludes its use in pre-eclampsia.

Isoflurane. This is the isomer of enflurane and is devoid of convulsant action. Uterine relaxation is comparable to that associated with halothane.[75] An important observation is that utero-placental blood flow is increased and fetal hypoxia and acidosis are absent when isoflurane, and also halothane, are used in concentrations up to $1.5 \times$ MAC.[76] Isoflurane and halothane $1.5 \times$ MAC anaesthesia may therefore actually benefit the fetus.

Some other influences on fetal and maternal welfare

The importance of an adequate placental blood flow is increasingly recognised in the fetal interest. The placenta lacks a mechanism for regulating its own circulation, which is therefore dependent directly upon the uterine artery blood flow and in turn upon maternal cardiovascular integrity. Fetal metabolic acidosis and hypoxia suggest an inadequate placental circulation. The influence of anaesthetic agents has been discussed. Other factors which can influence placental blood flow are maternal posture, operating time and maternal $PaCO_2$.

Maternal posture (caval occlusion)

In the supine position the inferior vena cava is normally compressed by the gravid uterus. There is always a small reduction in cardiac output and arterial pressure is maintained by vasoconstriction (concealed caval occlusion). In about 6 per cent of unanaesthetised mothers supine hypotension and bradycardia (revealed caval occlusion) develop and cardiac output falls by up to 50 per cent.[5] Revealed caval occlusion is commoner under anaesthesia. Both types of caval occlusion are liable to reduce placental blood flow. When Caesarean section is performed in the unmodified supine position the infant and the mother frequently develop a more severe metabolic acidosis and a lower PaO_2 than is the case when the table is tilted laterally.[77,78,79] A tilt to the left is preferred[80,81,82] and the mother should be in the tilted or full lateral position for 30 minutes before anaesthesia whenever possible.[93]

Operating time

Time, tilt and fetal acidosis are closely related at Caesarean section. When a lateral tilt is used then the time from the induction of anaesthesia to incision of the uterus is unrelated to the condition of the infant at birth, whereas the time from incision of the uterus to delivery of the child significantly influences the extent of fetal acidosis at delivery.[83,84] Here is confirmation that placental blood flow is usually adequate during light anaesthesia in the tilted position and that extraction of the child from the uterus should be performed expeditiously by a competent obstetrician.

Maternal PaO_2 and $PaCO_2$

Umbilical venous PO_2 is maximal when the maternal PaO_2 is about 40 kPa (300 mmHg); a value attained when the FIO_2 is about 66 per cent.[85] The use of 66 per cent of oxygen with nitrous oxide calls for supplementation if awareness is to be avoided.

Hyperventilation may harm the fetus. A maternal $PaCO_2$ between 2.15 and 2.85 kPa (17 and 20 mmHg) causes fetal metabolic and respiratory acidosis, explained by the reduction in placental blood flow which results from the vasoconstrictor response to hypocapnia and from the reduction in cardiac output associated with IPPV.[86] Normocapnia should be the aim. A $PaCO_2$ of 4 kPa (30 mmHg) is normal in pregnancy and it is not difficult to reduce the $PaCO_2$ to below 2.85 kPa (20 mmHg).

Awareness during anaesthesia

When unsupplemented 70:30 nitrous oxide and oxygen mixtures are used during Caesarean section, factual recall occurs in up to 9 per cent of patients.[87] If a higher FIO_2 is used in the fetal interest then awareness might be even more frequent. Supplementation is therefore essential. Intravenous supplements have proved disappointing and there is wide agreement on the use of low concentrations of volatile agents. 0.2 per cent of trichlorethylene or methoxyflurane reduce the incidence of awareness to 2.5 per cent when given with 66 per cent of oxygen.[84] Awareness occurs in well under 1 per cent of women if 0.5 per cent halothane is given with 50 per cent of oxygen[88] and a recent study suggests that 0.2 per cent halothane would suffice[89] while maintaining or increasing placental blood flow.[76]

REGIONAL ANALGESIA

Only three techniques need be considered, namely paracervical block, epidural analgesia and subarachoid analgesia.

Paracervical block

This simple technique of first stage analgesia involves the injection of 8–10 ml of local analgesic solution through each lateral fornix and relieves the pain of uterine contractions in up to 80 per cent of cases. Continuous fetal heart rate monitoring has shown that bradycardia occurs in from 20 to 50 per cent of cases, usually within 10 minutes of the injections and associated with fetal acidosis. The mechanism of this fetal hypoxia was thought to be depression of the fetal myocardium by the local analgesic drug. More recent work indicates that concentrations of drug in the fetal blood are not unduly high and that an impairment of the placental circulation is a more likely explanation[90] and may be due to a vasoconstrictor action of the local analgesic agent. The technique has been abandoned by most obstetricians.

Epidural analgesia

Lumbar epidural analgesia is by far the most effective method of pain relief in labour,[91,92,93] giving complete relief in over 80 per cent of cases and a useful measure of relief in most of the remainder. Although lumbar epidural analgesia has almost ousted caudal analgesia, most of the following discussion is applicable to either technique. Caudal analgesia does not allow 'selective' epidural analgesia with retention of perineal sensation and the success rate is substantially lower. The increasing use of epidural analgesia in labour is a major advance in obstetrics and in anaesthesia.

Safety depends upon skilled and experienced anaesthetists, obstetricians and midwives and above all upon the avoidance of caval occlusion in association with the extensive sympathetic blockade. The use of the lateral or tilted position at all times is of the utmost importance.[94] If caval occlusion is avoided and blood volume is maintained by intravenous fluids then placental blood flow is unchanged during epidural analgesia.[95] If hypotension occurs despite these measures then an intravenous injection of ephedrine 10 mg will restore blood pressure and utero-placental blood flow.[96]

Epidural analgesia minimises the increase in cortisol output which occurs in labours in which less effective forms of pain relief are used, suggesting that the stress of labour is also minimised.[97,98]

Epidural analgesia and the fetus
The progressive fetal metabolic acidosis which develops when the first stage of labour is managed with pethidine analgesia is absent when epidural analgesia is used.[36,99] If caval occlusion and hypotension are avoided there are no pathological alterations in fetal heart rate attributable to epidural analgesia.[99,100,101] Serious disturbances in heart rate are usually the result of hypotension or overstimulation with oxytocin. Maternal hyperventilation and hypocapnia in response to pain are abolished by epidural analgesia, with improvement in placental circulation and fetal acid base status.[36,86]

Neurobehavioural responses. In the newborn neurobehavioural responses are unimpaired after epidural analgesia with bupivacaine,[102] indicating that drug-induced depression is absent. When lignocaine or mepivacaine is used there is neonatal hypotonia, but reflexes are intact.[103] Bupivacaine is extensively bound to maternal plasma proteins and the fetal/maternal concentration ratio is approximately 0:3. Lignocaine and mepivacaine are less well bound to protein and plancental transfer is free. Chloroprocaine does not affect the infant because it is very rapidly hydrolysed by cholinesterase.[68]

Uterine action
If inco-ordinate uterine action is present then epidural analgesia is often followed by a more normal type of uterine action.[101,104] In normal labour the overall rate of cervical dilatation is unaffected by epidural analgesia. An epidural injection is sometimes followed by a cessation of uterine contractions for a few minutes, even in the claimed absence of caval occlusion.[101] Others have attributed this effect to hypotension or concealed caval occlusion.[105] Oxytocin can modify the responses to epidural analgesia.

Choice of local analgesic agent
Bupivacaine is the agent of choice for pain relief in labour because it is relatively safe,[106] long acting, associated with an acceptable incidence of motor block,[107] has a low fetal/maternal concentration ratio and does not affect neonatal neurobehavioural responses.[102]

   Etidocaine also has a low fetal/maternal concentration ratio, but is inferior to bupivacaine for the relief of pain in labour because of the high incidence of motor block.[107,108,109] Etidocaine 1 per cent is an excellent agent for Caesarean section.[110] Although chloroprocaine does not affect the infant,[64] its very short duration of action makes it inconvenient in use. Lignocaine, mepivacaine and prilocaine are agents of second choice for pain relief in labour because they are relatively short-acting, cause a relatively high incidence of motor block,[107] have high fetal/maternal concentration ratios and cause neonatal hypotonia.[103] Prilocaine causes maternal and fetal methaemogloblinaemia. Carbonated lignocaine disappointingly fails to reduce the incidence of unblocked segments.[93]

   The duration of pain relief with 0.25 per cent and 0.375 per cent bupivacaine and 1.5 per cent lignocaine is essentially the same and only 0.5 per cent and

0.75 per cent bupivacaine and 1 per cent etidocaine solutions substantially prolong analgesia while also increasing the incidence of motor block.[107] The addition of adrenaline to bupivacaine solutions does not prolong their action and does not decrease toxicity.

The problem of imperfect analgesia
Complete analgesia is achieved in over 80 per cent of mothers. In only 2 or 3 per cent is pain relief classed as unsatisfactory, so that about 15 per cent of women get useful but imperfect analgesia.[91,92,93] Technical difficulties and inappropriate posture are the principal causes of imperfect analgesia and are often reme-diable.[111,112] If more than 2 cm of catheter is left within the epidural space or the mother lies for long periods on one side then the incidence of unilateral blocks increases to 12 per cent[93] or even 21 per cent.[113] Unblocked spinal segments cause persistent pain, often in one groin, in 6 to 9 per cent of patients.[93,114] In more than 50 per cent of cases this pain can be relieved by a top-up injection given while the mother lies on her painful side.

Pain experienced while awaiting a top-up injection was, perhaps surprisingly found not to be an important cause of imperfect analgesia and it was confirmed that unilateral analgesia and unblocked segments were the main cause of imperfect pain relief.[112]

Epidural analgesia and the forceps delivery rate
The instrumental delivery rate associated with epidural analgesia ranges from an essentially normal 15 per cent or 20 per cent[115,116] to 60 per cent.[117] The incidence of malpositions of the fetal head is said to be not increased[115] or to be trebled, even when epidural analgesia is used solely for pain relief in the absence of obstetric pathology.[117] There were no apparent harmful effects upon the infants, even when rotational forceps deliveries were performed in 20 per cent of cases[117] but there is always a potential risk of trauma to mother and child with a difficult instrumental delivery.[30] A large increase in rotational and mid-cavity forceps is clearly undesirable and seems to be attributable to certain techniques of epidural analgesia and not to others. Although abnormalities such as inco-ordinate uterine action, pre-eclampsia and heart disease increase the forceps delivery rate[118] such abnormalities were absent in the Oxford series where the forceps rate was 60 per cent.[117]

Relaxation of the pelvic floor muscles by the use of 0.5 per cent bupivacaine solution appears to inhibit rotation of the fetal head.[117] The incidence of malpositions was not increased when 0.25 per cent bupivacaine was used.[115] The acceleration of labour with oxytocin promotes rotation and reduces the incidence of occipito-posterior positions in the second stage.[119] Perineal analgesia abolishes involuntary pushing and the use of a 'selective' block, confined to the lower thoracic and upper lumbar nerves results in spontaneous delivery in 80 per cent of cases.[116]

Indications for epidural analgesia
Most epidural blocks are given solely or primarily for pain relief in labour. A few are given before amniotomy,[127] or an epidural catheter may be inserted at

that time and the block 'activated' when labour becomes painful. Most anaesthetists await the onset of painful labour before performing the block. Epidural analgesia is given to between 10 and 70 per cent of mothers, where a service exists and a representative figure for an established service lies between 25 and 30 per cent.[70] Staffing shortages still prevent the establishment of an epidural service in some hospitals and a few obstetricians have themselves provided an epidural service.[120,121,122] While giving every credit to the high motives behind such services, it should be stated that the safety of an epidural service without a resident anaesthetist skilled in tracheal intubation has been questioned.

There are some specific indications for epidural analgesia and one or two situations where the use of this method is controversial.

Pre-eclampsia
Epidural analgesia reduces systolic and diastolic blood pressure by over 20 per cent on average in severe pre-eclampsia and the rises in arterial pressure which accompany painful contractions are avoided.[46] Forceps delivery is facilitated. Diazepam injections or a chlormethiazole infusion[45] are given to prevent convulsions. A plasma volume expander such as salt-poor albumin may be used to correct the hypovolaemia of severe pre-eclampsia[123] and central venous pressure monitoring will be helpful. An antihypertensive drug such as diazoxide or hydrallazine may be combined with epidural blockade for the control of hypertension. Early delivery is important and is the only cure for pre-eclampsia.

Heart disease
Pain and anxiety cause tachycardia, which may precipitate pulmonary oedema in patients with valvular lesions and effective analgesia is especially important for such mothers. Vasodilatation is often beneficial in heart failure, and especially in acute left ventricular failure, where hypertension causes 'forward impedence'[124,125] Epidural analgesia offers excellent pain relief, a reduction in peripheral resistance and optimal conditions for elective forceps delivery. The muscular efforts and the Valsalva effect associated with spontaneous delivery are potentially harmful.[126] Ergometrine increases arterial and central venous pressure and should be replaced by oxytocin.[22,24,26]

Labour after previous Caesarean section
Whatever the method of pain relief, there is always a risk of uterine rupture during labour when the uterus is scarred by previous surgery and the risk is greater where there is a possibility of overstimulation by oxytocin. Two questions arise from the use of epidural analgesia in these labours. Does epidural blockade further increase the risk of uterine rupture and does epidural analgesia hinder the diagnosis of uterine rupture by masking the pain?

Undoubtedly overstimulation with oxytocin has caused rupture during epidural analgesia[127] and experience suggests that the 'epidural sieve' permits the transmission of the more powerful impulses of the constant pain of uterine rupture.[128] Other signs of rupture include hypotension, tachycardia and the cessation of contractions and should be detectable under epidural analgesia and the risk of a truly 'silent' rupture is probably small. The decision to use epidural analgesia should take account of the indication for the previous Caesarean section. If cephalo-pelvic disproportion is absent, oxytocin doseage is carefully controlled and only a short labour is permitted then epidural analgesia may be used.[129,130] With these provisos, and with skilled and careful management of labour there seems no reason to think that epidural analgesia causes or in itself predisposes to uterine rupture.

Breech delivery
Far from being contraindicated for assisted breech delivery, epidural analgesia is now considered the technique of first choice.[131,132,133] The relaxed and pain-free condition of the mother allows a controlled delivery of the head, which is beneficial for the infant, especially if it is premature. The duration of the second stage is prolonged by about 10 minutes, but the percentage of breech extractions is not increased despite perineal analgesia. Premature expulsive efforts are abolished and the anaesthetist is no longer required to induce general anaesthesia in a struggling patient in the lithotomy position. The obstetrician must be skilled in breech delivery and prepared to perform Caesarean section at any time in labour.

The delivery of twins
As in breech delivery, so is epidural analgesia now seen by some authorities as advantageous for the delivery of twins.[134,135] Controlled, painless delivery is possible, whatever the presentation of each infant, and prompt delivery of the second twin is possible. Delay in delivery contributes substantially to the well recognised extra mortality among second twins. The risk for the first twin is no different from the risk for singleton fetuses also delivered under epidural analgesia.[134] Labour is not prolonged and the percentage of breech extractions is not increased.[135]

Caesarean section under epidural analgesia
There is a growing interest in the use of epidural analgesia for Caesarean section. In the United Kingdom a few centres now perform approximately 50 per cent of Caesarean sections under epidural block and in teaching centres in the U.S.A. epidural analgesia is replacing subarachnoid analgesia.[136]
    The advantages of epidural analgesia include:

1. No risk of death from pulmonary aspiration or failed intubation.[1,2]
2. No drug-induced neonatal depression if bupivacaine or etidocaine used.[102,103,110]
3. The awareness problem is eliminated.
4. Emotional satisfaction for the mother.
5. Fetal acid-base status normal if caval occlusion and hypovolaemia are prevented.

    Epidural analgesia requires time and is unsuitable if operation is urgent or if the patient does not willingly accept the technique. A perfect block from S5 to T6 is essential and cutaneous analgesia should be sought throughout this entire area. 20 ml or even 25 ml of 0.5 per cent bupivacaine or 1 per cent etidocaine are required.[110] Pain and nausea during uterine surgery can usually be eliminated if 10 ml of solution are injected in the sitting position and this position is maintained for 15 minutes. The remainder of the dose is given in the supine, tilted position.[137] Preloading with at least a litre of crystalloid fluid is important[138] and caval occlusion must be prevented. These measures reduce the incidence of hypotension to under 7 per cent.[139] Oxytocin should replace ergometrine to eliminate vomiting.[25,140]

The infant is usually active at birth. Apgar scores are high, TSR's are short and neurobehavioural responses are improved, although lignocaine causes hypotonia.[110,141,142,143] Fetal metabolic acidosis has been reported, but this is little greater than that which occurs under general anaesthesia and is probably the result of potentially preventable caval occlusion or hypovolaemia.[95] With impeccable technique the condition of the infant is likely to be better than is usual after general anaesthesia and this improved state is likely to be present for up to 48 hours. The problems which call for a high level of anaesthetic expertise are the maintenance of maternal and placental circulation and the attainment of a perfect block. The emotional satisfaction felt by the mother at the birth of her child is often justification in itself.

Spinal subarachnoid analgesia

A potential role for subarachnoid analgesia is in the form of a rapidly-acting single injection technique for forceps delivery. Saddle block and low spinal analgesia are extensively used for this purpose in the U.S.A. Pudendal nerve block is ineffective in about 50 per cent of patients[144] and there is a place for an effective substitute. The use of a 25 gauge needle and introducer almost eliminates postspinal headache and the role of caval occlusion and hypovolaemia in the production of hypotension are well understood.[5,138]

ACUPUNCTURE AND ELECTROANALGESIA

It is perhaps surprising that acupuncture has been rarely used in labour in China and in the Western world.[145] When 21 volunteer American women had acupuncture in childbirth, 19 of these mothers got no relief whatsoever.[145] Even if acupuncture were effective, the requirements for trained personnel and patient instruction would limit the applicability of the technique.

Low intensity currents of 8–10 mA with a frequency of 750–1000 Hz are passed through electrodes applied to the frontal and mastoid regions to provide electroanalgesia. Russian workers claim that most women obtain relief and that in 'a majority' of patients with inco-ordinate uterine action labour becomes more normal.[146] This is the recognised response in inco-ordinate labour to effective analgesia[101,104] and suggests that electroanalgesia is indeed effective. Detailed results of a well-conducted trial would be of interest. Electroanalgesia, like acupuncture, is presumed to be harmless to mother and child.

REFERENCES

1. Department of Health and Social Security (1975) *Report on Confidential Enquiries into Maternal Deaths in England and Wales 1970–72.* London: H.M.S.O.
2. Scottish Home and Health Department (1978) *A Report on an Enquiry into Maternal Deaths in Scotland 1972–75.* Edinburgh: H.M.S.O.
3. Peskett, W. G. H. (1973) Antacids before obstetric anaesthesia. A clinical evaluation of the effectiveness of mist. magnesium trisilicate, BPC. *Anaesthesia*, **28**, 509–513.
4. Chesley, L. C. & Duffus, G. M. (1971) Posture and apparent plasma volume in late pregnancy. *Journal of Obstetrics and Gynaecology of the British Commonwealth*, **78**, 406–412.
5. Lees, M. M., Scott, D. B., Kerr, M. G. & Taylor, S. H. (1967) Circulatory effects of the supine position in late pregnancy. *Clinical Science*, **32**, 453–465.
6. Baldwin, G. R., Moorthi, D. S., Whelton, J. A. & MacDonnell, K. F. (1977) New lung functions and pregnancy. *American Journal of Obstetrics and Gynecology*, **127**, 235–239.
7. Bevan, D. R., Holdcroft, A., Loh, H., MacGregor, W. G., O'Sullivan, J. C. & Sykes, M. K. (1974) Closing volume and pregnancy. *British Medical Journal*, **1**, 13–15.
8. Craig, D. B. & Toole, M. A. (1975) Airway closure in pregnancy. *Canadian Anaesthetists' Society Journal*, **22**, 665–672.
9. Holdcroft, A., Bevan, D. R., O'Sullivan, J. C. & Sykes, M. K. (1977) Airway closure and pregnancy. *Anaesthesia*, **32**, 517–523.
10. Templeton, A. & Kelman, G. R. (1976) Maternal blood-gases (Pao_2–Pao_2), physiological shunt and V_D/V_T in normal pregnancy. *British Journal of Anaesthesia*, **48**, 1001–1004.
11. Archer, G. W. & Marx, G. F. (1974) Arterial oxygen tension during apnoea in parturient women. *British Journal of Anaesthesia*, **46**, 358–360.
12. Huch, A., Huch, R., Lindmark, G. & Rooth, G. (1974) Maternal hypoxaemia after pethidine. *Journal of Obstetrics and Gynaecology of the British Commonwealth*, **81**, 608–614.
13. Myers, R. E., Stange, L., Joelson, I., Huzell, B. & Wussow, C. (1977) Effects upon the fetus of oxygen administration to the mother. *Acta obstetrica et gynecologica scandinavica*, **56**, 195–203.
14. Davison, J. S., Davison, M. C. & Hay, D. M. (1970) Gastric emptying time in late pregnancy and labour. *Journal of Obstetrics and Gynaecology of the British Commonwealth*, **77**, 37–41.
15. Nimmo, W. S., Wilson, J. & Prescott, L. F. (1975) Narcotic analgesia and delayed gastric emptying during labour. *Lancet*, **1**, 890–893.
16. Parry, E., Shields, R. & Turnbull, A. C. (1970) Transit time in the small intestine in pregnancy. *Journal of Obstetrics and Gynaecology of the British Commonwealth*, **77**, 900–901.
17. Spence, A. A., Moir, D. D. & Finlay, W. E. I. (1967) Observations on intragastric pressure. *Anaesthesia*, **22**, 249–256.
18. Lind, F. J., Smith, A. M., McIver, D. K., Coopland, A. T. & Crispin, J. S. (1968) Heartburn in pregnancy—a manometric study. *Canadian Medical Association Journal*, **98**, 571.
19. Dick, W., Ahnefeld, F. W., Milewski, P. & Schöch, G. (1977) Important clinical adaptation processes of women during pregnancy: Anesthesiologic considerations. *Journal of Perinatal Medicine*, **5**, 103–113.
20. Knight, R. J. (1977) Labour retarded by β-agonist drugs. A therapeutic problem in emergency anaesthesia. *Anaesthesia*, **32**, 639–641.
21. Weis, F. R. & Peak, J. (1974) Effects of oxytocin on blood pressure during anesthesia. *Anesthesiology*, **40**, 189–190.
22. Johnstone, M. (1972) The cardiovascular effects of oxytocic drugs. *British Journal of Anaesthesia*, **44**, 826–834.
23. Moir, D. D. & Amoa, A. B. (1978) Ergometrine or oxytocin? *British Journal of Anaesthesia* (in press).
24. Williams, C. V., Johnson, A. & Ledward, R. (1974) A comparison of central venous pressure changes in the third stage of labour following oxytocic drugs and diazepam. *Journal of Obstetrics and Gynaecology of the British Commonwealth*, **81**, 596–599.
25. Moodie, J. E. & Moir, D. D. (1976) Ergometrine, oxytocin and epidural analgesia. *British Journal of Anaesthesia*, **48**, 571–574.
26. Wassef, M. R., Lal, H. & Pleuvry, J. (1974) The cardiovascular effects of ergometrine in the experimental animal in vivo and in vitro. *British Journal of Anaesthesia*, **46**, 473–478.
27. Abouleish, E. (1976) Postpartum hypertension and convulsion after oxytocic drugs. *Current Researches in Anesthesia and Analgesia*, **55**, 813–815.
28. Beazley, J. M., Leaver, E. P., Morewood, J. H. M. & Bircumshaw, J. (1967) Relief of pain in labour. *Lancet*, **1**, 1033–1035.
29. Holdcroft, A. & Morgan, M. (1974) An assessment of the analgesic effect in labour of pethidine and 50 per cent nitrous oxide in oxygen (Entonox). *Journal of Obstetrics and Gynaecology of the British Commonwealth*, **81**, 603–607.

30. O'Driscoll, K. (1975) An obstetrician's view of pain. *British Journal of Anaesthesia*, **47**, 1053–1059.
31. Brackbill, Y., Kane, J., Manniello, R. S. & Abramson, D. (1974) Obstetric meperidine usage and assessment of neonatal status. *Anesthesiology*, **40**, 116–120.
32. Wiener, P. C., Hogg, M. I. J. & Rosen, M. (1977) Effects of naloxone on pethidine-induced neonatal depression. *British Medical Journal*, **2**, 228–231.
33. Moore, J. & Ball, H. G. (1974) A sequential study of intravenous analgesic treatment during labour. *British Journal of Anaesthesia*, **46**, 365–372.
34. Evans, J. M., Rosen, M., McCarthy, J. & Hogg, M. I. J. (1976) Apparatus for patient-controlled administration of intravenous narcotics in labour. *Lancet*, **1**, 17–18.
35. Richards, M. P. M. & Bernal, J. F. (1972) Effects of obstetric medication on mother-infant interaction and infant development. In *Psychosomatic Medicine in Obstetrics and Gynaecology*, ed. Morris, N. p. 303. Basel: Karger.
36. Pearson, J. F. & Davies, P. (1974) The effect of continuous lumbar epidural analgesia upon fetal acid-base status during the first stage of labour. *Journal of Obstetrics and Gynaecology of the British Commonwealth*, **81**, 971–974.
37. Koch, G. & Wandel, H. (1968) Effect of pethidine on the postnatal adjustment of respiration and acid-base balance. *Acta obstetrica et gynecologica scandinavica*, **47**, 27.
38. Hogg, M. I. J., Wiener, P. C., Rosen, M. & Mapleson, W. W. (1977) Urinary excretion and metabolism of pethidine and norpethidine in the newborn. *British Journal of Anaesthesia*, **49**, 891–899.
39. Stephen, G. W., Cooper, L. V. & Harvey, D. (1976) The effect of narcotic and narcotic-antagonist drugs in the newborn rabbit. *British Journal of Anaesthesia*, **48**, 635–638.
40. Campbell, D., Masson, A. H. B. & Norris, W. (1965) The clinical evaluation of narcotic and sedative drugs. 2. A re-evaluation of pethidine and Pethilorfan. *British Journal of Anaesthesia*, **37**, 199–207.
41. Girvan, C. B., Moore, J. & Dundee, J. W. (1976) Pethidine compared with pethidine-naloxone administered during labour. *British Journal of Anaesthesia*, **48**, 563–569.
42. Elder, M. G. & Crossley, J. (1969) A double blind trial of diazepam in labour. *Journal of Obstetrics and Gynaecology of the British Commonwealth*, **76**, 264–265.
43. Speight, A. N. P. (1977) Floppy-infant syndrome and maternal diazepam and/or nitrazepam. *Lancet*, **2**, 878.
44. Scher, J., Hailey, D. M. & Beard, R. W. (1972) The effect of diazepam on the fetus. *Journal of Obstetrics and Gynaecology of the British Commonwealth*, **79**, 635–638.
45. Duffus, G. M., Tunstall, M. E. & MacGillivray, I. (1968) Intravenous chlormethiazole in pre-eclamptic toxaemia in labour. *Lancet*, **1**, 335–337.
46. Moir, D. D., Victor-Rodrigues, L. & Willocks, J. (1972) Epidural analgesia during labour in patients with pre-eclampsia. *Journal of Obstetrics and Gynaecology of the British Commonwealth*, **79**, 465–469.
47. Wilson, J., Stephen, G. W. & Scott, D. B. (1969) A study of the cardiovascular effects of chlormethiazole. *British Journal of Anaesthesia*, **41**, 840–843.
48. Kullander, S. & Källen, B. (1976) A prospective study of drugs in pregnancy. II. Anti-emetic drugs. *Acta obstetrica et gynecologica scandinavica*, **55**, 105–111.
49. Kullander, S. & Källen, B. (1976) A prospective study of drugs in pregnancy. I. Psychopharmaca. *Acta obstetrica et gynecologica scandinavica*. **55**, 25–33.
50. Oullette, E. M., Rosett, H. L., Rosman, N. P. & Weiner, L. (1977) Adverse effects of maternal alcohol abuse during pregnancy. *New England Journal of Medicine*, **297**, 528–530.
51. Geber, W. F. & Schramm, L. C. (1975) Congenital malformations of the central nervous system produced by narcotic analgesics in the hamster. *American Journal of Obstetrics and Gynecology*, **123**, 705–713.
52. Davidson, J. T., Rubin, S., Eyal, Z. & Polliack, A. (1974) A comparison of the pulmonary response to the endotracheal instillation of 0.1 N hydrochloric acid and Hartmann's solution in the rabbit. *British Journal of Anaesthesia*, **46**, 127–132.
53. Downs, J. B., Chapman, R. L. Jr., Modell, J. H. & Hood, I. (1974) An evaluation of steroid therapy in aspiration pneumonitis. *Anesthesiology*, **40**, 129–135.
54. Holdsworth, J. D., Furness, R. M. B. & Roulston, R. G. (1974) A comparison of apomorphine and stomach tubes for emptying the stomach before general anaesthesia in obstetrics. *British Journal of Anaesthesia*, **46**, 526–529.
55. Brock-Utne, J. G., Rubin, J., Downing, J. W., Dimopoulos, G. E., Moshal, M. G. & Naicker, M. (1976) The administration of metoclopramide with atropine. *Anaesthesia*, **31**, 1186–1190.
56. Taylor, G. & Prys-Davies, J. (1966) Prophylactic use of antacids in the prevention of the acid-pulmonary-aspiration syndrome (Mendelson's syndrome). *Lancet*, **1**, 288–291.
57. Roberts, R. B. & Shirley, M. A. (1974) Reducing the risk of acid aspiration during Cesarean section. *Current Researches in Anesthesia and Analgesia*, **53**, 859–868.

58. Roberts, R. B. & Shirley, M. A. (1976) The obstetrician's role in reducing the risk of aspiration pneumonitis with particular reference to the use of oral antacids. *American Journal of Obstetrics and Gynecology*, **124**, 611–617.

59. Higgs, R. H., Smyth, R. D. & Castell, D. O. (1974) Gastric alkalinization. Effect on lower esophageal sphincter pressure and serum gastrin. *New England Journal of Medicine*, **291**, 486–490.

60. Lahiri, S. K., Thomas, T. A. & Hodgson, R. M. H. (1973) Single-dose antacid therapy for the prevention of Mendelson's syndrome. *British Journal of Anaesthesia*, **45**, 1143–1146.

61. Dudley, W. R. & Marshall, B. E. (1974) Steroid treatment for acid-aspiration pneumonitis. *Anesthesiology*, **40**, 136–141.

62. Akamatsu, T. J. & Bonica, J. J. (1977) Ketamine for obstetric delivery. *Anesthesiology*, **46**, 78.

63. Levinson, G., Shnider, S. M., Gildea, J. E. & De Lorimier, A. A. (1973) Maternal and fetal cardiovascular and acid-base changes during ketamine anaesthesia in pregnant ewes. *British Journal of Anaesthesia*, **45**, 1111–1115.

64. Downing, J. W., Mahomedy, M. C., Jeal, D. E. & Allen, P. J. (1976) Anaesthesia for Caesarean section with ketamine. *Anaesthesia*, **31**, 883–892.

65. Mahomedy, M. C., Downing, J. W., Jeal, D. E. & Coleman, A. J. (1976) Anaesthetic induction for Caesarean section with propanidid. *Anaesthesia*, **31**, 205–211.

66. Downing, J. W., Mahomedy, M. C., Coleman, A. J., Mahomedy, Y. H. & Jeal, D. E. (1974) Anaesthetic induction for Caesarean section. Althesin versus thiopentone. *Anaesthesia*, **29**, 689–695.

67. Chamberlain, J. H., Seed, R. G. F. L. & Chung, D. C. W. (1977) Effect of thiopentone on myocardial function. *British Journal of Anaesthesia*, **49**, 865–870.

68. Hodkinson, R., Marx, G. F., Kim, S. S. & Miclat, N. M. (1977) Neonatal neurobehavioural tests following vaginal delivery under ketamine, thiopental and extradural anesthesia. *Current Researches in Anesthesia and Analgesia*, **56**, 548–553.

69. Blogg, C. E., Simpson, B. R., Tyers, M. B., Martin, L. E. & Bell, J. A. (1975) Human placental transfer of AH8165. *Anaesthesia*, **30**, 23–29.

70. Cane, R. D. & Sinclair, D. M. (1976) The use of AH8165 for Caesarean section. *Anaesthesia*, **31**, 212–214.

71. Young, H. S. A., Clarke, R. S. J. & Dundee, J. W. (1975) Intubating conditions with AH8165 and suxamethonium. *Anaesthesia*, **30**, 30–33.

72. Corall, I. M., Ward, M. E., Page, J. & Strunin, L. (1977) Conditions for tracheal intubation following fazadinium and pancuronium. *British Journal of Anaesthesia*, **49**, 615–617.

73. Blitt, C. D., Petty, W. C., Alberternst, E. E. & Wright, B. J. (1977) Correlation of plasma cholinesterase activity and duration of action of succinylcholine during pregnancy. *Current Researches in Anesthesia and Analgesia*, **56**, 78–81.

74. Marx, G. F., Eckstein, K. L. & Halevy, S. (1973) Placental transmission and maternal and neonatal elimination of fluroxene. *Current Researches in Anesthesia and Analgesia*, **52**, 654–660.

75. Munson, E. S. & Embro, W. J. (1977) Enflurane, isoflurane and halothane and isolated human uterine muscle. *Anesthesiology*, **46**, 11–14.

76. Palahniuk, R. J. & Shnider, S. M. (1974) Maternal and fetal cardiovascular and acid-base changes during halothane and isoflurane anesthesia in the pregnant ewe. *Anesthesiology*, **41**, 462–472.

77. Ansari, I., Wallace, G., Clemetson, C. A. B., Mallikarjuneswara, V. R. & Clemetson, C. D. M. (1970) Tilt Caesarean section. *Journal of Obstetrics and Gynaecology of the British Commonwealth*, **77**, 713–721.

78. Crawford, J. S. Burton, M. & Davies, P. (1972) Time and lateral tilt at Caesarean section. *British Journal of Anaesthesia*, **44**, 477–484.

79. Downing, J. W., Coleman, A. J., Mahomedy, M. C., Jeal, D. E. & Mahomedy, Y. H. (1974) Lateral table tilt for Caesarean section. *Anaesthesia*, **29**, 696–703.

80. Drummond, G. B., Scott, S. E. M., Lees, M. M. & Scott, D. B. (1974) Effects of posture on limb blood flow in late pregnancy. *British Medical Journal*, **4**, 587–588.

81. Eckstein, K. L. & Marx, G. F. (1974) Aorto-caval compression and uterine displacement. *Anesthesiology*, **40**, 92–96.

82. Buley, R. J. R., Downing, J. W., Brock-Utne, J. G. & Cuerden, C. (1977) Right versus left lateral tilt for Caesarean section. *British Journal of Anaesthesia*, **49**, 1009–1014.

83. Crawford, J. S., Burton, M. & Davies, P. (1973) Anaesthesia for section: further refinements of a technique. *British Journal of Anaesthesia*, **45**, 726–731.

84. Crawford, J. S., James, F. M. III, Davies, P. & Crawley, M. (1976) A further study of general anaesthesia for Caesarean section. *British Journal of Anaesthesia*, **48**, 661–667.

85. Rorke, N. J., Davey, D. A. & Dutoit, H. J. (1968) Fetal oxygenation during Caesarean section. *Anaesthesia*, **23**, 585–596.

86. Levinson, G., Shnider, S. M., de Lorimier, A. & Steffenson, J. L. (1974) Effects of maternal hyperventilation on uterine blood flow and fetal oxygenation and acid-base status. *Anesthesiology*, **40**, 340–347.
87. Wilson, J. & Turner, D. J. (1969) Awareness during Caesarean section under general anaesthesia. *British Medical Journal*, **1**, 280–283.
88. Moir, D. D. (1970) Anaesthesia for Caesarean section. An evaluation of a method using low concentrations of halothane and 50 per cent of oxygen. *British Journal of Anaesthesia*, **42**, 136–142.
89. Latto, I. P. & Waldron, B. A. (1977) Anaesthesia for Caesarean section. Analysis of blood concentrations of halothane using 0.2 per cent or 0.65 per cent halothane with 50 per cent nitrous oxide in oxygen. *British Journal of Anaesthesia*, **49**, 371–378.
90. Liston, W. A., Adjepon-Yamoah, K. K. & Scott, D. B. (1973) Fetal and maternal lignocaine levels after paracervical block. *British Journal of Anaesthesia*, **45**, 750–754.
91. Crawford, J. S. (1972) The second thousand epidural blocks in an obstetric hospital practice. *British Journal of Anaesthesia*, **44**, 1277–1287.
92. Moore, J., Murnaghan, G. A. & Lewis, M. A. (1974) A clinical evaluation of the maternal effects of extradural analgesia for labour. *Anaesthesia*, **29**, 537–544.
93. Moir, D. D., Slater, P. J., Thorburn, J., McLaren, R. & Moodie, J. (1976) Extradural analgesia in obstetrics: a controlled trial of carbonated lignocaine and bupivacaine hydrochloride with or without adrenaline. *British Journal of Anaesthesia*, **48**, 129–135.
94. Weaver, J. B., Pearson, J. F. & Rosen, M. (1975) Posture and epidural block in pregnant women at term. *Anaesthesia*, **30**, 752–756.
95. Wallis, K. L., Shnider, S. M., Hicks, J. S. & Spivey, H. T. (1976) Epidural anesthesia in the normotensive pregnant ewe: effects on uterine blood flow and fetal acid-base status. *Anesthesiology*, **44**, 481–487.
96. Ralston, D. H., Shnider, S. M. & de Lorimier, A. A. (1974) Effects of equipotent ephedrine, metaraminol, mephentermine and methoxamine on uterine blood flow in the pregnant ewe. *Anesthesiology*, **40**, 354–370.
97. Buchanan, P. C., Milne, M. K. & Browning, M. C. K. (1973) The effect of continuous epidural blockade on plasma II-hydroxycorticosteroid concentrations in labour. *Journal of Obstetrics and Gynaecology of the British Commonwealth*, **80**, 974–977.
98. Jouppila, R., Hollmen, A., Jouppila, P., Kauppila, A. & Tuimala, R. (1976) The effect of segmental epidural analgesia on maternal ACTH, cortisol and TSH during labour. *Annals of Clinical Research*, **8**, 378–383.
99. Thalme, B., Belfrage, P. & Raabe, N. (1974) Lumbar epidural analgesia in labour 1. Acid-base balance and clinical condition of mother, fetus and newborn child. *Acta obstetrica et gynecologica scandinavica*, **53**, 27–35.
100. Maltau, J. M. (1975) The frequency of fetal bradycardia during selective epidural anesthesia. *Acta obstetrica et gynecologica scandinavica*, **54**, 357–361.
101. Raabe, N. & Belfrage, P. (1976) Epidural analgesia in labour IV. Influence on uterine activity and fetal heart rate. *Acta obstetrica et gynecologica scandinavica*, **55**, 305–310.
102. Scanlon, J. W., Ostheimer, G. W., Lurie, A. O., Brown, W. U., Weiss, J. B. & Alper, M. H. (1976) Neurobehavioral responses and drug concentrations in newborns after maternal epidural anesthesia with bupivacaine. *Anesthesiology*, **45**, 400–405.
103. Scanlon, J. W., Brown, W. U., Weiss, J. B. & Alper, M. H. (1974) Neurobehavioral responses of newborn infants after maternal epidural anesthesia. *Anesthesiology*, **40**, 121–128.
104. Moir, D. D. & Willocks, J. (1967) Management of inco-ordinate uterine action under continuous epidural analgesia. *British Medical Journal*, **3**, 396–400.
105. Schellenberg, J. C. (1977) Uterine activity during lumbar epidural analgesia with bupivacaine. *American Journal of Obstetrics and Gynecology*, **127**, 26–31.
106. Moore, D. C., Mather, L. E., Bridenbaugh, L. D., Balfour, R. I., Lysons, D. F. & Horton, W. G. (1976) Arterial and venous plasma levels of bupivacaine following peripheral nerve blocks. *Current Researches in Anesthesia and Analgesia*, **55**, 763–768.
107. Littlewood, D. G., Scott, D. B., Wilson, J. & Covino, B. G. (1977) Comparative anaesthetic properties of various local anaesthetic agents in extradural block for labour. *British Journal of Anaesthesia*, **49**, 75–79.
108. Bromage, P. R., Datta, S. & Dunford, L. A. (1974) Etidocaine: an evaluation in epidural analgesia for obstetrics. *Canadian Anaesthetists' Society Journal*, **21**, 535–545.
109. Edelist, G. & Perera, E. (1976) Comparison of etidocaine and lidocaine for obstetrical analgesia. *Canadian Anaesthetists' Society Journal*, **23**, 459–464.
110. Lund, P. C., Cwik, J. C., Gannon, R. T. & Vassallo, H. G. (1977) Etidocaine for Caesarean section—effect on mother and baby. *British Journal of Anaesthesia*, **49**, 457–460.
111. Doughty, A. (1975) Lumbar epidural analgesia—the pursuit of perfection. *Anaesthesia*, **30**, 741–751.

112. Moir, D. D., Thorburn, J. & Aitkenhead, A. (1977) Epidural 'top-ups by the clock': a clinical evaluation. *Anaesthesia*, **32**, 824.
113. Caseby, N. G. (1974) Epidural analgesia for the surgical induction of labour. *British Journal of Anaesthesia*, **46**, 747–751.
114. Ducrow, M. (1971) The occurrence of unblocked segments during continuous lumbar epidural analgesia for pain relief in labour. *British Journal of Anaesthesia*, **43**, 1172–1174.
115. Matouskova, A., Dottori, O., Forssman, L. & Victorin, L. (1975) An improved method of epidural analgesia with reduced instrumental delivery rate. *Acta obstetrica et gynecologica scandinavica*, **54**, 231–235.
116. Doughty, A. (1969) Selective epidural analgesia and the forceps rate. *British Journal of Anaesthesia*, **41**, 1058.
117. Hoult, I. J., MacLennan, A. H. & Carrie, L. E. S. (1977) Lumbar epidural analgesia in labour: relation to fetal malposition and instrumental delivery. *British Medical Journal*, **1**, 14–16.
118. Moir, D. D. & Willocks, J. (1968) Epidural analgesia in British obstetrics. *British Journal of Anaesthesia*, **40**, 129–138.
119. O'Driscoll, K. & Stronge, J. M. (1975) Active management of labour and occipito-posterior position. *Australian and New Zealand Journal of Obstetrics and Gynaecology*, **15**, 1–4.
120. Cooper, K., Vella, P. & Browning, D. (1972) Lumbar epidural analgesia given by obstetricians. *Journal of Obstetrics and Gynaecology of the British Commonwealth*, **79**, 144–148.
121. Brown, S. E. & Vass, A. C. R. (1977) An extradural service in a district general hospital. *British Journal of Anaesthesia*, **49**, 243.
122. Taylor, A. B. W., Abukhalil, S. H., El-Guindi, M. M., Tharian, B. & Watkins, J. A. (1977) Lumbar epidural analgesia in labour: a 24-hour service provided by obstetricians. *British Medical Journal*, **2**, 370–372.
123. Soffronoff, E. C., Kaufmann, B. M. & Connaughton, J. F. (1977) Intravascular volume determinations and fetal outcome in hypertensive diseases of pregnancy. *American Journal of Obstetrics and Gynecology*, **127**, 4–9.
124. Cohn, J. N. & Franciosa, J. A. (1977) Vasodilator therapy of cardiac failure (first of two parts). *New England Journal of Medicine*, **297**, 27–31.
125. Cohn, J. N. & Franciosa, J. A. (1977) Vasodilator therapy of cardiac failure (second part). *New England Journal of Medicine*, **297**, 254–258.
126. Weaver, J. B., Pearson, J. F. & Rosen, M. (1977) Response to a Valsalva manoeuvre before and after epidural block. *Anaesthesia*, **32**, 148–153.
127. Brudenell, M. & Chakravarti, S. (1975) Uterine rupture in labour. *British Medical Journal*, **2**, 122–123.
128. Crawford, J. S. (1976) The epidural sieve and MBC (minimal blocking concentration): an hypothesis. *Anaesthesia*, **31**, 1277–1280.
129. Cooper, K. (1972) In *Proceedings of the Symposium on Epidural Analgesia in Obstetrics*. Ed. Doughty, A. p. 82. London: Lewis.
130. Meehan, F. P., Moolgaoker, A. S. & Stallworthy, J. (1972) Vaginal delivery under caudal analgesia after Caesarean section and other major uterine surgery. *British Medical Journal*, **2**, 740–742.
131. Crawford, J. S. (1974) An appraisal of lumbar epidural blockade in patients with a singleton fetus presenting by the breech. *Journal of Obstetrics and Gynaecology of the British Commonwealth*, **81**, 867–872.
132. Bowen-Simpkins, P. & Fergusson, I. L. C. (1974) Lumbar epidural block and the breech presentation. *British Journal of Anaesthesia*, **46**, 420–424.
133. Donnai, P. & Nicholas, A. D. G. (1975) Epidural analgesia, fetal monitoring and the condition of the baby at birth with breech presentation. *Journal of Obstetrics and Gynaecology of the British Commonwealth*, **82**, 360–365.
134. James, F. M., Crawford, J. S., Davies, P. & Naiem, H. (1977) Lumbar epidural analgesia for labor and delivery of twins. *American Journal of Obstetrics and Gynecology*, **127**, 176–180.
135. Weekes, A. R. L., Cheridjian, V. E. & Mwanje, D. K. (1977) Lumbar epidural analgesia in labour in twin pregnancy. *British Medical Journal*, **2**, 730–732.
136. Hicks, J. S., Levinson, G. & Shnider, S. M. (1976) Obstetric anesthesia training centers in the U.S.A.—1975. *Current Researches in Anesthesia and Analgesia*, **55**, 839–845.
137. Moir, D. D. & Thorburn, J. (unpublished data).
138. Marx, G. F., Cosmi, E. V. & Wollman, S. B. (1969) Biochemical status and clinical condition of mother and infant at Caesarean section. *Current Researches in Anesthesia and Analgesia*, **48**, 986–993.
139. Baheti, D. K., Pandit, S. K., Devi, P. K. & Mirakhur, R. K. (1975) Epidural analgesia with left lateral tilt for Caesarean section. *Anaesthesia*, **30**, 396–401.

140. Milne, M. K. & Murray Lawson, J. I. (1973) Epidural analgesia for Caesarean section. *British Journal of Anaesthesia*, **45,** 1206–1210.
141. James, F. M., Crawford, J. S., Hopkinson, R., Davies, P. & Naiem, H. (1977) A comparison of general anesthesia and lumbar epidural analgesia for elective Cesarean section. *Current Researches in Anesthesia and Analgesia*, **56,** 228–235.
142. Palahniuk, R. J., Scatliffe, J., Biehl, D., Wiebe, H. & Sankaran, K. (1977) Maternal and neonatal effects of methoxyflurane, nitrous oxide and lumbar epidural anaesthesia for Caesarean section. *Canadian Anaesthetists' Society Journal*, **24,** 586–596.
143. Magno, R. (1976) Anesthesia for Cesarean Section. Thesis, University of Göteborg.
144. Scudamore, J. H. & Yates, M. J. (1966) Pudendal block—a misnomer? *Lancet*, **1,** 23–24.
145. Wallis, L. S., Shnider, S. M., Palahniuk, R. J. & Spivey, H. T. (1974) An evaluation of acupuncture analgesia in obstetrics. *Anesthesiology*, **41,** 596–601.
146. Persianinov, L. S. (1975) The use of electro-analgesia in obstetrics and gynecology. *Acta obstetrica et gynecologica scandinavica*, **54,** 373–384.

5. General anaesthesia and sedation for dentistry

J. A. Thornton

It is almost 140 years since the first general anaesthetic was administered to render a patient unconscious for a tooth to be painlessly extracted. Today the technique offered to many patients differs very little from that practised over a century ago. Many patients are managed seated upright in the dental chair, and many, despite the increasing availability of adjuvants, are subjected to hypoxic mixtures of nitrous oxide and oxygen. It can be fairly said that outpatient dental general anaesthetic practice is at the cross-roads. The declining numbers of general anaesthetics administered in dental schools has led to inevitable deficiencies in the training and experience of dental undergraduates in the art of dental anaesthesia. The lack of adequate instruction in basic medicine also increases the difficulties confronting the dental practitioner in selecting those patients at risk for outpatient general anaesthesia. The training of medical graduates in the art of dental anaesthesia is also unsatisfactory. Despite the efforts of the Faculty of Anaesthetists of the Royal College of Surgeons of England to include experience in outpatient dental anaesthesia as a part of the General Professional Training of the anaesthetist there is evidence that not all trainees are given this opportunity. The increasingly widespread use of controlled inhalational and intravenous methods of sedation, and the greater use of antibiotics, have led undoubtedly to a significant reduction in the number of general anaesthetics administered for dental purposes. Nevertheless the United Kingdom continues to stand out as a country where outpatient general anaesthesia is practised on a large scale, whereas in many other countries this practice has largely been abandoned. With the development of more sophisticated methods of general anaesthesia the suitability of the average dental surgery for this purpose is also being questioned.

INCIDENCE OF GENERAL ANAESTHESIA FOR DENTAL TREATMENT

Accurate estimates of the number of general anaesthetics administered for dental purposes are not readily available. However, the numbers of general anaesthetics administered for dental surgery in England and Wales within the National Health Service are published by the Dental Estimates Board, and the School Dental Service. Included in these numbers there may be an indeterminate proportion of patients who have received intravenous and inhalational sedative techniques. The number of general anaesthetics administered in the private sector is not known. There is however good evidence that the number of general anaesthetics administered per annum is diminishing[1] (Table 5.1). Between the years 1963 and 1973 the number of general anaesthetics administered within the aegis of the

NHS Dental Estimates Board fell by 18 per cent whilst the number of treatment courses rose by 54 per cent. A similar trend can be detected in the available figures for the School Dental Service where the number of general anaesthetics fell by 32 per cent between 1960 and 1970 and the attendances rose by 14 per cent. The decline in general anaesthesia for dental outpatients may be related in part to the unsatisfactory remuneration available from the Department of Health and Social Security. A reliable estimate for the number of general dental anaesthetics administered to outpatients in the public and private sectors in England and Wales during 1976 is in the region of 1.5 million.[2]

Table 5.1a General Dental Service, England and Wales

| | General anaesthetics estimates | | | |
	Total	Operator-administered	% Operator administered	All treatment courses
1963	1 439 330	374 830	26	16 064 733
1964	1 387 380	346 640	25	17 067 070
1965	1 322 980	319 240	24	17 669 795
1966	1 227 890	279 400	23	18 429 910
1967	1 287 520	265 640	21	19 410 683
1968	1 292 090	224 780	17	20 065 772
1969	1 238 570	200 620	16	20 225 583
1970	1 225 690	178 000	15	20 747 678
1971	1 217 950	164 930	14	22 038 056
1972	1 226 520	148 280	12	23 418 337
1973	1 176 820	132 970	11	24 756 190
1963–1973	− 18%	− 65%		+ 54%

Table 5.1b School Dental Service, England and Wales

	Attendances for treatment	General anaesthetics given	% of attendances with general anaesthetics
1960	3 125 428	530 700	17
1965	3 260 550	405 302	12
1970	3 563 411	358 382	10
1960–1970	+ 14%	− 32%	

MORTALITY AND MORBIDITY ASSOCIATED WITH DENTAL ANAESTHESIA

The most readily obtainable evidence on deaths associated with dental anaesthesia comes from the Office of Population Censuses and Surveys (Table 5.2). Since 1963 the number of deaths per annum in England and Wales has varied between 4 and 12. Between 1970 and 1976 the number has been between 7 and 12. Despite the dramatic decline in the number of general anaesthetics given for outpatient dental purposes over these years the death rate has increased and can give just cause for anxiety. Many factors may account for this increase in mortality rate. The increased use of potent adjuvants such as the intravenous agents and halothane and the decline in the training and experience of both medical and dental anaesthetists may account for a number of these deaths.

Posture

In 1957 Bourne[3] first drew attention to the vulnerability of the brain should cerebral perfusion fall with the patient seated upright in the traditional position in the dental chair. He suggested that fainting might occur and pass unnoticed during induction of anaesthesia. Continuous intra-arterial recordings of blood pressure in dental patients gave weight to his suggestion.

The possibility of cerebral hypoxia resulting from poor perfusion of the brain in the patients seated upright has persuaded many that the routine adoption of the horizontal posture would minimise such effects. However, the upright posture carries with it relative ease of access to the dentition and the claim, by some, that airway obstruction is less likely than in the horizontal posture. The

Table 5.2 Mortality in general anaesthesia for dental outpatients. Deaths associated with dental anaesthesia 1963–1976 England and Wales. Supplied by the Office of Population Censuses and Surveys.

	Hospital	Place of treatment		Not known	Total
		Surgery			
		General anaesthesia	Local analgesia		
1963	5	6	–	–	11
1964	4	4	–	–	8
1965	0	2	1	1	4
1966	2	5	1	1	9
1967	2	4	–	–	6
1968	4	5	1	–	10
1969	–	–	–	–	6
1970	5	4	–	3	12
1971	5	7	–	1	12
1972	7	2	1	–	10
1973	2	3	–	2	7
1974	4	6	–	2	12
1975	–	3	1	3	7
1976	1	6	1	1	9

chances of regurgitation and inhalation of stomach contents would appear to be greater in the horizontal posture particularly in the presence of respiratory obstruction and/or hiatus hernia. Coplans and Curson[4] reporting on an analysis of deaths noted that in 1974 a higher proportion of patients dying during outpatient dental anaesthesia had received their anaesthetics whilst lying in the horizontal posture. They suggested that this vindicated Tomlin's[5] comment that posture is seldom if ever causally related to the anaesthetic death and that the 1974 data indicated a conversion of dental anaesthetists to the use of the supine position for their patients.

Recently attention has been paid to the possibility of marked lability of the cardiovascular system in the dental outpatient and is has been suggested that this may account for a number of deaths. It is well recognised that a high degree of autonomic sympathetic hyperactivity prevails in the dental patient and is associated with raised plasma adrenaline concentrations.[6,7]

This usually manifests itself as tachycardia[6-15] with heart rates up to 200 beats per minute being reported. Dry mouth, vasoconstriction, sweating, nausea and hyperventilation are also frequently present and are further evidence of autonomic overactivity. However, it has not been fully appreciated that against this background of increased sympathetic activity there may be increased para-sympathetic tone.[7] Fainting, associated with increased vagal activity, has long been recognised accompanying exposure of subjects to stressful situations such as the sight of blood, instruments, and the general environment of the dental surgery,[17] but has usually been thought to be accompanied by bradycardia. Taggart and his colleagues[7] have demonstrated mean heart rates of 80–90 b.p.m. before induction of anaesthesia, and have claimed that these rates are lower than would be expected in other stressful situations (140–200 b.p.m.) suggesting that, despite elevation of plasma catecholamine levels, a degree of parasympathetic overactivity is also present. A further fall in heart rate to near normal or tranquil levels, within a minute of injection of local analgesic solution and drilling, during the height of an emotional challenge in the face of increasing anxiety and a rising plasma catecholamine level, suggests intense parasympathetic activity overriding greatly enhanced sympathetic activity. They found the heart rates to be significantly lower during the procedure in subjects who had received the β-adrenergic blocking agent oxprenolol when compared with a placebo, but as the difference was small strong vagal activity was likely.

This emotionally produced parasympathetic activity may arise in cortical autonomic areas and from stimulation of the anterior cyngulate gyrus.[18] The importance of having a tranquil patient cannot be overstressed and is of particular importance in reducing the incidence of ventricular fibrillation in patients with acute myocardial infarction presumably because of reduced sympathetic activity.[19] Although preoperative sedation by the oral route will do much to reduce patient anxiety it carries the disadvantage of prolonging recovery of street fitness after operation. Much can be done however by creating a tranquil environment, careful and sympathetic handling of the patient, and by keeping instruments out of sight. Drummond-Jackson[20] pioneered the introduction of controlled sedation by the intravenous route by introducing the 'minimal incremental technique' in 1965, and by doing so stimulated an awareness by the dental surgeon of the patient's predicament (see page 126). It is of interest to note that methohexitone, the agent employed by Drummond-Jackson, was associated with marked tachycardia.[21-25] With the loss of consciousness associated with induction of anaesthesia parasympathetic overactivity wanes and sympathetic tone tends to predominate. This high sympathetic tone is possibly the cause of the high incidence of dysrhythmias such as are associated with dental surgery under general anaesthesia.[8-15,26-44] Afferent impulses from the trigeminal nerve may stimulate sympathetic nerve centres in the medulla with the result that impulses reach the cardiac plexus via sympathetic tracts in the spinal cord.

This adrenergic stimulation increases the automaticity of pacemaker cells, changes conduction velocity, and predisposes to the development of ectopic rhythms. The presence of halothane anaesthesia may aggravate further this disturbance in heart rhythm by sensitising the heart to the action of adrenaline.[42,43] Ryder,[10] reviewing the findings of his own and other workers, found an incidence of dysrhythmias varying between 9 and 50 per cent. Ryder and Townsend[44] found that dysrhythmias occurred most frequently with halothane and trichlor-ethylene and significantly less frequently with divinylether and methoxyflurane and did not occur with methohexitone. The administration of atropine intra-venously before induction of anaesthesia increased the incidence of these dysrhythmias.[12,13,40,42] However, the intramuscular administration of atropine may be effective in preventing dysrhythmias.[40] The findings of Long and his colleagues[45a] who noted a decrease in the incidence of dysrhythmias in patients under cyclopropane anaesthesia following the intravenous administration of droperidol, prompted Bradshaw[40] to investigate the use of this drug as an anti-dysrhythmic agent during dental anaesthesia. The intravenous administration of 0.1 mg/kg droperidol prior to surgery failed to reduce the incidence of dysrhythmias. Rollason and Hall[11] found that the β-adrenergic blocking agent, practolol was effective in both the prevention and the treatment of these dysrhythmias, although they suggested that its routine use should await results of haemodynamic studies. Ryder and his colleagues[12] also found a worthwhile effect with practolol but not with atropine.

Local infiltration of lignocaine without adrenaline prior to extraction under general anaesthesia is effective in preventing dysrhythmias[45b] but Kaufman[9] found that this was only for operations on the upper and not the lower jaw. Patients receiving tricylic antidepressant drugs are at particular risk in relation to dental surgery.[46] Local analgesia with adrenaline and other vasoconstrictors may cause severe hypertension and the incidence of cardiac dysrhythmias is significantly increased in patients on this group of drugs when receiving halothane anaesthesia for exodontia. Alexander[47] has demonstrated that Althesin appears to protect against dysrhythmias.

The lability in heart rate and rhythm probably has no great importance in normal myocardial tissue but in subjects with ischaemic heart disease and myocarditis the consequences may be severe. This is a clear example where the pre-operative assessment can be of particular value in eliminating patients thought to be at risk. Lability of the blood pressure during general anaesthesia for exodontia in patients seated upright receiving nitrous oxide: oxygen 70:30 with halothane 1.5 per cent has also been demonstrated[15] but none of the changes could be regarded as of clinical relevance in the normal subject. A number of instances have been reported of patients dying under general anaesthesia where autopsy has subsequently demonstrated a cardio-myopathy.[48] Although difficult to detect clinically, anaesthetists should always be on the look out for this con-dition. Cardio-respiratory arrest is a real hazard of diabetic autonomic neuro-pathy[49] and is a further reason why diabetic patients should not receive out-patient general anaesthetics, in addition to the fact that because of starvation, drug therapy is sometimes difficult to control.

Hypoxia

Tomlin[5] has drawn attention to the very real difficulties in determining the true cause of death. Reporting an analysis of 46 out of 48 dental anaesthetic deaths occurring in England and Wales over a 6-year period he pointed out that 29 cases arose in dental surgery practice outside hospital. In these cases there was a strong suggestion that hypoxia was the most common single cause of death.

Pulmonary oedema was also a feature in a number of deaths and the possibility that this might be due to cardiac dysrhythmias, tachycardia and failure of the heart was considered. A particular feature was the number of deaths that occurred during the recovery period. Commenting on the matter of posture Tomlin[5] advises that . . . 'our prime concern should be to prevent hypoxia, and that the anaesthetist should adopt the technique that in his hands offers the best protection against this hazard, rather than adopting a technique which minimizes the hazard of cerebral hypo-perfusion at the risk of increasing the hazard of hypoxia'. For many years anaesthetists have relied upon the deliberate restriction of oxygen in the inspired mixture to facilitate the induction and maintenance of general anaesthesia with nitrous oxide. Vickers and Pask[50] have shown very clearly that there is no indication to administer less than 20 per cent oxygen when using nitrous oxide.

Even with the increasing use of adjuvants such as halothane, restriction of oxygen concentration is still practised[51] and this combination of hypoxia and halothane anaesthesia may account for some of the cardiac deaths associated with dental anaesthesia. In 1967 Nainby-Luxmore[52] drew attention to the inadequate performance of certain intermittent flow demand-type machines and more recently Hutchinson has made a similar study.[53] Some of the concentrations of oxygen delivered by these machines are particularly inaccurate when the patient is hyperventilating—a common occurrence during induction of anaesthesia. In certain instances the machines were found to deliver 100 per cent nitrous oxide despite the fact that the dial was set for mixtures containing oxygen. The BOC Walton Mark V and Cyprane AE machines proved to be the most reliable in terms of accuracy of performance. These two machines also incorporate oxygen failure warning devices and automatic cutouts permitting the entrainment of air should there be a failure of supply of one of the gases. More recently continuous flow machines have been introduced for dental anaesthetic purposes, and whilst permitting the visualisation of gas flows, they have however the disadvantage that precise and rapid control of the inspired mixture is not possible on a breath-by-breath basis. Holden[54] and Neill[55] have considered the place of these machines in dental anaesthetic practice. Others[56,57] have advocated the use of pre-mixed nitrous oxide:oxygen (Entonox). Airway obstruction has long been recognised as one of the greatest hazards of general anaesthesia and every care is taken in the selection of patients to ensure that airway integrity is maintained. Selection of patients prior to anaesthesia will eliminate those who are particularly at risk e.g. Ludwig's angina and glottic oedema. However, a degree of airway obstruction is almost inevitable during exodontia and can be minimised by careful attention to packing and cooperation between the dental surgeon and the anaesthetist.[58] Nevertheless, respiratory obstruction can occur and pass unnoticed by the anaesthetist as evidenced by a study of 50 patients, seated upright in the dental chair receiving 30 per cent oxygen with nitrous oxide and halothane. Six patients had falls in oxygen saturation of more than 3 per cent.[15] As the patients were breathing 30 per cent oxygen, gross reduction of alveolar ventilation must have occurred to have produced such a fall in oxygen saturation. When the recording technician alerted the anaesthetist of this fall in oxygen saturation re-adjustment of the jaw caused the oxygen saturation to rise to normal levels.

ANAESTHESIA FOR DENTAL EXTRACTION

Many methods are available for inducing and maintaining general anaesthesia for exodontia.[59] In general, techniques which rely solely on an intravenous method are difficult to use particularly in respect of achieving an even level of anaesthesia.[60] Surgical stimulation may provoke patient movement which calls for a further increment which itself may lead to respiratory depression in the absence of a surgical stimulus. Involuntary movements are particularly associated with the use of methohexitone and the newly introduced short acting agent etomidate (q.v.).

Cadle et al[61] have employed intermittent propanidid successfully for exodontia, whilst others[62,63] have used Althesin. Many anaesthetists employ an intravenous induction particularly in the adult and use nitrous oxide with or without halothane for maintenance. Others use an inhalational technique entirely,[64] finding nitrous oxide-oxygen-halothane a suitable combination. Methoxyflurane[65-68] and trichlorethylene[69] have been employed but carry the disadvantage of delayed recovery. The recently introduced halogenated ether, enflurane (Ethrane) which has a blood/gas solubility coefficient of 1.7 is ideally suited for outpatient general anaesthesia. Young[70] has found methohexitone followed by nitrous oxide-oxygen more suitable than propanidid or methohexitone alone, or propanidid followed by nitrous oxide-oxygen or nitrous oxide-oxygen-halothane.

Tracheal intubation

This is indicated when it is likely that surgery is to be prolonged, such as is possible with detailed conservation work, and anticipated difficulty with exodontia or because airway control is likely to be troublesome. A few anaesthetists employ endotracheal intubation routinely for outpatient dental anaesthesia even if the surgical procedure is relatively trivial. Endotracheal intubation is not without risk particularly in the hands of the inexperienced. Glottic oedema may follow and be a particular problem in the young. The use of suxamethonium to facilitate intubation can lead to muscle pains which can be of considerable severity in the ambulant patient.

MORBIDITY FOLLOWING DENTAL EXTRACTION

A number of studies have been carried out to assess the morbidity associated with exodontia. Muir and his colleagues[71] showed little difference in morbidity between those patients having general anaesthesia and those having local analgesia for their extractions. As might be expected the incidence of vomiting, giddiness and sleepiness on the day of operation were all significantly higher in those patients who have a general anaesthetic. Seventeen years before, Bishop and Potts[72] reported a 46 per cent incidence of cyanosis in their patients. This presumably because anaesthesia in 66 per cent of their patients was achieved by using nitrous oxide and oxygen alone. However, Muir et al[71] using nitrous oxide, oxygen, and intravenous adjuvants such as methohexitone, or inhalational agents such as halothane, witnessed no cyanosis in the 300 patients studied under general anaesthesia.

Fits

Jactitations are happily rarely witnessed today but were a frequent phenomenon when deliberate restriction of oxygen was employed to enhance the production of the anaesthetic state. Fits however are a very real hazard associated with the administration of methohexitone to patients with an epileptiform diathesis.[21,72,73] Convulsions have also been reported in association with propanidid,[74] Althesin[75] and ketamine[76] in subjects with a history of epilepsy.

Anaphylactoid reactions

The increasing use of intravenous induction agents such as propanidid and Althesin which are rapidly eliminated from the body, has been associated with a greater awareness of adverse reactions with these agents.[77-81] These reactions may vary from mild skin flushing to gross and widespread erythema, urticaria with profound cardiovascular collapse, and sometimes bronchospasm. The incidence of these reactions has been variously reported, with as low a frequency as 1 in 11 000 to 1 in 19 000[79] on the one hand, to 1 in 900 on the other.[80,81] The severity of such reactions is such that full resuscitation facilities together with the ability to rapidly infuse crystalloid solutions must be readily available in the dental surgery.

Other adverse reactions

Rarely angioneurotic oedema may arise in relation to the use of local analgesic agents.[82,83] Malignant hyperthermia, another rare condition, is becoming increasingly recognised as requiring prompt and efficient management. Cardiovascular collapse may arise from myocardial infarction and from adrenal cortical insufficiency in subjects who have been receiving steroid therapy within two months of anaesthesia and surgery.[84]

Return of street fitness

The increasing use of intravenous induction and sedative agents, some of which are relatively slowly eliminated from the body raises very real post anaesthetic problems for the safety of the patient and the public at large. Methohexitone, an agent commonly employed in dental outpatient anaesthetics has been shown to be relatively slowly eliminated from the body and to produce a recurrent sleep pattern on the electroencephalograph in the 24 hours following administration.[85] Propanidid[61] and Althesin,[63] being more rapidly broken down in the body, present less of a problem. Certain other intravenous agents such as benzodiazepines, and in particular diazepam, which is commonly employed for controlled intravenous sedation (*vide infra*), are slowly eliminated from the body. Indeed reappearance of active hypnotic metabolites may occur up to 8 hours following its administration and cause sleepiness in the patient.[86-88]

Many tests of recovery from anaesthesia have been devised to assess differing modalitites of function of the central nervous system.[89] Reliance should not be placed upon these tests as indicators of recovery to 'street-fitness'. As a general rule patients should be accompanied home by a responsible adult and not permitted to indulge in any activity which is potentially harmful to themselves or the public at large for 24 hours.

SURGERY FACILITIES

Perks[90] has drawn attention to the emergencies that may possibly arise in the dental surgery. These may include cardiovascular collapse of varying aetiology, grand mal, hypoglycaemia, angioneurotic oedema, acute respiratory obstruction, and reactions to drugs such as may occur when adrenaline is administered to a patient on tricyclic antidepressants. The surgery must be equipped to handle all these emergencies in an efficient and effective manner. The Standing Dental Advisory Committee for the Central Services Council, the Secretary of State for Social Services and the Secretary of State for Wales have stated that 'The safety of the patient demands that any surgery in which general anaesthetics are administered must be adequately equipped for dealing with emergencies'.[91] However, in the United Kingdom there is at present no requirement for either inspection of premises to ensure adequate anaesthetic, recovery and resuscitation facilities nor for the assessment of the training and experience of the dental anaesthetists.

In Canada[92,93] and certain parts of the USA[94,95] requirements are rigid and professional liability insurers require a relatively high premium for those administering general anaesthetics in the 'dental office' compared with those offering conscious sedation techniques. Young[96] in a survey of 300 dental surgeons found that 44 occurrences of cardiac arrest in patients or other persons had been experienced by them during their professional life time. Of these 44 cases of cardiac arrest 50 per cent recovered following resuscitation. None would doubt the necessity of training all dental surgeons in the principles of cardiopulmonary resuscitation. The problem arises as to what procedures are appropriate for a person, who is not medically qualified, and who does not have continuing day-to-day experience in such procedures as tracheal intubation and the evaluation of the electrocardiograph. A Report of a Working Party into Training in Dental Anaesthesia[97] suggested that the dental surgeon and his team of dental surgery assistants should be fully acquainted with the routine of cardiopulmonary resuscitation. The dental chair should be capable of being placed in the horizontal position even when there is a power failure. Ideally stores of oxygen should be such that flows of oxygen up to 10 litres/minute can be maintained for at least one hour.[90] All practices should establish close links with the local hospital resuscitation teams and the ambulance service, and access to the premises should permit the rapid removal to hospital of a patient undergoing resuscitation.

The provision of other facilities is less easy to be dogmatic about. In isolated parts of the country it could be argued that general anaesthesia should not be undertaken unless the anaesthetist is proficient in tracheal intubation, the use of the ECG and defibrillator. Full cover for all emergencies will require an experienced anaesthetist capable of setting up an intravenous infusion (angioneurotic oedema), using an ECG and defibrillator (cardiac arrest), carrying out tracheal intubation and even tracheostomy (respiratory obstruction). Provision of drugs should include all those likely to be required in the emergency situations likely to arise. Equipment should include laryngoscopes, tracheal tubes, airways, masks, and Air-Viva or Ambu-type resuscitation bags. Many would feel that general anaesthesia for dental surgery should now only take place in surgeries or health centres where adequate provision of resuscitation facilities are available. Some would even say that the present training of dental surgeons falls far short of what can be regarded as necessary for safe practice.

WHO IS THE DENTAL ANAESTHETIST OF THE FUTURE?[98]

Such is the concern about the inadequacies of training of dental anaesthetists that several working parties have addressed themselves to this problem over recent years.[97,99–101] All have recognised these deficiencies and have attempted to suggest ways of correcting them.

Windeyer and his colleagues[100] proposed that at least six months' attachment to anaesthetic departments should constitute part of the anaesthetist's training. Others[101,102] have suggested a higher qualification in dental anaesthesia. The recent report of the joint working party of the Faculties of Dental Surgery and Anaesthetists of the Royal College of Surgeons of England, the British Dental Association and the Association of Anaesthetists of Great Britain and Ireland, has suggested a recognised list of Dental Anaesthetists, entry to the list requiring the achievement of certain academic standards.[97] Experience of periods of attachment to anaesthetic departments has been varied. In Cardiff, Thompson[103] reports that such a scheme, though not intended to do so, has tended to discourage dental practitioners from subsequently practising general anaesthesia, whereas, in Manchester, Young[104] has reported to the contrary. With changes in attitudes within dental schools towards the teaching of dental undergraduates, and more critical selection of patients, it is likely that the number of patients presenting for general anaesthesia will further decline. This trend will be facilitated by the increasing use of antibiotics and the development of methods of controlled sedation.

Operator/Anaesthetist

The practice of the single operator/anaesthetist has been widely condemned. In 1975 a working party[1] stated very clearly that only under very exceptional circumstances could such practice be condoned.

The role of the dental surgeon in relation to controlled sedation is however rather different. If the dental surgeon and his team are adequately trained in the management of the unconscious subject and in resuscitation procedures, and his surgery is adequately equipped, it would seem reasonable for him to administer a drug with a wide margin of safety, 'titrating' the dosage to produce adequate sedation without loss of consciousness. Provided that verbal contact is maintained throughout the dental treatment, respiratory obstruction is unlikely to occur.

CONTROLLED SEDATION

The introduction of the 'minimal increment technique', using methohexitone, by Drummond-Jackson in 1965 helped to focus attention on the plight of the patient presenting for dental treatment. All patients have some degree of anxiety and in some this develops to a phobia. In order to ensure treatment of these patients' dental caries it may be necessary to resort to general anaesthesia. Most patients will respond by sympathetic understanding and careful handling. Whilst others require the administration of various drugs. Numerous techniques have been devised:

1. Minimal increment technique using intravenous methohexitone[20,23,24]
2. Diazepam[105-112]
3. Pethidine-pentobarbitone-hyoscine[113]
4. Diazepam-pentazocine[114,115]
5. Diazepam-methohexitone[116]
6. Alphaprodine-hydroxyzine-atropine-methohexitone[117]
7. Secobarbitone-pethidine-methohexitone[118]
8. Hydroxyzine-pethidine[119]
9. Alphaprodine-levallorphan-promethazine[120]
10. Methohexitone drip[120]
11. Neuroleptanalgesia[120]
12. Pentobarbitone-pethidine[120]
13. Pentazocine-cyclizine-atropine-methohexitone or propanidid[121]
14. Ketamine[120]
15. Nitrous oxide[122-126]
16. Methoxyflurane[125]
17. Flunitrazepam[127,128]
18. Althesin[129]
19. Propanidid[130]

Minimal increment technique[20]

This technique employs the methylated oxybarbiturate, methohexitone. It should be remembered that in common with all barbiturates there is a tendency' to lower the pain threshold with this drug and to increase the patients perception of pain. The high incidence of excitatory phenomena with this agent is another factor which makes sedation difficult to achieve. It is perhaps unfortunate that this drug should have been selected to develop a technique of controlled sedation, for agents subsequently introduced onto the market proved more suitable

Drummond-Jackson claimed that it was possible to achieve a state of 'ultra-light' anaesthesia, which was associated with amnesia, and lack of response to painful stimuli, without encroaching upon surgical anaesthesia with its inevitable association of loss of airway control. Two teams of research workers attempted to follow the method enunciated by Drummond-Jackson.[23,24] These workers found that it was extremely difficult to achieve this so-called ultra-light state without, from time to time, producing surgical anaesthesia. A significant incidence of hypoxaemia associated with loss of airway control was noted. It was also demonstrated that the laryngeal reflex was obtunded with the danger of inhalation of foreign material. Excitatory phenomena were frequent and a number of attacks of grand mal were reported. Tachycardia appeared to be a particular feature associated with the intravenous administration of methohexitone. Though a courageous attempt to control patient anxiety, it carried an unacceptable risk for the patient, particularly in the hands of the two research teams.[23-24]

Jørgensen technique[113]

This technique introduced by Professor Niels Jørgensen of Loma Linda University School of Dentistry in 1946 was a forerunner to the technique of minimal incremental methohexitone described by Drummond-Jackson. The technique involves the intravenous injection of 10 mg of pentobarbitone every thirty seconds until the patient seems relaxed and at ease (base-line dose).

Doses of 100 mg are seldom exceeded. As soon as the patient reports that he feels sleepy the injection is stopped and thirty seconds later 10 to 20 per cent of the base line dose is then injected. Another syringe containing pethidine 25 mg and hyoscine 0.32 mg diluted to 5 ml is then attached to the needle. A patient who requires 100 mg or more of pentobarbitone is given 25 mg of pethidine and correspondingly less if the patient requires less than 100 mg pentobarbitone. Amongst the disadvantages of this technique are the long induction time and exceedingly long recovery time. Many of the patients fall asleep and under these circumstances control of the airway cannot be guaranteed.

Diazepam[105–112]

The introduction of the benzodiazepine diazepam in 1968 was soon followed by its use in dentistry.[105–107] A dose of 0.3 mg/kg will produce anxiolysis in a high proportion of subjects, a number of whom will be rendered unconscious. Verrill[107] attempted to 'titrate' the degree of sedation by using the dropping of the eyelid to guide him to the 'end-point'. The added bonus associated with the intravenous administration of diazepam is the marked anterograde amnesia which is initially dense and tails off until at 30 minutes after injection is almost negligible.[131–133] It has been shown that the laryngeal reflex may be impaired when diazepam is administered intravenously[110] and loss of consciousness may be accompanied by loss of control of the airway and respiratory obstruction.[112]

Diazepam does not lower the pain threshold and there is some evidence that it may make the subject less sensitive to pain as the minimal alveolar concentration of halothane is reduced by 35 per cent.[134] However, other studies of individuals subjected to painful stimuli, suggest that a variable response may occur.[135] The effects on the respiratory system suggest that intravenous diazepam produces a dose dependent respiratory depression,[136–139] except in subjects with respiratory disorders where an impairment of the patient's ventilatory response to carbon dioxide challenge has been shown.[140] There have also been a number of reports of prolonged apnoea following the rapid administration of the drug, particularly in elderly patients.[141–144] In a dose of 0.2 mg/kg the effects on the cardiovascular system appear to be minimal[110,145] although Jenkinson et al[145] have shown a slight fall in cardiac output and stroke volume. Mild tachycardia is a feature of the intravenous administration of diazepam[110,112,145] and is thought to be due to central vagal inhibition.[146] Other workers have demonstrated coronary arterial vasodilatation,[147–150] Ikram and his colleagues[149] noting a 23 per cent increase in coronary blood flow in normal subjects and an increase of 73 per cent in patients with coronary arterial disease. Recovery of street fitness following intravenous diazepam is slow[112] and a recurrence of sleepiness some 6–8 hours after intravenous administration[151,153] has been associated with the reappearance of diazepam and its active metabolite desmethyl-diazepine[87] in the blood.

It has been suggested[151,152] that this results from an intra-hepatic circulation of diazepam but subsequent work has cast doubt on this possibility.[153,154] Although tiredness may remain for up to 24 hours after injection[108] Kortilla and Linnoila[88] have recommended that the subject should not indulge in any potentially harmful activity for at least 10 hours after its intravenous administration. Adiposity,[155] and liver disease[156] are other factors which may delay recovery from diazepam sedation. The recovery in aged patients appears to be similar to that in younger age groups.[156] Care must be taken to avoid accidental intra-arterial injection as there have been several reports indicating that the preparations of diazepam currently available may cause thrombosis and gangrene.[157] One of the greatest problems associated with the intravenous administration of diazepam is the almost prohibitive incidence of thrombophlebitis, even when the drug is injected into a large vein with a good blood flow.[158] Attempts have been made to produce other formulations in order to avoid the use of the two commonly employed solvents, 1 per cent propylene glycol and 50 per cent benzyl alcohol which are thought likely to cause the thrombophlebitis.[159] Burton and his colleagues[160] have suggested the use of Cremophor EL and they and Siebke et al[161] have claimed that the incidence of thrombophlebitis is negligible when using this latter preparation. Others[162,163] have advocated the use of oily emulsions and further dilution in intra-lipid.[163]

There is no doubt that the introduction of intravenous diazepam into conservative dentistry has brought relief of anxiety to many dental patients, proving valuable in anxious children.[164] However, the subject in whom sedation and anxiolysis are particularly required is the nervous teenager, amongst whom there is a small but significant proportion who do not respond and remain uncooperative.[165] MacDonald[166] and Healy et al[109] have found diazepam particularly useful in the handicapped. MacDonald[166] had good conditions in 82 per cent of spastics and 64 per cent of mentally retarded patients. The use of diazepam and methohexitone together in the same subject[167,168,169] is gaining in popularity. However Alexander[170] draws attention to the very real dangers of such a drug combination when the patient is breathing air. He found arterial oxygen tensions between 31 and 65 mmHg (4 and 8.5 kPa) indicating very severe hypoxaemia, even though some subjects were reacting to the painful stimulus of arterial puncture a situation which perhaps is similar to that pertaining during the preparation of a cavity. Patient awareness and movement does not, therefore, necessarily ensure that bodily functions are normal, a factor which is often forgotten by some dental practitioners. Others have suggested the combination of diazepam with potent narcotic analgesics such as pentazocine.[114-116,171] Clearly the injudicious administration of this drug combination may lead to loss of respiratory control and resulting hypoxaemia[172-176] and, for this reason, the two drugs should be given both slowly and separately, and verbal contact maintained throughout the procedure.

Finally it should be remembered that oral administration of diazepam can be useful in preparing a patient for dental treatment.[177-180] However general availability of diazepam should give rise to concern for not only have drug dependence and withdrawal symptoms been reported,[181] but there is also some evidence that maternal intake in the early stage of pregnancy may give rise to fetal abnormalities such as cleft palate.[182]

Flunitrazepam[127,128,158,183]

This benzodiazepine is miscible with water and is approximately ten times more potent than diazepam. Like diazepam anterograde amnesia follows the intravenous injection.[127,128,183] Conditions are similar to those produced by diazepam[128] but recovery of street fitness is said to take somewhat longer.[88] A dose of 0.014 mg/kg is recommended,[28] producing anxiolysis, sedation and amnesia without loss of consciousness.

Other intravenous techniques

Neuroleptanalgesia,[120] intermittent Althesin,[129] propanidid,[130] and ketamine[120] have all been employed with varying degrees of success. All require the presence of a trained anaesthetist in addition to the dental surgeon. The use of local analgesia in conjunction with these methods usually results in less intravenous agent being required.

However, loss of verbal contact can occur and can be associated with loss of airway control. Neuroleptanalgesia carries the problem of prolonged recovery, however, the availability of the narcotic antagonist naloxone, may permit modification of this technique for outpatient use. Ketamine[120] has also been employed, but it should be remembered that the laryngeal reflex can be depressed and inhalation of foreign material can take place. Respiratory obstruction can also occur during the dental procedure. The high incidence of dreams and the prolonged recovery make this agent unsuitable for use in outpatient dentistry unless recovery facilities are available which permit a quiet environment for several hours after use.

Relative analgesia[122-126]

Klock[123] and Tom[124] and more recently Langa[122] have employed nitrous oxide to produce sedation, analgesia, and amnesia. By employing relatively low concentrations of nitrous oxide Langa has been able to produce suitable conditions for outpatient dentistry whilst maintaining patient cooperation. The widespread application of relative analgesia undoubtedly reduces the need for general anaesthesia and intravenous sedation techniques. Relative analgesia can be administered by the dentist whilst at the same time maintaining patient cooperation.

The dental surgeon should, however, be trained to select patients on the basis of their medical history, to be capable of managing the unconscious patient and be able to carry out resuscitation when necessary. Verbal contact must be maintained throughout the time relative analgesia is being used.

Criteria for controlled sedation

In selecting a technique of controlled sedation certain basic requirements are necessary. The method must produce reliable sedation without loss of consciousness or patient cooperation. Amnesia is an added bonus. Conditions for dental surgery must be satisfactory and involuntary movement of the tongue, face and limbs must not occur. There must, at all times, be verbal contact between the patient and the dental surgeon. Under these circumstances the airway is unlikely to become obstructed. There must be minimal cardiovascular or respiratory depression. Recovery to street fitness must be rapid with preferably no side effects such as thrombophlebitis. Ideally the technique should have such a margin of safety as to permit the operator to induce and maintain the sedation. Of the intravenous techniques available, flunitrazepam, which appears in many ways to be similar to diazepam, but has the advantages that the incidence of thrombophlebitis is less, would appear to be the agent currently most suitable.

The combination of drugs is not without increased risk for the patient. Inhalational sedation with nitrous oxide possibly offers the greatest safety margin.

THE FUTURE

Greater emphasis should be placed at undergraduate level on teaching basic medicine and inculcating the discipline of patient selection, reserving for general anaesthesia only those patients who cannot be adequately treated under local analgesia with, or without, sedation. Dental undergraduate training should confine itself to management of the unconscious subject and resuscitation, and teaching methods of sedation. Under these circumstances the number of patients requiring general anaesthesia will diminish and such numbers will possibly be managed by medically qualified anaesthetists, and other interested dentists who have undergone special postgraduate training in dental anaesthesia.[184] Patients requiring general anaesthesia should be treated in premises where all the facilities for general anaesthesia and resuscitation are adequate and staff are properly trained for this work. The role of the dental surgeon in future is likely to develop around controlled sedation techniques. There will be continuing need for research into effective and safe means of controlled sedation.

REFERENCES

1. Report to Council of Working Party on the Operator/Anaesthetist in Dentistry (1975) British Dental Association. *British Dental Journal*, **138**, 355.
2. Dinsdale, R. C. W. & Dixon, R. A. (1978) Anaesthetic services to dental patients—England and Wales 1976. *British Dental Journal*, **144**, 271–279.
3. Bourne, J. G. (1957) Fainting and cerebral damage: a danger in patient kept upright during dental gas anaesthesia and after surgical operations. *Lancet*, **ii**, 499.
4. Coplans, M. P. & Curson, I. (1976) The effect of posture on dental anaesthetic mortality. *British Dental Journal*, **141**, 255.
5. Tomlin, P. J. (1974) Death in outpatient dental anaesthetic practice. *Anaesthesia*, **29**, 551–570.
6. Edmonson, H. D., Roscoe, B. & Vickers, M. D. (1972) Biochemical evidence of anxiety in dental patients. *British Medical Journal*, **iv**, 7–9.
7. Taggart, P., Hedworth-Whitty, R. & Carruthers, M. (1976) Observations on electrocardiogram and plasma catecholamines during dental procedures: the forgotten vagus. *British Medical Journal*, **ii**, 787–789.
8. Miller, J. R., Redish, C. H., Fish, C. & Oehler, R. C. (1970) Factors in arrhythmia during dental outpatient general anesthesia. *Anesthesia and Analgesia. Current Researches*, **49**, 701–706.
9. Kaufman, L. (1965) Cardiac arrhythmias in dentistry. *Lancet*, **ii**, 287.
10. Ryder, W. (1970) The electrocardiogram in dental anaesthesia. *Anaesthesia*, **25**, 46–62.
11. Rollason, W. N. & Hall, D. J. (1973) Dysrhythmias inhalational anaesthesia for oral surgery. Incidence and prevention and treatment with practolol. *Anaesthesia*, **28**, 139–145.
12. Ryder, W., Charlton, J. E. & Gorman, P. B. W. (1973) Oral atropine and practolol premedication in dental anaesthesia. *British Journal of Anaesthesia*, **45**, 745–749.
13. Thurlow, A. C. (1972) Cardiac dysrhythmias in outpatient dental anaesthesia in children. The effect of prophylactic intravenous atropine. *Anaesthesia*, **27**, 429–435.
14. Alexander, J. P., Bekheit, S. & Fletcher, E. (1972) Dysrhythmia and oral surgery II: Junctional Rhythms. *British Journal of Anaesthesia*, **44**, 1179–1182.

15. Al-Khishali, T., Padfield, A., Perks, E. R. & Thornton, J. A. (1978) Cardio-respiratory effects of nitrous oxide: oxygen: halothane anaesthesia administered to dental outpatients in the upright posture. *Anaesthesia*, **33**, 184.

16. Hemphill, B. (1975) Hypocapnia and dental anaesthesia. *British Dental Journal*, **138**, 123.

17. Carruthers, M. & Taggart, P. (1973) Vagotonicity of Violence. Biochemical and cardiac responses to violent films and television programmes. *British Medical Journal*, **3**, 384–389.

18. Breggin, P. R. (1964) The psycho-physiology of anxiety. *Journal of Nervous and Mental Diseases*, **139**, 558–568.

19. Nixon, P. G. F., Taylor, D. J. E., Norton, S. D. & Bromfield, M. (1968) A sleep regime for acute myocardial infarction. *Lancet*, **i**, 726–728.

20. Drummond-Jackson, S. L. (1966) SAAD views anaesthesia in Britain. *Anesthesia Progress*, **13**, 313.

21. Thornton, J. A. (1970) Methohexitone and its application in dental anaesthesia. *British Journal of Anaesthesia*, **42**, 255–261.

22. Christenson, G. R., Herbert, C. L. & Driscoll, E. J. (1961) Intravenous barbiturate anesthesia for dental outpatients. *Anesthesia and Analgesia. Current Researches*, **40**, 77.

23. Wise, C. C., Robinson, J. S., Heath, M. J. & Tomlin, P. J. (1969) Physiological responses to intermittent methohexitone for conservative dentistry. *British Medical Journal*, **2**, 540.

24. Mann, P. E., Matt, S. D., Dixon, R., Griffin, K. D., Perks, E. R. & Thornton, J. A. (1970) A minimal increment methohexitone technique in conservative dentistry. *Anaesthesia*, **26**, 3.

25. Shafto, C. E. (1969) Continuous intravenous anaesthesia for paediatric dentistry. *British Journal of Anaesthesia*, **41**, 407.

26. Alexander, J. P. (1971) Dysrhythmia and oral surgery. *British Journal of Anaesthesia*, **43**, 773–778.

27. Rollason, W. N. & Dundas, C. P. (1970) Incidence of cardiac arrhythmia during dental anaesthesia. *Progress in Anaesthiology*. (Proceedings of the 4th World Congress of Anaesthesiologists), p. 969. Amsterdam. Excestpa Medica Foundation.

28. Thurlow, A. C. (1969) Cardiac arrhythmias during outpatient dental extraction. *Proceedings of a Symposium on Methohexitone*, 1–2 May, 1969. p. 8. London. Eli Lilley and Company Ltd.

29. Ryder, W. (1971) Cardiac rhythm during dental anaesthesia. *Proceedings of the Royal Society of Medicine*, **64**, 82.

30. Kaufman, L. (1966) Cardiac arrhythmias during dental anaesthesia. *Proceedings of the Royal Society of Medicine*, **59**, 731.

31. Rollason, W. N. & Dundas, C. R. (1966) Recent developments in outpatient dental anaesthesia. *Acta anaesthesiologica Scandinavica*, Suppl. **24**, 207.

32. Fisch, C., Oehler, R. C., Miller, J. R. & Redish, C. H. (1969) Cardiac arrhythmias during oral surgery with halothane–nitrous oxide–oxygen anesthesia. *Journal of the American Medical Association*, **208**, 1839–1842.

33. Tolas, A. G., Allen, G. D., Ward, R. J., Kennedy, W. J. & Bonica, J. J. (1976) Comparison of effects of methods of induction of anaesthesia on cardiac rhythm. *Journal of Oral Surgery*, **25**, 54.

34. Tuohy, O. (1968) Cardiac arrhythmias during oral surgical procedures. *British Dental Journal*, **124**, 417.

35. Ryder, W. (1971) Cardiac rhythm during dental anaesthesia. *Proceedings of the Royal Society of Medicine*, **64**, 82.

36. Rollason, W. N. (1977) Cardiac arrhythmias during outpatient dental anaesthesia. *British Journal of Anaesthesia*, **49**, 637.

37. Forbes, A. M. (1966) Halothane, adrenaline and cardiac arrest. *Anaesthesia*, **21**, 22.

38. Shanahan, J. (1966) A dental anaesthetic death. *Lancet*, **i**, 717.

39. Driscoll, E. J., Christenson, G. R. & White, C. L. (1959) Physiologic studies in general anesthesia for ambulatory patients. *Oral Surgery, Oral Medicine and Oral Pathology*, **12**, 1496.

40. Bradshaw, E. G. (1976) Dysrhythmias associated with oral surgery. *Anaesthesia*, **31**, 13–17.

41. Ryder, W., Charlton, J. E. & Garman, R. B. W. (1971) Practolol and atropine premedication in dental anaesthesia. *Anaesthesia*, **26**, 508.

42. Johnstone, M. & Nisbet, H. I. A. (1961) Ventricular arrhythmia during halothane anaesthesia. *British Journal of Anaesthesia*, **33**, 9–16.

43. Johnstone, M. (1966) Cardiac arrhythmias during dental anaesthesia. *Lancet*, **i**, 881.

44. Ryder, W. & Townsend, D. (1974) Cardiac rhythm in dental anaesthesia. A comparison of five methods. *British Journal of Anaesthesia*, **46**, 760.

45a. Long, G., Dripps, R. D. & Price, H. L. (1967) Measurement of anti-arrhythmic potency of drugs in man: effects of dehydrobenzperidol. *Anesthesiology*, **28**, 318.

45b. Plowman, P. E., Thomas, W. J. W. & Thurlow, A. C. (1974) Cardiac dysrhythmias during dental anaesthesia for oral surgery. The effect of local blockade. *Anaesthesia*, **29**, 571.

46. Plowman, P. E. & Thomas, W. J. N. (1974) Tricyclic antidepressants and cardiac dysrhythmias during dental anaesthesia. *Anaesthesia*, **29**, 576.

47. Alexander, J. P. (1974) Arrhythmias and oral surgery. Induction of anaesthesia with althesin. *British Journal of Anaesthesia*, **46**, 770.
48. Green, R. A. & Coplans, M. P. (1973) In *Anaesthesia and Analgesia in Dentistry*. p. 279. London. H. K. Lewis.
49. Page, M. McB., & Watkins, P. J. (1978) Cardiorespiratory arrest and diabetic autonomic neuropathy. *Lancet*, **i**, 14–16.
50. Vickers, M. D. & Pask, E. A. (1966) Less than 20 per cent oxygen or not? *Anaesthesia*, **21**, 92 and 261.
51. Dinsdale, R. C. W. (1978) Personal communication.
52. Nainby-Luxmore, R. C. (1967) Some hazards of dental gas machines (The report of a survey). *Anaesthesia*, **22**, 545.
53. Hutchinson, R. I. (1975) The accuracy and efficiency of general anaesthetic machines in dental practice. *British Dental Journal*, **138**, 187.
54. Holden, G. G. P. (1976) Survey of relative analgesia and anaesthetic machines. *SAAD Digest*, **3**, 8–15 and 36–41.
55. Neill, I. (1975) The accuracy and efficiency of general anaesthetic machines in dental practice. *British Dental Journal*, **139**, 420.
56. Bracken, A., Brookes, R. C. & Goldman, V. (1968) New equipment for dental anaesthesia using premixed gases and halothane. *British Journal of Anaesthesia*, **40**, 903.
57. Rollason, W. N. & Dundas, C. R. (1969) Portable dental anaesthetic machine for premixed nitrous oxide/oxygen. *Anaesthesia*, **24**, 96.
58. Green, R. A. & Coplans, M. P. (1973) In *Anaesthesia and Analgesia in Dentistry*. pp 123–128. London. H. K. Lewis.
59. Young, J. V. I. (1975) General anaesthesia for ambulant dental patients. *British Journal of Hospital Medicine*, **16**, 441–448.
60. Christenson, G. R., Herbert, C. L. & Driscoll, E. J. (1961) Intravenous barbiturate anesthesia for dental outpatients. *Anesthesia and Analgesia. Current Researches*, **40**, 77.
61. Cadle, D. R., Boulton, T. B. & Swaine, M. S. (1968) Intermittent intravenous anaesthesia for outpatient dentistry. A study using propanidid. *Anaesthesia*, **23**, 65.
62. Ducailar, J., Rioux, J. & Virapin, P. (1972) Dental care under ambulant general anaesthesia with CT 1341. *Annales de l'anesthesiologie Française*, **13**, 487.
63. Rollason, W. N., Fidler, K. & Hough, J. M. (1974) Althesin in outpatient dental anaesthesia. *British Dental Journal Anaesthesia*, **46**, 881.
64. Goldman, V. (1968) Inhalation anaesthesia for dentistry in the chair. *British Journal of Anaesthesia*, **40**, 155.
65. Meyer, R., Allen, G. D. & Hooley, J. R. (1966) Methoxyflurane in outpatient oral surgery. *Oral Surgery, Oral Medicine and Oral Pathology*, **21**, 594.
66. McDowell, J. F. (1968) Clinical comparison of Methoxyflurane and halothane anesthesia for dental survey. *Anesthesia and Analgesia. Current Researches*, **47**, 425.
67. Wilkes, C. H. W. (1966) Methoxyflurane in dental anaesthesia. *British Dental Journal*, **121**, 195.
68. Allen, W. A. (1974) An alternative to halothane. *British Dental Journal*, **137**, 154.
69. Boston, F. K. (1956) Trichlorethylene in dental anaesthesia. *Anaesthesia*, **11**, 37–39.
70. Young, T. M. (1974) Anaesthesia for dental extraction: A comparison of various techniques in the author's hands. *Anaesthesia*, **29**, 614–623.
71. Muir, V. M. J., Leonard, M. & Haddaway, E. (1976) Morbidity following dental extracts. A comparative study of local analgesia and general anaesthesia. *Anaesthesia*, **31**, 171–180.
72. Bishop, C. & Potts, H. W. (1961) Complications of outpatient dental anaesthesia. *British Dental Journal*, **111**, 235.
73. Rose, J. G. M., Bourne, J. G. & Goldman, V. (1969) Methohexitone and epilepsy. *British Dental Journal*, **126**, 203.
74. Baron, D. W. (1974) Propanidid in epilepsy. *Anaesthesia*, **291**, 445–447.
75. Uppington, J. (1973) Epileptiform convulsions with althesin. *Anaesthesia*, **28**, 546–550.
76. Lees, D. E. & McNamara, T. (1977) Ketamine induced hyperthermia. Post-ictal or malignant? *Anesthesiology*, **47**, 390–391.
77. Bissett, W. L. K. (1967) Hypotension following propanidid. *British Dental Journal*, **122**, 131.
78. Schofield, E. & Jepson, P. D. (1970) Propanidid Anaesthesia. *British Dental Journal*, **122**, 207.
79. Clarke, R. S. J., Dundee, J. W., Garrett, R. T., McArdle, G. K. & Sutton, J. A. (1975) Adverse reactions to intravenous anaesthetics. A survey of 100 reports. *British Journal of Anaesthesia*, **47**, 575–585.
80. Fisher, M. McD. (1975) Severe histamine mediated reactions to the intravenous drugs used in anaesthesia. *Anaesthesia and Intensive Care*, **3**, 180–197.
81. Evans, J. M. & Keogh, J. A. M. (1977) Adverse reactions to intravenous anaesthetic induction agents. *British Medical Journal*, **2**, 735–736.

82. Aldrett, J. A. & Narang, R. (1975) Deaths due to local analgesia in dentistry. *Anaesthesia*, **30**, 685–686.
83. Ravindranathan, N. (1975) Allergic reaction to lignocaine. *British Dental Journal*, **138**, 101–102.
84. Plumpton, F. S., Besser, G. M. & Cole, P. V. (1969) Cortico-steroid therapy and surgery. 2—The management of steroid cover. *Anaesthesia*, **24**, 12–18.
85. Doenicke, A. & Kugler, J. (1965) Electrical brain function during emergency time after methohexitone and propanidid anaesthesia. *Acta anaesthesiologica Scandinavica Suppl.*, **17**, 99.
86. Eustace, P. W., Hailey, D. M., Cox, A. G. & Baird, E. S. (1975) Biliary excretion of diazepam in man. *British Journal of Anaesthesia*, **47**, 983.
87. Ghonheim, M. M., Mewlad, T. S. P. & Ambre, J. (1975) Plasma levels of diazepam and mood ratings. *Anesthesia and Analgesia. Current Researches*, **54**, 173.
88. Kortilla, K. & Linnoila, M. (1974) Skills related to driving after intravenous diazepam, flunitrazepam and droperidol. *British Journal of Anaesthesia*, **46**, 961.
89. Dixon, R. A. & Thornton, J. A. (1973) Tests of recovery from anaesthesia and sedation: intravenous diazepam in dentistry. *British Journal of Anaesthesia*, **45**, 207–215.
90. Perks, E. R. (1977) The diagnosis and management of sudden collapse in dental practice. *British Dental Journal*, **143**, 196–200, 235–237, 307–310.
91. The Standing Dental Advisory Committee for the Central Health Services Council, the Secretary of State for Social Services and the Secretary of State for Wales (1972) *'Emergencies in Dental Practice'*. H.M.S.O.
92. Treloar, E. J. & Gardner, C. W. (1975) Inspection of general anaesthetic facilities in dental offices. *Canadian Anaesthetists' Society Journal*, **22**, 241.
93. Treloar, E. J. (1967) An outpatient anaesthetic service: standards and organisation. *Canadian Anaesthetists' Society Journal*, **14**, 596.
94. Klein, S. L., Wollman, H. & Cohen, D. W. (1977) The responsibility of the speciality of Anesthesiology to the profession of Dentistry. *Anesthesiology*, **47**, 294.
95. Seldin, H. M. (1969) General anesthesia for Ambulatory patients in office oral surgery. *Anesthesia and Analgesia. Current Researches*, **48**, 10.
96. Young, T. M. (1975) Questionnaire on the need for resuscitation in the dental surgery. *Anaesthesia*, **30**, 391–401.
97. Report of Working Party into Teaching in Dental Anaesthesia. Faculty of Anaesthetists and Faculty of Dental Surgery. Royal College of Surgeons of England 1978.
98. Bramley, P. A., Dinsdale, R. C. W., Padfield, A., Perks, E. R., Thornton, J. A. & Wilkes, E. (1974) Who is the Dental Anaesthetist of the Future? *British Dental Journal*, **136**, 355–356.
99. Report on Joint Sub Committee of the Standing Medical and Dental Advisory Committees of the Central Health Services Council (1977) H.M.S.O.
100. Windeyer, B. (1969) Report of the Windeyer Committee. *British Dental Journal*, **128**, 295.
101. Report of Board of Studies. London University (1977).
102. Rollason, W. N. (1978) Personal Communication.
103. Thompson, P. W. (1978) Personal Communication.
104. Young, T. M. (1977) Postgraduate experience with general anaesthesia. *British Dental Journal*, **143**, 371.
105. Brown, P. R. H., Main, D. M. G. & Lawson, J. I. M. (1968) Diazepam in dentistry. Report on 108 patients. *British Dental Journal*, **125**, 498.
106. Rattray, I. J. (1968) Observations on the use of diazepam in general dental practice. *British Dental Journal*, **125**, 495.
107. O'Neil, R. & Verrill, P. J. (1969) Intravenous diazepam in minor oral surgery. *British Journal of Oral Surgery*, **7**, 12.
108. Baird, E. S. & Flowerdew, G. D. (1970) Intravenous diazepam in conservative dentistry. *British Dental Journal*, **128**, 11.
109. Healy, T. E. J., Edmonson, H. D. & Hall, N. (1970) The use of intravenous diazepam during dental surgery in the mentally handicapped patient. *British Dental Journal*, **128**, 22.
110. Healy, T. E. J., Robinson, J. S. & Vickers, M. D. (1970) Physiological responses to intravenous diazepam as a sedative for conservative dentistry. *British Medical Journal*, **3**, 10.
111. Healy, T. E. J., Lautch, H., Hall, N., Tomlin, P. J. & Vickers, M. D. (1970) Interdisciplinary study of diazepam sedation for outpatient dentistry. *British Medical Journal*, **3**, 13.
112. Dixon, R. A., Day, C. D., Eccersley, P. S. & Thornton, J. A. (1973) Intravenous diazepam in dentistry: monitoring results from a controlled clinical trial. *British Journal of Anaesthesia*, **45**, 202–206.
113. Jørgensen, N. (1953) Premedication in dentistry. *S. California State Dental Association*, **21**, 1.
114. Parsons, J. D. & Main, D.M.G. (1973) Pentazocine and diazepam in dentistry. *SAAD Digest*, **2**, 93.
115. Brown, P. R. H., Main, D. M. G. & Wood, N. (1975) Intravenous sedation in dentistry. A study of 55 cases using pentazocine and diazepam. *British Dental Journal*, **139**, 59.

116. Foreman, P. (1966) Intravenous Sedation: A technique for the routine dental treatment of the apprehensive ambulant patient. *Anaesthesia Progress*, **13**, 218.
117. Shane, S. M. (1966) Intravenous amnesia for total dentistry in one sitting. *Journal of Oral Surgery*, **24**, 27.
118. Berns, J. (1963) 'Twilight sedation'—a substitute for lengthy office intravenous anesthesia. *Journal Connecticut State Dental Association*, **37**, 1.
119. Abramson, A. (1958) Hydroxyzine as an adjunct to local anesthesia. *Journal S. California Dental Association*, **26**, 26.
120. Shane, S. M. (1975) Principles of sedation, local and general anesthesia in dentistry. Springfield Illinois. C. C. Thomas.
121. Kurland, P. (1968) A new technique for dental analgesia. *British Dental Journal*, **125**, 302.
122. Langa, H. (1957) Analgesia for modern dentistry. *New York Journal of Dentistry*, **27**, 228.
123. Klock, H. J. (1951) 'Analgesia'. A technique of supplementation anesthesia in oral surgery. *Anesthesia and Analgesia. Current Researches*, **30**, 151.
124. Tom, A. (1956) An innovation in technique for dental gas. *British Medical Journal*, **1**, 1085.
125. Edmunds, D. H. & Rosen, M. (1975) Inhalation sedation for conservative dentistry. A comparison between nitrous oxide and methoxyflurane. *British Dental Journal*, **139**, 398–402.
126. Young, T. M., O'Mullane, D. M. & Warren, N. V. (1976) Inhalation sedation (Relative Analgesia). *British Dental Journal*, **141**, 34.
127. Dundee, J. W., George, K. A., Vadarajan, C. R., Clarke, R. S. J. & Nair, S. K. G. (1976) Anaesthesia and amnesia with flunitrazepam. *British Journal of Anaesthesia*, **48**, 266.
128. Thornton, J. A. & Martin, V. C. (1976) Flunitrazepam in dental outpatients. *Anaesthesia*, **31**, 297.
129. Dixon, R. A., Atkinson, R. E., Kenyon, C., Lamb, D., Thornton, J. A. & Woodhead, S. (1976) Subanaesthetic dosage of althesin as a sedative for conservative dentistry. A controlled trial. *British Journal Anaesthesia*, **48**, 431–439.
130. Cossham, P. & Dixon, R. A. (1973) Subanaesthetic dosage of propanidid for dentistry. A controlled clinical trial. *British Journal Anaesthesia*, **45**, 269.
131. Clarke, P. R. F., Eccersley, P. S., Frisby, J. P. & Thornton, J. A. (1970) The amnesic effect of diazepam (Valium). *British Journal of Anaesthesia*, **42**, 690.
132. D'Hollander, A. A., Monteny, E., Dewachter, B., Sanders, M. & Dubois-Primo, J. (1974) Intubation under topical supraglottic analgesia in unpremedicated and non-fasting patients: Amnesic effects of subhypnotic doses of diazepam and Innovar. *Canadian Anaesthetists' Society Journal*, **21**, 467.
133. Brown, S. S. & Dundee, J. W. (1968) Clinical studies of induction agents XXV: Diazepam. *British Journal of Anaesthesia*, **40**, 108.
134. Perisho, J. A., Buechel, D. R. & Miller, R. D. (1971) The effect of diazepam (valium) on MAC requirement in man. *Canadian Anaesthetists' Society Journal*, **18**, 536.
135. Hall, S. M., Whitwam, J. G. & Morgan, M. (1974) Effect of diazepam on experimentally induced pain thresholds. *British Journal of Anaesthesia*, **46**, 50–53.
136. Dalem, J. E., Evans, H. L., Banas, J. S., Brooks, H. L., Parakos, J. A. & Dexter, L. (1969) The hemodynamic and respiratory effects of diazepam. *Anesthesiology*, **30**, 259–263.
137. Weaver, D. C. & Dalen, J. E. (1969) The effects of diazepam. *Anesthesiology*, **31**, 196.
138. Catchlove, R. F. H. & Kafer, E. R. (1971) The effects of diazepam on ventilatory response to carbon dioxide and on steady state gas exchange. *Anesthesiology*, **34**, 9–13.
139. Pearce, C. (1974) The respiratory effects of diazepam supplementation of spinal anaesthesia in elderly males. *British Journal of Anaesthesia*, **46**, 439–441.
140. Catchlove, R. F. H. & Kafer, E. R. (1971) The effects of diazepam on respiration in patients with obstructive pulmonary disease. *Anesthesiology*, **34**, 14–18.
141. Hall, S. C. & Ovassapian, A. (1977) Apnoea after intravenous diazepam therapy. *Journal of the American Medical Association*, **238**, 1052.
142. Greenblatt, D. J. & Koch-Weser, J. (1973) Adverse reactions to intravenous diazepam: a report from Boston Collaborative drug surveillance program. *American Journal of Medical Science*, **226**, 261–266.
143. Clinical Anesthesia Conference (1971) Unexpected responses following diazepam. *New York State Journal of Medicine*, **71**, 578–580.
144. Hellewell, J. (1968) Induction of anaesthesia with diazepam. In *Diazepam in Anaesthesia*. p. 47. Bristol. J. Wright.
145. Jenkinson, J. L., Macrae, W. R., Scott, D. B. & Gould, J. F. (1974) Haemodynamic effects of diazepam used as a sedative for oral surgery. *British Journal of Anaesthesia*, **46**, 294–297.
146. Keim, K. L. & Sigg, E. B. (1973) Vagally mediated cardiac reflexes and their modulation by diazepam and pentobarbitone. *Neuropharmacology*, **12**, 319–325.
147. Abel, R. M., Reis, R. L. & Staroscik, R. N. (1970) Coronary vasodilation following diazepam (Valium). *British Journal of Pharmacology*, **38**, 620–631.

148. Abel, R. M., Reis, R. L. & Staroscik, R. N. (1970) The pharmalogical basis of coronary and systemic vasodilator actions of diazepam (Valium). *British Journal of Pharmacology*, **39,** 261.
149. Ikram, H., Rubin, A. P. & Jewkes, R. F. (1973) Effect of diazepam on myocardial blood flow of patients with and without coronary artery disease. *British Heart Journal*, **35,** 626.
150. Bloor, C. M. & Leon, A. S. (1973) Coronary and systemic hemodynamic effects of diazepam (Valium) in the unanesthetized dog. *Chemical Pathology and Pharmacology*, **6,** 1043.
151. Baird, E. S. & Hailey, D. M. (1972) Delayed recovery from a sedative : correlation of the plasma levels of diazepam with clinical effects after oral and intravenous administration. *British Journal of Anaesthesia*, **44,** 803.
152. Van De Kleijn, E., Van Rossum, J., Muskens, E. & Rijutjes, N. (1971) Pharmocokinetics of diazepam in dog, mice and humans. *Acta Pharmacologica Toxicologica*. (suppl.) 3 (kbh) **29,** 109.
153. Eustace, P. W., Hailey, D. M., Cox, A. G. & Baird, E. S. (1975) Biliary excretion of diazepam in man. *British Journal of Anaesthesia*, **47,** 983.
154. Mahon, W. A., Inaba, T., Umeda, T., Tsutsumi, E. & Stone, R. (1976) Biliary elimination of diazepam in man. *Clinical Pharmacology and Therapeutics*, **19,** 443–450.
155. Kanto, J. H., Pihajamaki, K. K. & Iisalo, E. U. M. (1974) Concentration of diazepam in adipose tissue of children. *British Journal of Anaesthesia*, **46,** 168.
156. Klotz, U., Avant, G. R., Hoyumpa, A., Schenker, S. & Wilkinson, G. R. (1975) The effect of age and liver disease on the disposition and elimination of diazepam in adult man. *Journal of Clinical Investigation*, **55,** 347–359.
157. Gould, J. D. M. & Lingam, S. (1977) Hazards of intra-arterial diazepam. *British Medical Journal*, **2,** 298.
158. Hegarty, J. E. & Dundee, J. W. (1977) Sequelae after intravenous injection of three benzodiazepines—diazepam, lorazepam and flunitrazepam. *British Medical Journal*, **ii,** 1384–1385.
159. Graham, C. W., Pagano, R. R. & Katz, R. L. (1977) Thrombophlebitis after intravenous diazepam—can it be prevented? *Anesthesia and Analgesia. Current Researches*, **56,** 409–413.
160. Burton, G. W., Lenz, R. J., Thomas, T. A. & Midda, M. (1974) Cremophor EL as a diluent for diazepam. *British Medical Journal*, **3,** 258.
161. Siebke, H., Ellertsen, R. R. & Linde, B. (1976) Reactions to intravenous injections of diazepam. *British Journal of Anaesthesia*, **48,** 1187.
162. Von Aardel, O., Mebius, C. & Mossberg, T. (1976) Diazepam in emulsion form for intravenous usage. *Acta anaesthesiologica Scandinavica*, **20,** 221.
163. Thorn-Alquist, A-M. (1977) Parenteral use of diazepam in an emulsion formulation. A clinical study. *Acta anaesthesiologica Scandinavica*, **21,** 400–404.
164. Healy, T. E. J. & Hamilton, M. C. (1971) Intravenous diazepam in the apprehensive child. *British Dental Journal*, **30,** 25.
165. Carmichael, A. F. & MacDonald, A. G. (1968) Diazepam. *British Dental Journal*, **125,** 480.
166. MacDonald, A. G. (1970) The use of diazepam for conservative dentistry in handicapped children. *Anaesthesia*, **25,** 127.
167. Kurland, P. (1975) Diazepam and methohexitone. *British Dental Journal*, **138,** 159.
168. Mandiwall, H. (1975) Diazepam and methohexitone. *British Dental Journal*, **138,** 43.
169. Hudson, M. W. P. (1974) Diazepam and methohexitone. *British Dental Journal*, **137,** 459.
170. Alexander, J. P. (1975) Drug combinations for anaesthesia. *British Medical Journal*, **2,** 505.
171. Kurland, P. (1968) A new technique for dental analgesia. *British Dental Journal*, **125,** 302.
172. Cohen, R., Finn, H. & Steen, S. N. (1969) Effect of diazepam and meperidine, alone and in combination on response to carbon dioxide. *Anesthesia and Analgesia. Current Researches*, **48,** 353–355.
173. Zsigmond, E. K., Flynn, K. & Martinex, O. A. (1974) Diazepam and meperidine on arterial blood gases in healthy volunteers. *Journal of Clinical Pharmacology*, **14,** 377.
174. Schoenfeld, A., Goldman, J. A. & Levy, E. (1974) Pentazocine and diazepam analgesia for minor gynaecological operations. *British Journal of Anaesthesia*, **46,** 385–386.
175. Gasger, J. C. & Bellville, J. W. (1976) The respiratory effects of hydroxyzine, diazepam and pentazocine in man. *Anaesthesia*, **31,** 718.
176. Dixon, R. H., Tilton, B. E. & Briggs, B. D. (1970) A comparison of the sedative and cardiorespiratory effects of diazepam and pentazocine premedication. *Anesthesia and Analgesia. Current Researches*, **49,** 546–550.
177. Baird, E. S. & Curson, I. (1970) Orally administered diazepam in conservative dentistry. *British Dental Journal*, **128,** 25.
178. Kurland, P. (1968) Diazepam. *British Dental Journal*, **125,** 524.
179. Gamble, J. A. S., Dundee, J. W. & Assaf, R. A. E. (1975) Plasma diazepam levels after single dose oral and intramuscular administration. *Anaesthesia*, **30,** 164.
180. Assaf, R. A. E., Dundee, J. W. & Gamble, J. A. S. (1975) The influence of the route of administration on the clinical action of diazepam. *Anaesthesia*, **30,** 152.

181. Patch, V. D. (1974) The dangers of diazepam, as a street drug. *New England Journal of Medicine*, **290,** 807.
182. Saxen, I. & Saxen, L. (1975) Association between maternal intake of diazepam and oral clefts. *Lancet*, **2,** 498.
183. Stovner, J., Endresen, R. & Österud, A. (1973) Intravenous anaesthesia with a new benzodiazepine R05-4200. *Acta anaesthesiologica Scandinavica*, **17,** 163–169.
184. Hutton, A. M., Wedley, J. R. & Seed, R. F. (1978) Teaching of anaesthesia to dentists. *British Dental Journal*, **144,** 35–39.

6. Sodium nitroprusside

Peter Cole

Although the use of sodium nitroprusside (SNP) during anaesthesia and in the Intensive Care Unit has only been developed in the past ten years, the compound is by no means new to science. It was first synthesised by Playfair as long ago as 1849[1] and its hypotensive properties in man were described by Johnson in 1929.[2] It was not until 1955, however, that Page reported on its clinical usefulness in the management of severe hypertension.[3] In 1962, Moraka[4] in the U.S.A., first described the use of the drug to induce hypotension during anaesthesia and in 1968 the drug was introduced to this country in a paper delivered to the Anaesthetic Research Society.[5] Taylor, Styles and Lamming described the use of SNP during anaesthesia in a large series of patients in 1970 and commented favourably on the drug.[6] Since that time there have been many other reports, mostly favourable, describing the use of nitroprusside both as a hypotensive agent and for the reduction of peripheral vascular resistance. It is interesting that since the advent of the drug, induced hypotension during anaesthesia has become a popular technique in the U.S.A. where previously normotensive anaesthesia was almost mandatory.

PHYSICAL AND CHEMICAL PROPERTIES

In this country, until recently, the reddish-brown crystals of nitroprusside were made up in hospital pharmacies as an orange coloured solution usually containing 100 mg of the drug in 10 ml of sterile water. Doubts have been cast on the long term stability of this solution,[7] but three samples supplied to us by Professor Holmi, University of the West Indies, and stored in amber vials for the previous three years were shown to have maintained their original concentration and to contain no free cyanide. Roche Pharmaceuticals have neatly side-stepped this potential problem by freeze-drying their commercial compound ('Nipride') and presenting it as 50 mg of dry powder in a sealed ampoule. For clinical use the contents of one or two of these can be instantly dissolved and made up in 500 ml of isotonic saline or 5 per cent dextrose to give solutions of 100 or 200 μg/ml. These dilute solutions are, however, unstable. If they are exposed to bright daylight there is a 10 per cent decrease in potency after 3 hours and after 48 hours as much as 50 per cent of the active drug is lost.[8] If the bottles or bags are protected from the light, this loss becomes negligible (Fig. 6.1). A useful warning sign of undue breakdown of the drug is the appearance of a blue colour—Prussian Blue (Ferric Ferrocyanide). Such solutions should immediately be rejected.

In clinical practice, solutions of the drug in dextrose are to be preferred to those in saline because:

1. They are probably more stable
2. They are more suitable for use in the coronary care unit
3. The 'Prussian Blue' reaction occurs earlier.

PHARMACOLOGY

Sodium Nitroprusside is a powerful 'direct' smooth muscle relaxant—between 50 and 1000 times more potent than nitrites.[2] This action is specific to the blood vascular system. The exact mode of action of the drug is uncertain, although Needleman has postulated that it and similar drugs act through a common inter-mediate vaso-dilatation site, which involves sulphydryl (SH) groups bound to the smooth muscle membrane.[9] The active unit is probably the iron-nitroso group Fe-NO.[3]

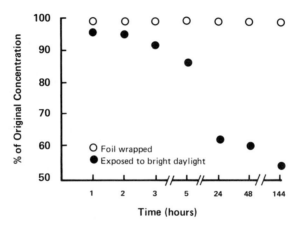

Fig. 6.1   Breakdown of infusion solutions of nitroprusside when exposed to or protected from bright daylight. Covering with tin-foil or a black velvet bag is a convenient method and should be used if the infusion is expected to exceed three hours.

When infused, SNP produces profound arterial hypotension, the degree of which can easily be titrated against the drip rate. The onset of hypotension is rapid, usually within one minute of administration. Reversal is always spontaneous when the drug is discontinued. Arterial pressure usually returns to pre-hypotensive levels within six minutes, provided, of course, any blood loss has been replaced. Vasopressors are never required. The drug acts mainly on the arterial system (resistance vessels) and less on the venous system (capacitance vessels), whereas autonomic ganglion blockers act equally on both systems—this implies that SNP has less effect on central venous pressure and venous return to the heart is more easily maintained. Wildsmith and his co-workers reported a mean fall in CVP of 2.8 mmHg during infusion of SNP in patients breathing halothane[10] and Styles reported falls around 2 mmHg.[11] However, Simpson et al reported no significant change in dogs on IPPV after relatively large bolus doses of the drug.[12] The author has observed no significant change in CVP in man during clinical anaesthesia when SNP is infused.

There is, again, some disagreement about the changes in cardiac output induced by the drug although it is certain that it has no direct effect upon the myocardium.[13,14] In the experimental animal, Ross and Cole demonstrated large increases in cardiac output which were largely unaffected by previous β-adrenergic blockade.[15] Other authors have reported no significant change,[16] or even small falls,[14] but these workers included halothane in their anaesthetic techniques. In man, most authors agree that cardiac output is maintained during infusion of SNP whether conscious or anaesthetised.[13,17] In fact, Wildsmith[10] and Lawson[18] reported a 20 per cent rise during anaesthesia with spontaneous ventilation. Thus as a hypotensive agent nitroprusside is unique since both IPPV with halothane and ganglion blockade diminish cardiac output during anaesthesia.[19] The principal action of ganglion blockers is loss of tone of capacitance vessels to produce 'venous pooling'. Thus positioning of the patient so that the operative site is uppermost is of paramount importance. This is much less critical with SNP and 'bloodless' surgery can be carried out effectively with the patient supine.[18]

Maintenance of cardiac *output* implies adequate tissue-flow despite falls in perfusion pressure and coronary flows have been shown to increase in dogs during infusion of the drug.[15] In man, during anaesthesia, the ECG shows no evidence of ischaemic changes despite large falls in arterial pressure.[20] Renal blood flow also increases—the drug produces dilatation of the renal vessels[3] and an early use of the drug was to facilitate renal angiography.[4]

Of particular interest to the anaesthetist is the effect of induced hypotension on cerebral blood flow. Under normal circumstances this flow is independent of perfusion pressure within wide limits i.e. the brain exhibits autoregulation. However, if the systolic pressure falls below about 60 mmHg, autoregulation fails and cerebral blood flow tends to fall, at least during hypotension induced by trimetaphan.[21] During SNP induced hypotension, cerebral blood flows appear to be essentially constant down to cerebral perfusion pressures of around 30 mmHg.[22] This is thought to be due to the abolition of the cerebral autoregulating mechanism by nitroprusside. The increase in flow inevitably has an effect upon intracranial pressure and under moderate hypotension (with the dura closed) it may rise. More importantly, intracranial pressure may also rise in the immediate post-operative period when arterial pressure has returned to normal but auto-regulation has not.[23]

METABOLISM[12]

In the literature there have been strange accounts of the breakdown of SNP, including the invocation of an erythrocytic enzyme 'thiocyanate oxidase' which probably does not exist.[24] A simplified version of the metabolism of the drug is shown in Figure 6.2. On entering the plasma, nitroprusside is quickly broken down by the sulphydryl (SH) groups present in sulphur-containing amino acids. Most of the HCN released immediately enters the red cell which acts as a 'cyanide sink' and where, in clinical concentrations at least, it appears to have little adverse effect.[25] Smith and Kruszyna suggest that SNP breakdown actually occurs in the red cell and that some of the cyanide forms cyanmethaemoglobin with methaemoglobin as an intermediary.[26] We have shown that the initial rise in plasma cyanide concentrations after infusion of SNP precedes that in the red cell, and this suggests that at least some occurs outside.[12] However it arrives there, the cyanide in the red cell is slowly released and is rapidly removed from the plasma by conjugation with thiosulphate to form thiocyanate. This reaction is catalysed by the mitochondrial enzyme rhodanese, found mainly in the liver and kidneys. The plasma thiocyanate rises slowly and for this reason is a poor indicator of SNP overdose during short term infusions. It is invaluable, however, when monitoring toxicity during long term infusion of the drug and is a relatively easy estimation for the average clinical laboratory. Thiocyanate is excreted unchanged in the urine. A small amount of cyanide is excreted by combining with B_{12} (hydroxycobalamin) to form cyanocobalamin. This is the basis of the suggestion that SNP overdose could be treated with a large dose of B_{12}. Unfortunately it would require about 2.5 g of this drug to combine with all of the cyanide derived from 100 mg of nitroprusside!

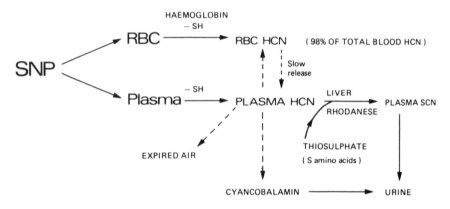

Fig. 6.2 Simplified diagram of current concept of nitroprusside metabolism. At the end of the infusion about 98 per cent of the cyanide liberated from the SNP is found in the red cells from which it is slowly released. The half-life of the plasma cyanide is about 30 min.

TOXICOLOGY

There have unfortunately been five reports of severe metabolic acidosis or cardiovascular collapse after infusion of SNP. Three of these patients eventually died (Table 6.1). In all these cases, the patients received large doses of nitroprusside and all the authors described progressive 'resistance' to the hypotensive effect of the drug. Davies has suggested that this abnormal response may be related to deficiencies in the cyanide detoxicating mechanism resulting in accumulation of cyanide.[27] Why cyanide accumulation should produce 'resistance' is not clear, since cyanide itself relaxes vasoconstrictor tone.[28] Further examination of these cases reveals that most of the patients were relatively young and resistance to hypotensive drugs is well described in young patients.[29] It is usually associated with the development of tachycardia mediated by the baroreceptor response, which is particularly active in younger, fitter patients. Thus, induced hypotension becomes progressively more difficult to achieve, and attempts to overcome this by 'pushing' the drug can result in doses of SNP high enough to produce a dangerous rise in plasma cyanide levels. It is highly probable that these patients were suffering from acute cyanide poisoning.[30]

High plasma cyanide levels exert their toxic effect by inhibition of tissue oxygenation i.e. 'histotoxic hypoxia'. Normal metabolism of pyruvate is thus inhibited and plasma lactate rises. Metabolic acidosis is therefore an inevitable consequence of nitroprusside overdose.[12] The minimum lethal dose of SNP for

Table 6.1   Some details of published reports of toxic effects of sodium nitroprusside. The last column indicated our estimate of the possible level of plasma cyanide reached by each patient. The minimum lethal level is about 10 μmol/l for short exposures

Reference	Dose of SNP	Details	Estimated plasma cyanide (μmol/l)
Persheau et al[53]	130 mg (3 mg/kg or 10.1 μmol/kg)	14 yr old male infused over 5 h—severe reversible acidosis	6.8
Macrae & Owen[54]	250 mg (4.2 mg/kg or 14 μmol/kg)	42 yr old female infused over 90 min—severe reversible acidosis	9.3
Merrifield & Blundell[55]	750 mg (2mg/kg/h or 20 μmol/kg in 3h)	20 yr old male infused over 5 h—fatal	13.0 after 3 h infusion 22.0 after 5 h infusion
Davies et al[56]	400 mg (10 mg/kg or 33.6 μmol/kg)	14 yr old male infused over 80 min—fatal	22.0
Jack[57]	750 mg (approx. 11 mg/kg or 37 μmol/kg)	39 yr old male infused over 30 min—fatal	24.0

short infusions is about 200–300 mg in the average patient.[26] This has been confirmed by McDowell in baboons.[31] The author has administered SNP during anaesthesia to over 500 patients, most receiving a total of less than 20 mg. Used in this manner the therapeutic ratio is of the order of 10–15:1 and nitroprusside becomes a relatively safe drug. However, if the patient is suffering from a condition which affects normal cyanide metabolism e.g. Lebers optic atrophy or tobacco amblyopia, nitroprusside should not be used. It should also be avoided in patients with renal or hepatic failure.

Treatment of overdose
Overdose with nitroprusside is usually manifested by progressive cardiovascular collapse during administration or the persistance of hypotension after withdrawal of the drug. Care must be taken that fluid replacement has been adequate. The presence of severe and progressive metabolic acidosis confirms the diagnosis. The initial treatment of choice is the administration of 25 ml of 50 per cent sodium thiosulphate intravenously over a period of 3–5 minutes. If no improvement occurs 20 ml (300 mg) of cobalt edetate should be injected at a rate of 1 ml/second.

CLINICAL USE

Despite many favourable reports on the use of sodium nitroprusside for the production of a 'dry field' during routine procedures, the author is of the opinion that the drug has few real advantages over more conventional techniques. Satisfactory conditions for plastic, facio-maxillary or orthopaedic surgery can usually be provided more easily and simply with autonomic ganglion blockade or IPPV with halothane. If however, the surgeon requires a particularly bloodless field or the blood pressure to be varied during the procedure, use of SNP is easily justified.

Recommended procedure[30]

After induction, all patients should be artificially ventilated with at least 33 per cent oxygen using tubocurarine as a relaxant. Anaesthesia can be supplemented with halothane if necessary. Sodium nitroprusside should be administered as a *separate* infusion of 100 or 200 μg/ml in 5 per cent dextrose. This can be inserted directly into the 'flash-ball' of the normal drip set, but 'T' piece and two-way tap systems should not be used. The drip-rate is most easily adjusted by some form of electronic drip controller although a 'Dial a Flow' has been found satisfactory. The infusion should be protected from the light if procedures lasting more than three hours are contemplated. The maximum safe dose on the basis of 1.5 mg/kg should be calculated and never exceeded. Direct measurement of the arterial pressure is mandatory.

The initial response to infusion of the drug should be carefully observed and the drip rate immediately slowed if the pressure starts to fall abruptly. Occasionally, it may be necessary to vary the drip rate a little to achieve the desired pressure but once a plateau is achieved it is usually easy to maintain. If at this stage, or at any time during the procedure, adequate hypotension becomes difficult to maintain, the drug should not be 'pushed'. It is preferable to increase the halothane concentration or control the tachycardia which is almost invariably present with small doses of a β-adrenergic blocker. One should beware of administering a disproportionate amount of SNP in the early stages of the anaesthetic. Positioning the patient so that the operative field is uppermost can be helpful but is by no means absolutely necessary.[18] The drip bottle should be removed from the theatre as soon as it is no longer required.

Neurosurgery

Sodium nitroprusside has now become the agent of choice for the induction of hypotension during neurosurgery, particularly for cerebral aneurysms and arterio-venous malformations.[32–34] The surgical approach to the lesion is usually con-ducted under normal or slightly reduced pressure but it can rapidly be reduced to perhaps 60 mmHg systolic or even lower during the actual surgical manipu-lation. Haemostasis can then be ensured under direct view by allowing the pressure to rise. In the event of a sudden haemorrhage the pressure can again quickly be reduced.

During prolonged periods of hypotension and with the patient in the steep head-up position, no significant change in arterial oxygenation, base deficit or cardiac output has been observed.[35] The longest period of induced hypotension with the drug has been reported by Siqueira and colleagues.[36] They describe a period of nine and a quarter hours, with the mean arterial pressure between 30 and 50 mmHg for the removal of a large arteriovenous malformation. This prodigious feat of endurance by all concerned was accomplished using a total dose of just 24 mg of nitroprusside. In general, although results appear to be similar whether induced hypothermia or SNP-induced hypotension is used for aneurysm surgery, there is little doubt that the latter technique is easier and more convenient.[37]

Phaeochromocytoma

Despite previous treatment with both α- and β-adrenergic blocking agents, handling of the tumour prior to clamping the adrenal vein can result in potentially catastrophic rises of arterial pressure. Although phentolamine is often effective at first, tachyphylaxis is a major disadvantage.[38] Sodium nitroprusside, however, seems to be effective at this time and resistance does not develop. After tumour removal, persistent hypotension has been described; this is probably due to loss of vasomotor tone in capacitance vessels and can be exacerbated if longer acting hypotensive agents or phentolamine were employed earlier in the operation.[39] Csanky-Treels has described a case where, after a fall of arterial pressure to 70 mmHg on removal of the tumour, the pressure then rose to 190/100 mmHg. The presence of further chromaffin tissue was suspected and only after three more tumours had been removed did the pressure stabilise at around 130/90 mmHg without SNP.[40]

Aortic surgery

During surgery for co-arctation or aortic aneurysm, the systolic pressure may rise to above 200 mmHg when the aorta is cross-clamped. This can easily be controlled with SNP. The infusion is stopped immediately prior to unclamping and the surgeon can be instructed to release the clamp *slowly* when the pressure starts to rise.

Cardiopulmonary bypass

SNP can be useful during cardiopulmonary bypass in patients undergoing open-heart surgery when a rising perfusion pressure develops due to vasoconstriction. However doubt has recently been cast on the efficacy of this manoeuvre,[41] particularly during hypothermia. It has also been employed to improve ventricular action in the immediate post bypass period by decreasing the afterload.

INTENSIVE CARE

The use of sodium nitroprusside to control severe hypertension has a much longer history than its use during anaesthesia. In fact, it was introduced for this purpose during the early 1950s in the U.S.A. It is interesting to note that only since the drug has been used during anaesthesia has there been a significant revival in its use in the Intensive and Coronary Care Units. Whilst in anaesthesia it has principally been used to reduce arterial pressure, in the Intensive Care Unit its range of use has been greatly extended—often to decrease peripheral vascular resistance without a significant degree of accompanying hypotension.

During long-term therapy, overdose may be avoided by monitoring plasma thiocyanate. Levels exceeding 1.7 mmol/l (10 mg per cent) should be avoided. The only significant toxic effect reported has been the development of hypothyroidism in a patient with severely impaired renal function who received the drug for 21 days.[42]

Severe hypertension

SNP is the most rapidly acting and consistently effective agent at present available for the management of acute hypertensive crises.[43] It is effective even where other agents have failed and is often administered to control the acute phase together with longer acting agents such as hydralazine or diazoxide. It can then slowly be withdrawn as they take effect.[44] It is particularly indicated when the hypertension is producing other pathology e.g. encephalopathy, intracranial haemorrhage or dissecting aneurysm. We have recently treated a patient at St. Bartholomew's Hospital with dissecting aneurysm using SNP infusion for a total period of 12 days. Eventually the aneurysm spontaneously re-entered at femoral level. The cause of the hypertension was treated by means of unilateral nephrectomy and the patient made a successful recovery. He received a total dose of 2.6 g SNP during this period, his highest plasma cyanide was 0.80 μmol/l and highest plasma thiocyanate 880 μmol/l.

Excessively high arterial pressure is also a problem after coronary artery surgery: about one third of such patients are affected. Nitroprusside infusion has become an accepted method of management and needs to be continued for about eight hours.[45]

Improvement of cardiac function

Franciosa et al described a series of eight patients with acute myocardial infarction and cardiogenic shock.[46] Cardiac output increased by about 10 per cent with an infusion rate, merely sufficient to drop the mean arterial pressure by an average of 16 mmHg. Their left ventricular filling pressures were halved, cardiac work appeared to decrease and there was significant clinical improvement in their shocked state. There seems to be a considerable measure of agreement that infusion of nitroprusside can reduce both the pre- and after-load of the failing heart.[47] It does this by dilatation of peripheral resistance vessels with, perhaps, relaxation of capacitance vessels.[48,49] The drug has been used to treat all forms of refractory heart failure and often appears to relieve pulmonary hypertension at the same time. This may be a result of decreased left atrial pressure but it has been suggested that the drug itself reduces pulmonary vascular resistance by direct action.[50]

Ergot overdose

Ergotamine tartrate is widely used in the treatment of migraine. Overdose with this drug produces intense peripheral vasoconstriction; ischaemia and gangrene can follow, which may necessitate limb amputation. Although most methods of treatment of this condition appear ineffective, a recent report of its successful management by nitroprusside infusion is encouraging.[51]

Renal vasodilatation

In 1929, Johnson achieved dilatation of the isolated perfused renal artery of the dog with nitroprusside.[2] This was further investigated by Page who described falls in both renal perfusion pressures and renal vascular resistance during infusion of the drug.[3] However, a more recent study of renal blood flow in intact man described a *decrease* when the mean arterial pressure had fallen by 44 per cent using SNP under general anaesthesia.[58]

Cerebral vasospasm

Spasm of cerebral arteries occurs both after operative treatment of cerebral aneurysm and after subarachnoid haemorrhage. To date, there are no reports of the use of SNP in man to treat this condition but it has been reported effective in relaxing artificially induced vascular spasm in the baboon.[52] Continuous infusion of SNP into the temporal artery, in amounts insufficient to cause systemic cardiovascular effects, produces sustained increases in cerebral blood flow of about 31 per cent in the goat. Extrapolation of these results to man would not necessarily produce similar results, because spasm after subarachnoid haemorrhage is often long established and may be considerably more difficult to treat.

SUMMARY

Sodium nitroprusside is a potent, rapid-acting hypotensive agent administered by intravenous infusion. It acts by peripheral vasodilatation and reduction in peripheral resistance by a direct action on the vessel wall. Its hypotensive action is evanescent. On withdrawal of the drug, the pressure always returns to normal spontaneously. No patient has been reported to be completely refractory and tolerance and tachyphylaxis are rare.

The main clinical uses of this drug are as a hypotensive agent and to produce a fall in peripheral resistance. The drug has been used during anaesthesia, in the management of severe hypertension, and for the treatment of refractory cardiac failure, particularly after acute myocardial infarction.

REFERENCES

1. Playfair, L. (1849) On the nitroprussides: a new class of salts. *Proceedings of the Royal Society*, **5**, 846–847.
2. Johnson, C. C. (1929) The actions and toxicity of sodium nitroprusside. *Archives Internationales de Pharmacodynamie et Thérapie*, **35**, 480–496.
3. Page, I. H., Corcoran, A. C., Dustan, H. P. & Koppanyi, T. (1955) Cardiovascular actions of sodium nitroprusside in animals and hypertensive patients. *Circulation*, **11**, 188–198.
4. Moraca, P. P., Bitte, E. M., Hale, D. E., Wasmuth, C. E. & Poutasse, E. F. (1962) Clinical evaluation of sodium nitroprusside as a hypotensive agent. *Anesthesiology*, **23**, 193–199.
5. Jones, G. O. M. & Cole, P. (1968) Sodium nitroprusside as a hypotensive agent. *British Journal of Anaesthesia*, **40**, 804–805.
6. Taylor, T. H., Styles, M. & Lamming, A. J. (1970) Sodium nitroprusside as a hypotensive agent in general anaesthesia. *British Journal of Anaesthesia*, **42**, 859–863.
7. Schumacher, G. E. (1966) Sodium nitroprusside injection. *American Journal of Hospital Pharmacy*, **23**, 532.
8. Vesey, C. J. & Batistoni, G. A. (1977) The determinations and stability of sodium nitroprusside in aqueous solutions. *Journal of Clinical Pharmacy*, **2**, 105–117.

9. Needleman, P., Jakschik, B. & Johnson, E. M. (1973) Sulfhydryl requirement for relaxation of vascular smooth muscle. *Journal of Pharmacology and Experimental Therapeutics*, **187**, 324–331.
10. Wildsmith, J. A. W., Marshall, R. L., Jenkinson, J. L., Macrae, W. R. & Scott, D. B. (1973) Haemodynamic effects of sodium nitroprusside during nitrous oxide/halothane anaesthesia. *British Journal of Anaesthesia*, **45**, 71–74.
11. Styles, M., Coleman, A. J. & Leary, W. P. (1973) Some haemodynamic effects of sodium nitroprusside. *Anesthesiology*, **38**, 173–176.
12. Simpson, P. J., Adams, L., Vesey, C. J. & Cole, P. V. (1978) Some physiological and metabolic effects of sodium nitroprusside and cyanide. *British Journal of Anaesthesia*. (In press)
13. Rowe, G. G. & Henderson, R. H. (1974) Systemic and coronary haemodynamic effects of sodium nitroprusside. *American Heart Journal*, **87**, 83–87.
14. Adams, A. P., Clarke, T. N. S., Edmonds-Seal, J., Foex, P., Prys-Roberts, C. & Roberts, J. G. (1974) The effects of sodium nitroprusside on myocardial contractility and haemodynamics. *British Journal of Anaesthesia*, **46**, 807–817.
15. Ross, G. & Cole, P. V. (1973) Cardiovascular actions of sodium nitroprusside in dogs. *Anaesthesia*, **28**, 400–406.
16. Michenfelder, J. D. & Theye, R. A. (1977) Canine systemic and cerebral effects of hypotension induced by haemorrhage, trimetaphan, halothane or nitroprusside. *Anesthesiology*, **46**, 188–195.
17. Schlant, R. C., Tsagaris, T. S. & Robertson, R. J. (1962) Studies on the acute cardiovascular effects of intravenous sodium nitroprusside. *American Journal of Cardiology*, **9**, 51–59.
18. Lawson, N. W., Thompson, D. S., Nelson, C. L., Flacke, J. W. & North, E. R. (1976) Sodium nitroprusside induced hypotension for supine total hip replacement. *Anesthesia and Analgesia, Current Researches*, **55**, 654–659.
19. Jordan, W. S., Graves, C. L., Boyd, W. A., Uedal, I. & Roberts, T. S. (1971) Cardiovascular effects of three technics for inducing hypotension during anaesthesia. *Anesthesia and Analgesia, Current Researches*, **50**, 1059–1068.
20. Simpson, P., Bellamy, D. & Cole, P. (1976) Electrocardiographic studies during hypotensive anaesthesia using sodium nitroprusside. *Anaesthesia*, **31**, 1172–1178.
21. Stoyka, W. W. & Schutz, H. (1975) The cerebral response to sodium nitroprusside and trimetaphan controlled hypotension. *Canadian Anaesthetists' Society Journal*, **22**, 275–283.
22. Ivankovich, A. D., Miletich, D. J., Albrecht, R. F. & Zahed, B. (1976) Sodium nitroprusside and cerebral blood flow in the anaesthetised and unanaesthetised goat. *Anesthesiology*, **44**, 21–26.
23. Turner, J. M., Powell, D., Gibson, R. M. & McDowall, D. G. (1977) Intracranial pressure changes in neurosurgical patients during hypotension induced with sodium nitroprusside or trimetaphan. *British Journal of Anaesthesia*, **49**, 419–425.
24. Vessey, C. J. & Wilson, J. (1978) Red cell cyanide. *Journal of Pharmacy & Pharmacology*, **30**, 20–26.
25. Krapez, J. R., Vesey, C. J. & Cole, P. V. (1978) The effects of sodium nitroprusside and cyanide on haemoglobin function. (In preparation)
26. Vesey, C. J., Cole, P. V. & Simpson, P. J. (1976) Cyanide and thiocyanate concentrations following sodium nitroprusside infusion in man. *British Journal of Anaesthesia*, **48**, 651–659.
27. Davies, D. W., Greiss, L., Kadar, D. & Steward, D. J. (1975) Sodium nitroprusside in children: observations on metabolism during normal and abnormal responses. *Canadian Anaesthetists' Society Journal*, **22**, 553–560.
28. Barcroft, H. (1973) The effect of cyanide, of circulatory arrest and of activity on intrinsic vasoconstrictor tone in blood vessels. *Journal of Physiology*, **232**, 111p.
29. Tyrrell, M. F. (1974) Hypotension. In *Scientific Foundations of Anaesthesia* ed. Scurr, C. & Feldman, S. B., p. 162. London: Heinemann.
30. Cole, P. V. (1978) The safe use of sodium nitroprusside. *Anaesthesia*, **33**, 473–477.
31. McDowall, D. G., Keaney, N. P., Turner, J. M., Lane, J. R. & Okudu, Y. (1974) The toxicity of sodium nitroprusside. *British Journal of Anaesthesia*, **46**, 327–332.
32. Siegal, P., Moraca, P. P. & Green, J. R. (1971) Sodium nitroprusside in the surgical treatment of cerebral aneurysms and arteriovenous malformations. *British Journal of Anaesthesia*, **43**, 790–795.
33. Aitken, R. R. (1974) Hypotension in the operative treatment of intracranial aneurysm. *Proceedings of the IVth European Congress of Anaesthesiology*, Madrid, 779–782.
34. Lewelt, W., Moszynski, K., Trojanowski, T. & Brzozowski, S. (1975) Controlled arterial hypotension during neurosurgical operations. *Anaesthesia, Resuscitation and Intensive Therapy*, **3**, 325–328.
35. Stoelting, R. K., Viegas, O. & Campbell, R. L. (1977) Sodium nitroprusside produced hypotension during anaesthesia and operation in the head-up position. *Anesthesia and Analgesia, Current Researches*, **56**, 391–394.
36. Siqueira, E. B. & Behnia, R. (1976) Prolonged, profound hypotension produced safely with sodium nitroprusside. *Surgical Neurology*, **6**, 169–172.

37. Adams, C. B. T., Loach, A. B. & O'Laoire, S. A. (1976) Intracranial aneurysms: analysis of results of microneurosurgery. *British Medical Journal*, **2**, 607–609.
38. El-Nagger, M., Suerte, E. & Rosenthal, E. (1977) Sodium nitroprusside and lidocaine in the anaesthetic management of pheochromacytoma. *Canadian Anaesthetists' Society Journal*, **24**, 353–360.
39. Katz, R. L. & Wolf, C. E. (1971) Pheochromocytoma. In *Highlights of Clinical Anesthesiology* ed. Mark, L. C. & Ngai, S. H. pp. 55–65. New York: Harper & Row.
40. Csanky-Treels, J. C., Lawick Van Pabst, W. P., Brands, J. W. J. & Stamenkovic, L. (1976) Effects of sodium nitroprusside during the excision of phaechromocytoma. *Anaesthesia*, **31**, 60–62.
41. Evans, P. J. D., Ruygrok, P., Seelye, E. R. & Harris, E. A. (1977) Does sodium nitroprusside improve tissue oxygenation during cardiopulmonary bypass? *British Journal of Anaesthesia*, **49**, 799–803.
42. Nourok, D. S., Glassock, R. J., Solomon, D. H. & Maxwell, M. H. (1964) Hyperthyroidism following prolonged sodium nitroprusside therapy. *American Journal of Medical Sciences*, **248**, 129–138.
43. A. M. A. Committee on Hypertension (1974) The treatment of malignant hypertension and hypertensive emergencies. *Journal of the American Medical Association*, **228**, 1673–1679.
44. Katz, R. L. & Wolf, C. E. (1971) Sodium nitroprusside for controlled hypotension and hypertensive emergencies. In *Highlights of Clinical Anesthesiology*, ed. Mark, L. C. & Ngai, S. H.
45. Viljoen, J. F., Estafanous, F. G. & Tarazi, R. C. (1976) Acute hypertension immediately after coronary artery surgery. *Journal of Thoracic and Cardiovascular Surgery*, **71**, 548–550.
46. Franciosa, J. A., Guiha, N. H., Limas, C. J., Rodriguera, E. & Cohn, J. N. (1972) Improved left ventricular function during nitroprusside infusion in acute myocardial infarction. *Lancet*, **1**, 650–654.
47. Chatterjee, K., Parmley, W. W., Ganz, W., Forrester, J., Walinsky, P., Crexells, C. & Swan, H. J. C. (1973) Haemodynamics and metabolic responses to vasodilator therapy in acute myocardial infarction. *Circulation*, **48**, 1183–1193.
48. Guiha, N. H., Cohn, J. N., Mikulic, E., Franciosa, J. A. & Limas, C. J. (1974) Treatment of refractory heart failure with infusion of nitroprusside. *New England Journal of Medicine*, **291**, 587–592.
49. Harshaw, C. W., Crossman, W., Munro, A. B. & McLaurin, L. P. (1975) Reduced systemic vascular resistance as therapy for severe mitral regurgitation of valvular origin. *Annals of Internal Medicine*, **83**, 312–316.
50. Knapp, E. & Gmeiner, R. (1977) Reduction of pulmonary hypertension by nitroprusside. *International Journal of Clinical Pharmacology and Biopharmacy*, **15**, 75–80.
51. Carliner, N. H., Denune, D. P., Finch, C. S. Jr. & Goldberg, L. I. (1974) Sodium nitroprusside treatment of ergotamine-induced peripheral ischaemia. *Journal of the American Medical Association*, **227**, 308–309.
53. Persheau, R. A., Modell, J. H., Bright, R. N. & Shirley, P. D. (1977) Suspected sodium nitroprusside induced cyanide intoxication. *Anesthesia and Analgesia, Current Researches*, **56**, 533–536.
54. Macrae, W. R. & Owen, M. (1974) Severe metabolic acidosis following hypotension induced with sodium nitroprusside. *British Journal of Anaesthesia*, **46**, 795–797.
55. Merrifield, A. J. & Blundell, M. D. (1974) Toxicity of sodium nitroprusside. *British Journal of Anaesthesia*, **46**, 324.
56. Davies, D. W., Kadar, D., Steward, D. J. & Munro, I. R. (1975) A sudden death associated with the use of sodium nitroprusside for induction of hypotension during anaesthesia. *Canadian Anaesthetists' Society Journal*, **22**, 547–552.
57. Jack, R. D. (1974) Toxicity of sodium nitroprusside. *British Journal of Anaesthesia*, **46**, 952.
58. Birch, A. A. & Boyce, W. H. (1977) Changing renal blood flow following sodium nitroprusside in patients undergoing nephrectomy. *Anesthesia and Analgesia, Current Researches*, **56**, 102–109.

7. Controlled ventilation

J. C. Stoddart

At the present time the aspects of controlled ventilation which are arousing the greatest interest are:

1. The indications for the use of Positive End Expiratory Pressure, or Controlled Positive Airway Pressure (PEEP, CPAP etc.)
2. The place of Intermittent Mandatory Ventilation (IMV) in 'weaning' patients from ventilator therapy
3. The value of High Frequency Positive Pressure Ventilation (HFPPV), particularly during tracheal and pulmonary operations
4. The need for and methods of sterilising ventilatory equipment.

In a review of this nature only a small fraction of the papers which have appeared can be discussed. Many of the opinions quoted are conflicting and all the reviewer can do is attempt to present a balanced selection, but in some instances no final analysis is possible. Throughout, two points should be borne in mind by the reader. In the first place, the results of experiments which are performed upon healthy animals or on man under ideal circumstances cannot automatically be transferred to sick patients with unpredictably varying pulmonary mechanics. It is probably true to state that any machine which can safely produce a sine-wave ventilatory pattern with a variable respiratory rate and minute volume will adequately ventilate any healthy patient. The variants of the sine-wave which are discussed in the remainder of this section are intended for patients with abnormal pulmonary mechanics.

Secondly, the respiratory system must not be considered in isolation. At several points in the succeeding section, attention is focussed upon the effects of controlled ventilation upon other bodily systems. In some instances it is necessary to weigh the more obvious advantages of a particular type of ventilation against some of its less obvious but no less important disadvantages.

POSITIVE END EXPIRATORY PRESSURE

Many synonyms have been given to the ventilatory pattern which maintains a positive pressure throughout the expiratory phase but PEEP is probably that which is most widely used. Although the term is in everyday use at present, when ventilatory therapy was introduced the idea was anathema. At that time the guidelines for the design of an ideal ventilator included safety and simplicity, but almost every writer agreed that a ventilator which generated a low mean intrathoracic pressure was desirable. It was recognised that intermittent positive pressure ventilation (IPPV) reduced the venous return, cardiac output and pulmonary blood flow.[1,2] Ventilators were therefore designed to have a low inspiratory to expiratory time ratio and to generate gas-flow patterns which achieved a desirable tidal volume with the minimum rise in intrathoracic pressure. It was realised that with IPPV the mean intrathoracic pressure was inevitably positive but this was regarded as an acceptable penalty for adequate ventilation.

For a brief period the use of negative expiratory pressure (NEEP) was popular particularly for patients with diseased or narrowed air passages. It was initially believed that this would increase the expiratory gas flow rate and then by generating a negative intrathoracic pressure increase the venous return. It soon became apparent that this belief was ill-founded and recent work[3] has confirmed that NEEP has little or no place in ventilator therapy. It is of interest to note that in healthy dogs, it has been reported that although NEEP did not affect respiratory gas exchange, it did improve renal function, whereas IPPV did not and PEEP actively interfered with renal blood flow, glomerular filtration rate and urine secretion.[4] However NEEP is unlikely to regain popularity as a diuretic for healthy dogs.

Many workers have experimented with different applied wave forms and gas flow rates in an attempt to find the ideal pattern for IPPV. In 1957 Pask[5] demonstrated with the aid of a simple model the existence of frequency dependent compliance. He showed that when the 'patient' had narrowed airways but normally compliant lungs a slow inspiratory flow rate achieved the most effective ventilation whereas a rapid gas flow rate was more satisfactory for a 'patient' with normal airways but lower lung compliance. This parallels the clinical problem of the patient with unevenly distributed respiratory disease. For such a patient a compromise ventilatory pattern has to be accepted. In a series of papers which reported clinical investigations on a variety of patients, Johansson and Löftström[6,7,8,9] showed that although a pattern of decelerating gas flow improved pulmonary compliance it also increased the dead space and they concluded that an accelerating inspiratory flow rate was best overall. Bake and his colleagues[10] demonstrated that for healthy seated patients, at low gas flow rates most of the gas was distributed to the lower parts of the lung but when the gas flow was increased to 15 litres per second (which is frequently achieved during IPPV) all parts of the lung were equally ventilated. Other workers[11] showed that a slowly accelerating wave form achieved the most effective ventilation for a patient with chronic airways obstruction. However, Johansson, in the final paper of the series quoted above[9] said that most of the characteristics of a particular gas flow are lost during the passage through the airways and are not transmitted to the oesophagus or the central vessels.

Positive pressure breathing was first used in aviation medicine and interest in its clinical use evolved slowly. Linde, Shumanns and Ellman[12] investigated the cardiocirculatory effects of PEEP on normal volunteers and showed that it reduced cardiac output and did not change the transmural pulmonary artery pressure gradient which suggested that it would not be helpful in the treatment of pulmonary oedema.

However, in 1969 Ashbaugh and his co-workers[13] reported that PEEP induced radiographic evidence of improvement in acute pulmonary oedema and it was for this purpose that it was originally used in clinical practice, although Ashbaugh doubted its overall benefit and stated that it may simply prolong the survival of patients who ultimately died of pulmonary fibrosis.

In the same year Uzawa and Ashbaugh[14] showed that when haemorrhagic pulmonary oedema was produced experimentally by the infusion of oleic acid into dogs, those animals ventilated with a positive end-expiratory pressure recovered more quickly than those given IPPV. All of the animals survived, which suggested that the model did not mimic the clinical situation, and the authors stated that the hazards of PEEP could outweigh their benefits, particularly in those animals 'with comparatively normal lungs'. A fall in cardiac output was the major problem encountered and this has been the most widely quoted disadvantage of PEEP.[14,15]

When utilised in the treatment of clinical pulmonary oedema the results have been both unpredictable and variable. Esteban and his colleagues[16] treated with PEEP eight consecutive patients who had pulmonary oedema. In none was there any improvement in the radiographic appearance and in two cases there was no improvement in arterial oxygenation. In the other six cases PEEP of from 10–20 cmH_2O marginally but not significantly improved the alveolar to arterial Po_2 gradient.

Noble, Kay and Obdrzalek[17] used a double indicator method to measure the volume of lung water. They showed that PEEP below 16 cm water did not reduce lung water and that at pressures greater than this, lung water was increased. They showed that PEEP could increase the FRC and arterial oxygen tension marginally, but did not assess its effects upon oxygen transport. The pulmonary artery pressure, which rose as oedema was induced, did not change with the application of PEEP, which reinforced the observations referred to earlier[12] that transmural pressure is not affected by increasing airway pressure.

Another paper by Obdrzalek and his colleagues[18] showed that PEEP could slow but not prevent the onset of experimentally induced pulmonary oedema. They showed that there was a reduction in the percentage of blood shunted through oedematous areas and that the animals' cardiac output and oxygen consumption were both reduced. Similar results were recorded by Dueck, Wagner and West.[19] These authors also showed that when the level of end expiratory pressure exceeded 15 cm water, gas exchange was further impaired and the dead space volume increased.

Although much of the foregoing evidence is conflicting, there is little doubt that IPPV with or without PEEP is the most effective form of oxygen therapy which can be applied at normal ambient atmospheric pressure. The additive effects of PEEP must be regarded as uncertain. Caldini, Leith and Brennan[20] reviewed its effects and reported results which suggested that far from improving pulmonary oedema PEEP could increase interstitial and alveolar water. They quoted the results of Shirley and his co-workers[21] which suggested that PEEP 'stretched' the alveolar membranes, opening pores and allowing both protein and water to leak into the alveoli.

These latter opinions are in agreement with those of the reviewer who has on many occasions observed the development of pulmonary oedema while patients were receiving IPPV and has failed impressively to remove it with the aid of PEEP.

One of the as-yet unsolved problems of respiratory therapy is intractable hypoxaemia. This can be defined as a situation in which the patient's arterial oxygen tension is dangerously low (perhaps less than 7 kPa) when the patient is given 100 per cent oxygen by IPPV. Great interest has been focussed on evidence which suggested that PEEP could increase the functional residual capacity (FRC) and the arterial oxygen tension of patients with this condition.[22,23,24] In some instances the FRC was shown to rise linearly with the mean airway pressure[25] and it was believed that PEEP splinted the alveoli and reduced their tendency to collapse. Other workers had shown that rapid deflation of the lung was accompanied by an equally rapid fall in arterial oxygen tension, probably due to atelectasis.[26,27] The same group believed that hypoxia associated with atelectasis could be reversed by periodic hyperinflation of the lungs (sighing)[28] but others showed that hypoxia could only be reversed if the lungs were inflated to a pressure of 40 cm H_2O sustained for 40 seconds.[29] A similar effect could be achieved by the constant use of IPPV with large tidal volumes, of the order of 15 ml/kg body weight.[30] This will be referred to again later.

Conditions which are associated with a reduction in FRC include the infant and adult respiratory distress syndromes (RDS) and interstitial pulmonary oedema. The terminology of adult RDS is unsatisfactory because whereas some clinicians believe this to be identical with 'shock lung'[31,32] others would include patients with infected pulmonary oedema and those with respiratory failure due to sepsis and acid aspiration pneumonia.

There have been several reviews of the use of PEEP in intractable hypoxia recently and it is difficult to untangle the varying opinions.[33,34,35] Most of the reviewers believe that PEEP has a place in the treatment of this condition but they usually point out that although the arterial oxygen tension may rise by a variable amount after PEEP is applied the patient's cardiac output may fall to such an extent that the amount of oxygen carried to the tissues ($\dot{Q} \times$ Oxygen saturation) may fall.[36,37,38,39] In two papers Civetta and his colleagues[40,14] suggested that the effects of PEEP on cardiac output in the very sick patient are minimal, implying that respiratory disease in some way protects the patient's cardiovascular system, possibly by a 'damping' action. Colgan and co-workers[42] also stated that in spite of causing a fall in cardiac output in some patients, it could be beneficial even in patients suffering from a low cardiac output state if the mixed venous oxygen tension was below 3.5 kPa (25 mmHg).

In another paper from the Harvard group[43] it was shown that if PEEP was applied to patients who did not really need it, as defined earlier, the cardiac output dropped markedly, particularly if the patients were hypovolaemic, and only relative overtransfusion could compensate for these ill effects. This raises the theoretical problem of circulatory overload and the development of pulmonary oedema when PEEP is released. Other workers[44] showed that for patients undergoing surgical procedures under general anaesthesia, the use of large tidal volumes were as good as or better than PEEP. Although it is difficult to imagine a clinical situation in which such a technique would be tried, Aalto-Setala, Heikonen and Salorine[45] showed that during one-lung anaesthesia, IPPV caused a smaller fall in cardiac output than did PEEP.

It is widely believed that reduced production of surfactant is a major factor in the development of the neonatal and adult respiratory distress syndrome and may be the principal cause of the fall in FRC which is observed in these conditions. It is therefore of interest that two groups found that the use of PEEP was associated with an increased production and reduced inactivation of surfactant.[46,47] Many experienced clinicians believe that PEEP is the greatest advance in the treatment of the neonatal respiratory distress syndrome since IPPV was first instituted.[34,48,49] In spite of this enthusiasm a cautionary note was struck by Stevens in 1976[50] when, in a review of the benefits of PEEP he maintained that it had not significantly improved the survival of patients suffering from the respiratory distress syndrome. Another group of workers[51] suggested that any improvement in arterial oxygenation which was produced with the aid of PEEP might be due to the reversal of true intracardiac shunts. This same group showed that PEEP increased the patient's dead space and $Paco_2$, observations which have been made by others.[19,39] West[52] confirmed that PEEP tended to overventilate areas of the lung which were already well ventilated, thus increasing the ventilation:perfusion ratio. It may be possible to correct an increase in the physiological dead space by increasing the tidal volume, but this may not correct the V/Q disturbance and $AaPo_2$ tension difference.

At the beginning of this section it was stated that one of the first harmful effects of PEEP which was recognised was a reduction in the cardiac output. Since its introduction PEEP has been used to treat patients suffering from almost every kind of pulmonary disease and certain contraindications to its use have now emerged.

In 1972 Sugermann, Rogers and Miller[53] stated that PEEP should not be used to treat patients with chronic obstructive airways disease while others simply said that its beneficial effects were not obvious.[54] Ashbaugh and Petty[55] later suggested that it should not be used in the treatment of status asthmaticus. In the same paper the authors stated that if the lungs were healthy the disadvantages of PEEP outweighed any possible advantage and other authors have emphasised the same point. McMahon, Halprin and Sieker[56] stated that in their experience PEEP was of no value in patients with pneumonia, which is to be anticipated in view of the underlying pathological process.

Kumar and his co-workers wrote in 1970[57] that out of 8 patients treated with PEEP 4 developed a pneumothorax which required treatment. In this paper the figures which were given for the patients' arterial oxygen tension before PEEP was applied showed that the lowest Pao_2 on an Fio_2 of 1 was 20 kPa (150 mmHg). This suggests that by present standards these patients would not have received PEEP. A later publication from the same group[58] reviewing a larger series suggested that the incidence of pulmonary barotrauma was no higher in the patients given PEEP (11 per cent) than in those treated with IPPV alone (10 per cent). On the other hand, Kao and Tierney[59] showed that 10 cm H_2O of PEEP could predispose to alveolar rupture and air embolism in the absence of overt pneumothorax. They suggested that cerebral air embolism could be a common but unrecognised cause of coma in patients receiving ventilator treatment.

Renal failure often develops in acutely ill patients, many of whom will be undergoing controlled ventilation. Continuous positive pressure breathing was first used to overcome the problems of high altitude hypoxia in aviation and it is interesting to note that in 1947, Drury, Henry and Goodman[60] reported that it was accompanied by a temporary reduction in urine output. Sladen, Laver and Pontoppidan[61] showed that both fluid retention and pulmonary oedema could occur during the clinical use of PEEP. Pontoppidan, Geffin and Loewenstein[62] later found that PEEP increased aldosterone secretion, which could cause sodium and water retention. Other workers showed that PEEP impaired all aspects of renal function; it not only reduced renal blood flow but also caused the creatinine clearance and hourly urine output to fall.[63] In 1977 Baratz, Philbin and Patterson[64] reported that animal experiments suggested that continuous positive pressure breathing could increase the secretion of antidiuretic hormone. If this series of results is considered with those which were quoted earlier it is hard to escape the conclusion that PEEP is absolutely contraindicated in the treatment of pulmonary oedema.

A miscellaneous although nonetheless important group of apparently harmful effects of PEEP completes this section. In the first place it has been shown to reduce portal blood flow[65] which among other things could have harmful effects upon albumin synthesis and the activity of the hepatic reticulo-endothelial system. Intracranial pressure rises in parallel with the mean intrathoracic pressure[66] which could give rise to cerebral oedema, and in patients with poor cardiac output, cerebral ischaemia.

Pulmonary wedge pressure measurement is frequently used as an index of left atrial function during the resuscitation of the acutely ill patient and it has been shown that this correlation is lost if PEEP is used.[67,68] The importance of pulmonary oxygen toxicity during long term ventilatory treatment is still in dispute, and the 'safe' concentration of oxygen is not really known[69,70] but it has been shown that PEEP hastens the onset of oxygen toxicity in experimental animals given 100 per cent oxygen.[71]

In spite of the conflicting nature of the evidence presented above many clinicians believe that PEEP has an important part to play in practice although it is probable that as awareness of its disadvantages grows, its place will be more rigidly defined. In any case it is vital to monitor as many aspects of the patient's response to PEEP as possible whenever it is used. The minimum number of investigations which must be performed routinely include; alveolar to arterial, arterial and mixed venous oxygen tension measurement, ideally together with the total oxygen consumption so that the tissue oxygen delivery and cardiac output can be measured; hourly urine output and urinalysis, to determine sodium excretion and glomerular filtration rate, together with scrupulous attention to fluid balance; frequent chest radiography and the measurement of the chest diameter, to facilitate the recognition of pneumothorax and progressive air trapping.

If this system of monitoring is adhered to whenever PEEP is used its true place in ventilatory treatment will soon be established.

INTERMITTENT MANDATORY VENTILATION

Many clinicians have stated that it is frequently difficult to 'wean' patients away from long term or intermediate term ventilatory treatment. Others consider that with rare exceptions, patients will gladly dispense with such treatment as soon as they are physically and psychologically ready to do so. This disagreement has resulted in the search for a method of 'weaning' patients who would otherwise remain ventilator dependent. The use of triggered ventilators was an early answer to this problem. In this system the patient was attached to a ventilator which was set to give a low but safe minute volume, and he was expected to demand more by triggering a ventilator which had either a magnetic or barometric valve governing its respiratory rate. The best triggering systems could be set to respond to either a low or high inspiratory effort, and the tidal volume which was delivered depended upon the pressure setting of the ventilator. Triggered ventilators were, in the main, a curse, because they allowed anxious patients to breathe out of phase with the ventilatory pattern selected by the observer and such patients often sounded as if they were in battle with a machine gun. The difference between triggered ventilation and intermittent mandatory ventilation (IMV) is difficult to define. In one a pre-determined low minute volume is set while the patient is expected to demand any extra he may need. In the other, the same applies. The basic difference is that IMV can be used with volume cycling ventilators. In any case weaning patients from ventilators may take time, and there is no way at present to decide whether IMV, triggered ventilation or mandatory minute volume (MMV) shortens or improves the safety and efficiency of this period.[72] Although IMV was mentioned in earlier publications it is likely that the paper by Downs and his co-workers[73] first reviewed the subject in depth. It was hoped that by designing a circuit which could produce on demand exactly the same gas mixture, tidal volume and cycling pressure as the patient had previously received by IPPV, the patient would regain his respiratory confidence and readily re-establish spontaneous ventilation. This appeared to be the case, but as mentioned earlier, the decision as to whether or not a patient is ready to breathe spontaneously is not yet a quantifiable one. The following year Downs, Block and Vennan[74] suggested that for patients with chronic obstructive airways disease the use of IMV made weaning easier than their previous method which was simply to disconnect the patient and see what happened. By 1974 Desautels and Bartlett[75] were able to review several different methods of producing IMV but still could not state an obvious indication for its use. A further modification introduced by Feeley and his colleagues[76] suggested that patients should be weaned from IPPV by way of spontaneous breathing through a circuit which included a PEEP valve.

The problem was well reviewed by Hodgkin, Bowser and Barton in 1976[77] who suggested that weaning should be by stages from controlled ventilation, via a pressure cycling ventilator with a triggered demand valve to spontaneous breathing. Halberman and co-workers[78] were of a similar opinion but in addition described a series of measurements which, they believed, allowed the observer to decide that a patient was ready for weaning. These included the patients vital capacity, which should be at least 1 litre, and the maximum force generated during inspiration against a closed system. This paper implied that patients who were ready to breathe spontaneously were recognisable clinically. No investigator has yet shown that the system of allowing a patient to breathe for a few minutes at a time while under constant supervision is any less satisfactory than the other weaning methods. Two recent papers from Northwick Park[79,80] concentrate more upon the technical than upon the practical aspects of IMV and MMV. These simply increase the confusion of the reader by failing to distinguish clearly the real advantages of IMV over triggered ventilation and MMV over controlled ventilation. Hewlett, Platt and Terry[80] make the point that mandatory minute volume is less than satisfactory if the patient has a high spontaneous respiratory rate. This was of course the major problem associated with the use of triggered ventilation. Provided that the patient knows what is expected of him, has the correct psychological preparation for it and is not under the influence of depressant drugs, he will breathe if he is able.

It is difficult not to summarise the subject by saying the evidence for the need, effect and benefits IMV and its variants has not yet been established. Hopefully work in progress may clarify this by the time the subject is next reviewed.

HIGH FREQUENCY POSITIVE PRESSURE VENTILATION (HFPPV)

The technique which is described in this section is a method of producing ventilation with positive end expiratory pressure which may have advantages over the other methods described. Like many other new techniques in anaesthesia, it is not new in conception but is in its development and assessment. High frequency positive pressure ventilation is a variant of the 'ether insufflation technique' introduced by Meltzer in 1910.[81] This had a high degree of popularity until it was ousted by the technique of endotracheal intubation which is used today. A more recent development of the technique was introduced by Sanders in 1967[82] when he described the injector device which has found such a useful place in bronchoscopy under general anaesthesia. In 1971 Jonzon and his co-workers[83] described the use of HFPPV in a series of animal experiments. Their technique consisted of the insertion of a high flow, narrow bore insufflation tube down the centre of an endotracheal tube. The flow down the insufflator was interrupted by a solenoid valve at intervals which could be varied between 55–110 times per minute and the intrathoracic pressure was controlled by a variable orifice in the side of the endotracheal tube (Fig. 7.1). They noted that satisfactory gas exchange was obtainable with fewer deleterious effects on the animals' dead space volume, blood pressure and urine output than when IPPV was used. They also stated that the incidence of atelectasis was reduced. The intrathoracic pressure was positive throughout the ventilatory cycle with HFPPV and could be varied by adjusting the expiratory valve leak. In a later series of investigations on normal animals[84] the group showed that HFPPV had fewer harmful circulatory effects than had CPAP. In 1974 Heijman and Sjöstrand[85] reported some preliminary results of treatment of patients suffering from the infant respiratory distress syndrome. They compared the use of HFPPV with CPAP in this condition and concluded that HFPPV was at least as satisfactory as CPAP from the standpoint of gas exchange and was easier to manage for the nursing staff. They stated that the treatment could be applied without the need for sedation and an additional advantage over CPAP was the facility with which tracheobronchial suction could be performed. The insufflated gas mixture was fully humidified.

The surgical treatment of tracheal lesions has always presented a major problem to the anaesthetist. Erikson and his co-workers[86] showed that with the aid of HFPPV, satisfactory operating conditions and gas exchange were achieved during the resection of a tracheal stenosis. The method entailed the passage of an endotracheal tube proximal to the stenosed area and an insufflation tube distal to it. It was possible to freely mobilise both ends of the trachea after resection of the stenosed segment and the HFPPV apparatus presented no problems.

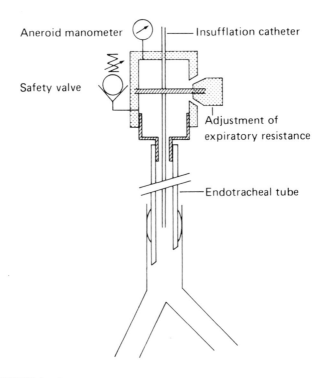

Aneroid manometer

Insufflation catheter

Safety valve

Adjustment of expiratory resistance

Endotracheal tube

Fig. 7.1   The HFPPV circuit.

Although at present this technique appears to be used in very few centres, it seems to have many advantages over existing methods and, being relatively simple to apply, deserves wider investigation and use.

VENTILATORY EQUIPMENT AS VECTORS OF INFECTION

Ventilators and anaesthetic equipment are frequently used for patients whose underlying disease and reduced resistance guarantees that sepsis will play a major part in their illness. It is not therefore surprising that such equipment has frequently been blamed for the dissemination of infection. It is probable that the first serious attempt to clarify this problem was made by Stark, Green and Pask in 1962.[87] They showed that it was very difficult to contaminate such equipment unless a massive amount of a pure growth of a pathogenic organism was deliberately introduced into it. They also showed that simple washing of tubing and expiratory valves was all that was required to achieve safety in re-use.

Later, Helliwell and co-workers[88] reviewed the theoretical and practical aspects of the problem and concluded that although they could not establish that ventilatory equipment was a source of cross infection they recommended that for safety's sake it should be sterilised between patients. Williams and his co-workers[89] reviewed the whole aspect of hospital-acquired infection and concluded that they could not incriminate ventilatory apparatus as a vector of cross infection but nevertheless were cautious in their recommendation that sterilisation of such equipment was advisable.

It was realised that the humidifier was a potential source of cross infection and Kohn[90] suggested that this and other possible infection sources should be sterilised by pasteurisation. In 1973 a naturally cautious leader in the British Medical Journal[91] concluded that although it was difficult to identify or quantitate the transfer of pulmonary sepsis through infected respiratory apparatus, this was a theoretically potent hazard and steps should be taken to prevent it. Teres and his co-workers[92] showed quite clearly that wash-hand basins and sinks were a more important cause of cross infection in a general intensive therapy unit (ITU) than ventilatory equipment. Nevertheless, the search for the ideal method of sterilising such equipment goes on. Ethylene oxide, vaporised alcohol, formalde-hyde and hydrogen peroxide are widely used.[93] Most bacteriologists believe that autoclaving presents the only complete answer to the problem, whether or not it is a real one. Holdcroft and her co-workers[94] suggested that the best way around the problem was to prevent its occurrence, with the aid of heated bacterial filters. This is an eminently sensible suggestion which has not yet been improved upon, although it may eventually turn out to be superfluous. Reviews of the potential problem by Perea and co-workers[95] and by Gaya[96] still conclude that the prevention or treatment of contamination of apparatus is desirable. Du Moulin and Saubermann[97] suggest that social cleanliness is all that is required, and the normal practice in the anaesthetic room implies that this is so. It is impossible without the use of disposable equipment to remove the risk of cross infection entirely but except in obviously contaminated cases it is probably not necessary. However, in the ITU, ventilators should either be sterilised by the least obnoxious, explosive or destructive means possible or be protected by bacterial filters from contamination. Autoclaving, the use of ethylene oxide and hydrogen peroxide aerosols are the most satisfactory choices available. In anaesthetic practice, humidifiers, external tubing and connectors must be changed between patients if there is obvious risk of cross infection (tuberculosis, bronchiectasis, staphylococcal pneumonia). In the ITU this should be done daily. All ventilatory equipment should be monitored for bacterial contamination at frequent short intervals according to a pre-determined schedule, which is rigidly adhered to.

As a postscript to this section it is interesting to note that Paegle and his co-workers[98] found that the bacterial flora of the respiratory tract and large intestine of animals which were exposed to 100 per cent oxygen for many hours was changed from a predominantly gram positive or commensal type to a pre-dominance of Pseudomonas species. The significance or otherwise of this obser-vation is at present in doubt, although it must be added to the increasing volume of data which concerns the importance of gram negative infections in critically ill patients.

CHOICE OF VENTILATORS

With so many automatic ventilators on the market the problem of selection is a difficult one. The basic requirements of a ventilator are:

1. It must be safe and reliable
2. It should give audible and visual warning of airway obstruction, power failure and disconnection
3. It should be easy to understand and use
4. Its controls should permit independent alteration of respiratory rate, tidal volume and inspiratory gas flow rate
5. It should be easily cleaned and sterilised
6. It should provide adequate humidification
7. It should be quiet and unobtrusive in use
8. It should be economical to purchase, use and maintain.

Although the requirement for short term ventilation in the operating theatre may be less stringent than those of the ITU the same general ideals should be adhered to. In many circumstances the last requirement is the overriding one as the maintenance and servicing of respiratory equipment may be a costly business.

Many users will no doubt add another requirement to those listed above, namely, that positive end-expiratory pressure valves and the facility for intermittent mandatory ventilation be added. In the large majority of cases such requirements are superfluous and in the writer's experience, simplicity, safety and reliability are much more important. During long term ventilation patients are usually under the care of nursing staff with a variable degree of mechanical expertise, and the more complicated the ventilator, the greater the bewilderment for the nurse and the danger for the patient. Each large hospital should possess at least one ventilator which can produce every conceivably desirable permutation of flow, pressure, wave form and patient demand, both for therapeutic and educational purposes, but this should be under the constant care and observation of the doctor who chooses to use it, and who must be prepared to monitor its effects in the ways outlined above.

Many anaesthetists do not use a humidifier during procedures in the operating theatre but there is evidence that they can be beneficial for the patient both by keeping his airways moistened and his cilia active, and by helping to maintain his body temperature.[99] If it is decided to add a heated humidifier to the anaesthetic machine or ventilator, it is important to determine that it is electrically safe to do so, and to ensure that the ventilator's valves are not blocked or damaged by the increased amount of water vapour in the circuit.

Tho commonest fault which arises during ventilatory therapy is disconnection in the patient circuit and a simple circuit failure alarm should be an integral part of every ventilator. It is frequently stated that alarm systems reduce the level of vigilance and lead to complacency. This may be so, but during long term treatment the attendant often has other things to do for the patient that may distract him from the ventilatory system and a moments lack of attention can have unfortunate results. The need for an alarm system is less acute in the operating theatre where the patient is under constant surveillance. Sophisticated alarms that have upper and lower pressure limits or which include a pneumotachograph are both too expensive and too temperamental for everyday use.

REFERENCES

1. Cournand, A., Motley, M., Weikö, L. & Richards, D. W. (1948) Physiological studies on the effects of intermittent positive pressure breathing on cardiac output in man. *American Journal of Physiology*, **152**, 162–167.
2. Morgan, B. C., Martin, W. E., Horrein, T. F., Crawford, E. W. & Gunteroth, W. G. (1966) Hemodynamic effects of intermittent positive pressure respiration. *Anesthesiology*, **27**, 584–590.
3. Scott, D. B., Stephen, G. W. & Davie, I. T. (1972) Haemodynamic effects of a negative (subatmospheric) pressure expiratory phase during artificial ventilation. *British Journal of Anaesthesia*, **44**, 171–174.
4. Bevan, D. R. & Gammanpilot, S. (1977) Is NEEP dead? *Anaesthesia*, **32**, 405–406.
5. Pask, E. A. (1957) Carbon dioxide homeostasis in anaesthesia. *British Medical Bulletin*, **14**, 27–30.
6. Johansson, H. (1975) Effects of different inspiratory flow patterns on thoracic compliance during respirator treatment. *Acta Anaesthesiologica Scandinavica*, **19**, 89–95.
7. Johansson, H. (1975) Effects on breathing mechanics and gas exchange of different inspiratory gas flow patterns in patients undergoing respirator treatment. *Acta Anaesthesiologica Scandinavica*, **19**, 19–27.
8. Johansson, H. & Löftström, J. B. (1975) Effects on breathing mechanics and gas exchange of different inspiratory gas flow patterns during anaesthesia. *Acta Anaesthesiologica Scandinavica*, **19**, 8–18.
9. Johansson, H. (1975) Effects of different gas flow patterns on central circulation during respirator treatment. *Acta Anaesthesiologica Scandinavica*, **19**, 96–103.
10. Bake, B., Wood, L., Murphy, B., Macklem, P. T. & Milic-Emili, J. (1974) Effect of inspiratory flow rate on regional distribution of inspired gas. *Journal of Applied Physiology*, **37**, 8–17.
11. Jones, R. L., Overton, T. R. & Sproule, B. J. (1977) Frequency dependence of ventilation distribution in normal and obstructed lungs. *Journal of Applied Physiology: Respiratory, Environmental and Exercise Physiology*, **42**, 548–553.
12. Linde, L. M., Simmons, D. H. & Ellman, E. L. (1961) Pulmonary hemodynamics during positive pressure breathing. *Journal of Applied Physiology*, **16**, 664–666.
13. Ashbaugh, D. G., Petty, T. L., Bigelow, D. B. & Harris, T. M. (1969) Continuous positive pressure breathing in the adult respiratory distress syndrome. *Journal of Thoracic and Cardiovascular Surgery*, **57**, 31–40.
14. Uzawa, T. & Ashbaugh, D. G. (1969) Continuous positive pressure breathing in acute hemorrhagic pulmonary edema. *Journal of Applied Physiology*, **26**, 427–432.
15. Ashbaugh, D. G., Bigelow, D. B., Petty, T. L. & Levine, B. E. (1967) Acute respiratory distress in adults. *Lancet*, **2**, 319–323.
16. Esteban, A., de Elio, F. S., Ancillo, P., Gomez-Acebo, E. & Cerda, E. (1973) Continuous positive pressure ventilation in the management of eight cases of pulmonary oedema. *British Journal of Anaesthesia*, **45**, 1070–1074.
17. Noble, W. H., Kay, W. C. & Obdrzalek, S. (1975) Lung mechanics in hypervolemic pulmonary edema. *Journal of Applied Physiology*, **38**, 681–687.
18. Obdrzalek, J., Kay, J. C. & Noble, W. H. (1975) The effects of continuous positive pressure ventilation on pulmonary oedema: gas exchange and lung mechanics. *Canadian Anaesthetists' Society Journal*, **22**, 399–409.
19. Dueck, R., Wagner, P. D. & West, J. B. (1977) Effects of positive and expiratory pressure on gas exchange in dogs with normal and edematous lungs. *Anesthesiology*, **47**, 359–366.
20. Caldini, P., Leith, J. D. & Brennan, M. J. (1975) Effect of continuous positive pressure ventilation (CPPV) on edema formation in dog lung. *Journal of Applied Physiology*, **39**, 672–679.
21. Shirley, H. H., Wolfram, C. G., Wasserman, K. & Mayerson, H. S. (1957) Capillary permeability to macromolecules: stretched pore phenomenon. *American Journal of Physiology*, **190**, 189–193.
22. McIntyre, R. W., Laws, A. K. & Ramachandran, P. R. (1969) Positive expiratory pressure plateau: improved gas exchange during mechanical ventilation. *Canadian Anaesthetists' Society Journal*, **16**, 477–480.

23. Don, H. F., Craig, D. B., Wahba, W. M. & Canture, J. G. (1971) The measure of gas trapped in the lungs at FRC and the effects of posture. *Anesthesiology*, **35**, 582–586.

24. Craig, D. B. & McCarthy, D. S. (1972) Airway closure and lung volumes during breathing at maintained airway positive pressure. *Anesthesiology*, **36**, 540–543.

25. Alexander, J. I., Spence, A. A., Parikh, R. K. & Stuart, B. (1973) The role of airway closure in post-operative hypoxaemia. *British Journal of Anaesthesia*, **45**, 34–40.

26. Laver, M. B., Morgan, J., Bendixen, H. H. & Radford, E. P. (1964) Lung volume, compliance and arterial oxygen tensions during controlled ventilation. *Journal of Applied Physiology*, **19**, 725–733.

27. Bendixen, H. H., Hedley Whyte, J. & Laver, M. B. (1965) Impaired oxygenation in surgical patients during general anaesthesia with controlled ventilation: A concept of atelactasis. *New England Journal of Medicine*, **269**, 991–996.

28. Hedley Whyte, J., Laver, M. B. & Bendixen, H. H. (1964) Effects of changes in tidal ventilation on physiological shunting. *American Journal of Physiology*, **206**, 891–896.

29. Nunn, J. F., Bergman, N. A. & Coleman, A. J. (1965) Factors influencing the arterial oxygen tension during anaesthesia with artificial ventilation. *British Journal of Anaesthesia*, **37**, 898–914.

30. Hedley Whyte, J., Pontoppidan, H. & Morris, M. J. (1966) The relationship of alveolar to tidal ventilation during respiratory failure in man. *Anesthesiology*, **27**, 218–219.

31. Eiseman, B. & Ashbaugh, D. (1968) Pulmonary effects of non-thoracic trauma. *Journal of Trauma*, **8**, 899–911.

32. Dowd, J. & Jenkins, L. C. (1972) The lung in shock: a review. *Canadian Anaesthetists' Society Journal*, **19**, 309–316.

33. Downes, J. J. (1976) CPAP and PEEP: a perspective. *Anesthesiology*, **44**, 1–5.

34. Stokke, D. B. (1976) Review: artificial ventilation with positive and expiratory pressure (PEEP). *European Journal of Intensive Care Medicine*, **2**, 77–85.

35. Gilston, A. (1978) The effects of PEEP on arterial oxygenation. *Intensive Care Medicine*, **3**, 267–271.

36. Colgan, F. J., Barrow, R. & Fanning, G. (1971) Constant positive pressure breathing and cardiorespiratory function. *Anesthesiology*, **34**, 145–151.

37. Philbin, D. M., Patterson, R. W. & Baratz, R. A. (1972) Continuous positive pressure ventilation and oxygen delivery. *British Journal of Anaesthesia*, **44**, 667–670.

38. Colgan, F. J., Barrow, R. E., Fanning, G. L. & Marocco, P. P. (1972) The cardiorespiratory effects of constant and intermittent positive pressure breathing. *Anesthesiology*, **36**, 344–349.

39. Suter, P. M., Fairley, H. B. & Isenberg, M. D. (1975) Optimum end expiratory airway pressure in patients with acute respiratory failure. *New England Journal of Medicine*, **292**, 284–289.

40. Civetta, J. M., Bares, T. A. & Smith, L. O. (1975) Optimal PEEP and intermittent mandatory ventilation in the treatment of acute pulmonary failure. *Respiratory Care*, **20**, 551.

41. Civetta, J. M., Flor, R. J. & Smith, L. O. (1976) Aggressive treatment of acute respiratory insufficiency. *Southern Medical Journal*, **69**, 749–751.

42. Colgan, F. J., Nichols, F. A. & De Weese, J. A. (1974) Positive end expiratory pressure, oxygen transport and the low output state. *Anesthesia and Analgesia; Current Researches*, **53**, 538–543.

43. Quist, J., Pontoppidan, H., Wilson, R. S., Loewenstein, E. & Laver, M. B. (1975) Hemodynamic responses to mechanical ventilation with PEEP: the effect of hypovolaemia. *Anesthesiology*, **42**, 45–53.

44. Vissick, W. D., Fairley, H. B. & Hickey, R. F. (1973) The effects of tidal volume and end-expiratory pressure on pulmonary gas exchange during anaesthesia. *Anesthesiology*, **39**, 285–289.

45. Aalto-Setälä, M., Hleinonen, J., & Salorine, Y. (1975) Cardiothoracic function during thoracic anaesthesia: a comparison of two lung ventilation and one lung ventilation with and without PEEP. *Acta Anaesthesiologica Scandinavica*, **19**, 287–295.

46. Bulhain, W. J., Brody, J. S. & Fischer, A. B. (1972) Effect of artificial airway obstruction on elastic properties of the lung. *Journal of Applied Physiology*, **33**, 589–593.

47. Wyszogrodski, I., Kyei-Aboagye, K., Taensch, H. W. J. & Avery, M. E. (1975) Surfactant inactivation by hyperventilation: conservation by end expiratory pressure. *Journal of Applied Physiology*, **38**, 461–466.

48. Inkster, J. S. (1976) Paediatric anaesthesia and intensive care. *Recent Advances in Anaesthesia 12.* Eds. Langton Hewer, C. and Atkinson, R. S., p. 77. Edinburgh: Churchill Livingstone.

49. Corbet, A. J. S., Ross, J. A., Beandry, P. H. & Stern, L. (1975) Effect of positive pressure breathing on ADN_2 in hyaline membrane disease. *Journal of Applied Physiology*, **38**, (1) 33–38.

50. Stevens, P. M. (1976) The effect of continuous positive pressure on survival of patients with refractory hypoxaemia. *Bulletin of European Respiratory Physiopathology*, **12**, 125–131.

51. Stahlman, M., Shepherd, F. M., Young, W. C., Grey, J. & Blankenship, W. (1966) Assessment of the cardiovascular status of infants with hyaline membrane disease; in, *The Heart and Circulation in the Newborn and Infant.* Ed. Cassells, D. E. p. 121–129. Chicago, Grune and Stratton.

52. West, J. B. (1974) Blood flow to the lungs and gas exchange. *Anesthesiology*, **41**, 124–138.
53. Sugerman, H. J., Rogers, R. M. & Miller, L. D. (1972) Positive end expiratory pressure: indication and physiological considerations. *Chest*, **62**, 86–93.
54. Esteban, A., de Elio, F. J., Cerda, E., Gomez-Acebo, E. & Ancillo, P. (1974) Blood gas changes with different end expiratory pressures in patients with chronic bronchitis. *British Journal of Anaesthesia*, **46**, 159–164.
55. Ashbaugh, D. G. & Petty, T. L. (1973) Positive end expiratory pressure: physiology indications and contraindications. *Journal of Thoracic and Cardiovascular Surgery*, **65**, 165–172.
56. McMahon, S. M., Halprin, G. M. & Sieker, H. O. (1973) Positive end expiratory pressure in severe arterial hypoxemia. *American Review of Respiratory Disease*, **108**, 526–532.
57. Kumar, A., Falke, K. S., Geffin, B., Aldredge, C. F., Laver, M. B., Loewenstein, E. & Pontoppidan, H. (1970) Continuous positive pressure ventilation in acute respiratory failure. *New England Journal of Medicine*, **283**, 1430–1436.
58. Kumar, A., Pontoppidan, H., Falke, K. S., Wilson, R. S. & Laver, M. B. (1973) Pulmonary barotrauma during mechanical ventilation. *Critical Care Medicine*, **1**, 181–186.
59. Kao, D. K. & Tierney, D. F. (1977) Air embolism with positive pressure ventilation of rats. *Journal of Applied Physiology; Respiratory Environmental and Excercise Physiology*, **42**, 368–371.
60. Drury, D. R., Henry, J. P. & Goodman, J. (1947) The effects of continuous pressure breathing on kidney function. *Journal of Clinical Investigation*, **26**, 945–951.
61. Sladen, A., Laver, M. B. & Pontoppidan, H. (1968) Pulmonary complications and water retention in prolonged mechanical ventilation. *New England Journal of Medicine*, **279**, 448–451.
62. Pontoppidan, H., Geffin, B. C. & Loewenstein, E. (1972) Acute respiratory failure in the adult. *New England Journal of Medicine*, **287**, 690–697.
63. Hale, S. V., Johnson, E. E. & Hedley Whyte, J. (1974) Renal hemodynamics and function with continuous positive pressure ventilation in dogs. *Anesthesiology*, **41**, 452–457.
64. Baratz, R. A., Philbin, D. M. & Patterson, R. W. (1977) Plasma antidiuretic hormone and urinary output during continuous positive pressure breathing in dogs. *Anesthesiology*, **34**, 510–513.
65. Johnson, E. E. & Hedley Whyte, J. (1972) Continuous positive pressure ventilation and portal flow in dogs with pulmonary edema. *Journal of Applied Physiology*, **33**, 385–390.
66. Aidinis, S. J., Lafferty, J. & Shapiro, H. M. (1976) Intracranial responses to PEEP. *Anesthesiology*, **45**, 275–281.
67. Lozman, J., Powers, S. R., Older, T., Dutton, R. E., Roy, R. S., English, M., Marco, M. & Eckert, C. (1974) Correlation of pulmonary wedge and left atrial pressures. *Archives of Surgery*, **109**, 270–274.
68. Kane, P. B., Man, R. L., Ashkenazi, J., Neville, J. F., Hanson, E. L. & Webb, R. W. (1976) The effects of PEEP and left atrial pressure on the correlation between pulmonary artery wedge pressure and left atrial pressure. *British Journal of Anaesthesia*, **48**, 272–276.
69. Pratt, P. P. (1974) Pathology of pulmonary oxygen toxicity. *American Review of Respiratory Diseases*, **110**, 54–63.
70. Sevitt, S. (1974) Threshold for oxygen pneumonitis. *Journal of Clinical Pathology*, **27**, 21–29.
71. Liland, A. E., Zapol, W. M., Quist, J., Nash, G., Skoskiewitch, M., Pontoppidan, H., Lowenstein, E. & Laver, M. B. (1976) Positive airway pressure in lambs spontaneously breathing air and oxygen. *Journal of Surgical Research*, **20**, 85–92.
72. Feeley, T. W. & Hedley Whyte, J. (1975) Weaning from controlled ventilation and supplemental oxygen. *New England Journal of Medicine*, **292**, 903–906.
73. Downs, J. B., Klein, E. F., Desautels, D., Modell, J. H. & Kirby, R. R. (1973) Intermittent mandatory ventilation: a new approach to weaning patients from mechanical ventilators. *Chest*, **64**, 331–339.
74. Downs, J. B., Block, A. J. & Vennum, K. B. (1974) Intermittent mandatory ventilation in the treatment of patients with chronic obstructive pulmonary disease. *Anesthesia and Analgesia; Current Researches*, **53**, 437–439.
75. Desautels, D. & Bartlett, J. L. (1974) Methods of administering intermittent mandatory ventilation (IMV). *Respiratory Care*, **19**, 187–192.
76. Feeley, T. W., Saumaurez, R., Klick, J. M., McNabb, T. G. & Stillmann, J. J. (1975) Positive end expiratory pressure in weaning patients from controlled ventilation. *Lancet*, **2**, 725.
77. Hodgkin, J. E., Bowser, M. A. & Burton, G. G. (1976) Respiratory weaning, from; *The Lung in the Critically Ill Patient*, Ed. Shoemaker, W. C. pp. 105–109. Baltimore. Williams and Wilkins.
78. Hilberman, M., Kamm, B., Lamy, M., Dietrich, H. P., Martz, K. & Osborne, J. J. (1976) An analysis of potential physiological predictors of respiratory adequacy following cardiac surgery. *Journal of Thoracic and Cardiovascular Surgery*, **71**, 711–720.
79. Lawler, P. G. P. & Nunn, J. F. (1977) Intermittent mandatory ventilation. *Anaesthesia*, **32**, 138–147.

80. Hewlett, A. M., Platt, A. S. & Terry, V. G. (1977) Mandatory minute volume. *Anaesthesia*, **32,** 163–169.
81. Meltzer, S. J. (1910) The method of respiration by intra-tracheal insufflation, its practical availability in medicine and surgery. *Medical Record*, **77,** 477–489.
82. Sanders, R. D. (1967) Two ventilating attachments for bronchoscopes. *Delaware Medical Journal*, **39,** 170–174.
83. Jonzon, A., Oberg, P. A., Sedin, G. & Sjöstrand, U. (1971) High frequency positive pressure ventilation by endotracheal insufflation. *Acta Anaesthesiologica Scandinavica* Suppl. **43,** 1–43.
84. Jonzon, A., Sedin, G. & Sjöstrand, U. (1973) High frequency positive pressure ventilation (HFPPV) applied to small lung ventilation and compared with spontaneous respiration and continuous positive airway pressure (CPAP) *Acta Anaesthesiologica Scandinavica* Suppl. **53,** 25–36.
85. Heijman, K. & Sjöstrand, U. (1974) Treatment of the respiratory distress syndrome—a preliminary report. *Opuscula Medica*, **19,** 235–244.
86. Eriksson, I., Nilsson, L. G., Nordstrom, S. & Sjöstrand, U. (1975) High frequency positive pressure ventilation (HFPPV) during transthoracic resection of tracheal stenosis and during pre-operative bronchoscopic examination. *Acta Anaesthesiologica Scandinavica*, **19,** 113–119.
87. Stark, D. C. C., Green, C. A. & Pask, E. A. (1962) Anaesthetic machines and cross infection. *Anaesthesia*, **17,** 12–17.
88. Helliwell, P. J., Laws, M. E., Newman, T. H. & Williams, S. R. (1965) The cleaning, disinfecting and sterilising of anaesthetic equipment at Guys Hospital. *Anaesthesia*, **20,** 334–339.
89. Williams, S. R., Blowers, R., Garrod, L. P. & Spooter, R. A. (1966) Hospital Infection. London. Lloyd Luke 2nd Ed.
90. Kohn, J. (1970) A waste trap sterilising method. *Lancet*, **2,** 550–552.
91. Leading Article (1973) Disinfecting ventilators. *British Medical Journal*, **1,** 625.
92. Teres, D., Schweers, P., Bushnell, L. S., Hedley Whyte, J. & Feingold, D. S. (1973) Sources of Pseudomonas aeruginosa infection in a respiratory/surgical intensive therapy unit. *Lancet*, **1,** 415–417.
93. Stoddart, J. C. (1973) Gram negative infections in the ICU. *Critical Care Medicine*, **2,** 17–22.
94. Holdcroft, A., Lumley, J. & Gaya, H. (1973) Why disinfect ventilators? *Lancet*, **1,** 240–241.
95. Perea, E. J., Criado, A., Moreno, M. & Avello, F. (1975) Mechanical ventilators as vehicles of infection. *Acta Anaesthesiologica Scandinavica*, **19,** 180–186.
96. Gaya, H. (1976) Infection control in intensive care. *British Journal of Anaesthesia*, **48,** 9–14.
97. du Moulin, G. C. & Saubermann, A. J. (1977) The anesthesia machine and circle system are not likely to be sources of bacterial contamination. *Anesthesiology*, **47,** 353–358.
98. Paegle, R. D., Tewarin, R. P., Bernhard, W. N. & Peters, E. (1975) Microbial flora of the larynx, trachea and large intestine of the rat after long term inhalation of 100 per cent oxygen. *Anesthesiology*, **44,** 287–290.
99. Lewis, D. G. & Mackenzie, A. (1972) Cooling during major vascular surgery. *British Journal of Anaesthesia*, **44,** 859–864.

8. Monitoring

C. B. Franklin

A comprehensive review of advances in monitoring is beyond the capacity of a single author and certainly could not be encompassed in the space of a few pages. For these reasons the content of this chapter is restricted to a review of the contemporary 'state of the art' as seen through the eyes of the author and some observations on the application of computers in patient monitoring routines.

The term monitoring, which is derived from the Latin transitive verb moneo, embraces a wide range of activities connected with the detection of change and the prediction of events. In a clinical sense it is normally associated with the collection of information in order to assess function and also to give warning of life threatening situations. It includes clinical assessment, instrumental measurement of physiological variables, laboratory investigations, and in some instances procedures involving the use of X-ray apparatus or other equipment which can only be used in specially designed accommodation. However, the activities which are of immediate interest are instrumental measurement of physiological variables carried out during the course of treatment in an intensive care unit or throughout the administration of an anaesthetic, and those aspects of data handling associated with the derivation of indices of function or the assembly of related items of information as an aid to the recognition of trends.

A monitor is an instrument which is connected to a patient in order to *detect and measure* change in physiological variables with facilities to display measurements either as a meter reading or as a waveform. Also, it should have a built in alarm mechanism which can be set by the user and a number of socket outlets to permit connection to recording apparatus or to a computer and in some instances for the transmission of signals to remote display equipment. Patient connection is made by sensors applied directly to the patient or through a transducer which is connected to the patient by means of a fluid or gas filled tube. And in order to measure parameters such as core temperature, direct intravascular and extradural pressure, an invasive procedure has to be performed in order to make the necessary connection.

The function of a monitor is to convert small electrical signals produced by the patient or arising from changes in the sensing device into measurements or waveforms which can be readily understood and used by the clinician in the immediate care of the patient. The majority of instrumental monitoring routines are concerned with the assessment of the function of the circulation as a transport system. Indeed with a few notable exceptions the use of monitoring instruments is confined to the measurement of parameters which are used in the assessment of those physiological processes which collectively make up the oxygen pathway from the atmosphere to the tissues and in particular those functions which are concerned with the transfer of oxygen in the lungs and the distribution of oxygenated blood to the tissues.

A monitoring system may be no more than a single instrument along with the appropriate sensing device or patient connection. More commonly, however, it is made up of a selection of equipment mounted in a suitable console (Fig. 8.1) which may be linked to a secondary display situated at a distance from the patient or connected on-line to a computer.

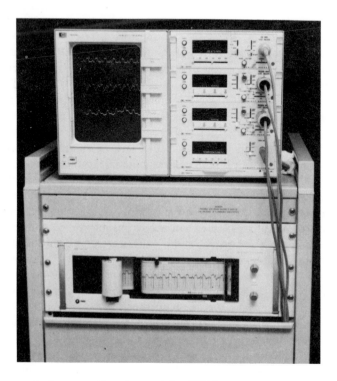

Fig. 8.1   *Mobile monitoring system.* Console containing ECG/heart rate, temperature, arterial and venous pressure, modules and four channel oscilloscope, mounted on a trolley with a built-in single channel recorder. (Hewlett Packard)

The increased employment of instrumental monitoring techniques in recent years is the result of the development of simple reliable instruments which will stand up to the rigours of prolonged use in a busy intensive care unit or operating theatre suite and also because of the introduction of new methods of treatment which can only be carried out safely when vital processes are being kept under close observation. The most important recent innovations in monitoring routines have been the application of Doppler ultrasound techniques for the measurement of systemic arterial blood pressure, the introduction of the flow-directed balloon-tipped pulmonary artery catheter,[1] and the development of small high speed analogue-digital computers.

The benefits of instrumental monitoring routines are the ability to obtain information which cannot be measured in any other way and reduction of demands on nursing staff when frequent recording of measurements is necessary. Also, monitoring instruments can be useful as warning devices when used under carefully controlled conditions.

PLANNING MONITORING ROUTINES

Monitoring is based on *careful detailed interpretation of a limited number of measurements* and the important decisions to be made when planning monitoring routines are deciding *what* is to be measured and *how* the measurements are to be made.

From the practical standpoint monitoring can be divided into making measurements for the immediate control of treatment and the derivation of indices of function using standard formulae to allow a more detailed analysis of the condition of the patient. The choice of measurements will be influenced by the experience of the individual clinician, the measuring instruments available, and the possible risks to the patient of any associated invasive procedures. In the majority of instances sufficient information can be obtained by clinical assessment making full use of the five senses and simple monitoring aids. However, in the management of patients with cardiac disease who are undergoing major surgery or in seriously ill patients with multiple medical disorders, even in the absence of cardiac disease, satisfactory control of treatment is only possible with more elaborate monitoring routines. In such circumstances it may be necessary to monitor a comprehensive selection of *circulatory*, *respiratory*, and *metabolic* parameters at least until the immediate danger to the patient has passed.

Monitoring the circulation

The correct distribution of oxygenated blood to the tissues depends on adequate circulating blood volume, optimal cardiac performance, and normal peripheral vascular resistance.

On *most* occasions the ECG, systemic arterial blood pressure, and clinical assessment of tissue perfusion provide sufficient information to assess the circulation. A more detailed analysis requires measurement of right and left heart pressures, cardiac output determination, estimation of arterial and mixed venous blood gases, and haemoglobin estimation. Information obtained from these measurements combined with surface area can then be used for the derivation of indices of right and left ventricular stroke work, pulmonary and systemic vascular resistance, oxygen availability and oxygen consumption.

Heart rhythm and rate

Measurement of the electrical activity of the heart forms the basis of dysrhythmia detection and in the majority of instances it is also used for the instrumental measurement of heart rate. Peripheral pulse monitors based on detection of alterations in the intensity of light reaching a photoelectric cell are also used for measurement of heart rate but they tend to be unreliable when the blood pressure is low even when local hyperaemia is produced at the site of attachment.

The use of the ECG to observe heart activity is normally based on a single lead system using self adhesive electrodes placed in positions on the chest wall which permit easy application of defibrillator paddles in an emergency and the electrodes are connected to the monitor by wires. The quality of the ECG signal depends on the siting of the electrodes, the removal of grease from the skin with ether, methylated spirit, and the use of conducting jelly or paste to ensure good electrical contact. Difficulties in maintaining electrodes in position for long periods of time due to perspiration reducing the effectiveness of the adhesive can be a source of irritation to staff and frequent detachment of electrodes can undermine confidence in ECG alarm systems. A more or less satisfactory alternative for use during anaesthetics is a dry back plate electrode which can be inserted under the patient, but when the quality of the ECG display is important for the safety of the anaesthetised patient it is preferable to use needle electrodes.

ECG display is an integral part of most monitoring systems and in coronary care units the heart activity is frequently the only parameter which is monitored. In these units amplified signals are usually relayed to a multichannel oscilloscope and automatic dysrhythmia detection instruments at a central station where one nurse can observe several traces without disturbing the patients. Central monitoring stations have no practical value in other types of intensive care unit because patients in such units usually require close supervision and the information is normally *only* needed at the bedside.

Visual inspection of the individual ECG complex has been made easier since the introduction of oscilloscopes with storing or freezing options and it is hoped that computer based techniques for automatic dysrhythmia detection which are being evaluated will improve the arrangements for long term monitoring of heart activity in coronary care units. Heart rate is usually displayed as a meter reading but some of the newer oscilloscopes incorporate a speedometer type bar graph display (Fig. 8.2).

Blood pressures

Systemic arterial blood pressure is a valuable index of cardiac output and peripheral vascular resistance. *On most occasions* this measurement can be made by an indirect method, but when frequent readings are required either because of persistent hypotension or when sudden changes are taking place direct measurement using an intravascular pressure line is often essential.

Central venous pressure is widely used as an index of circulating blood volume and also of cardiac performance. However, the usefulness of this measurement is limited because it basically reflects the function of the right ventricle, which in some circumstances does not parallel the function of the left ventricle,[2,3] and for this reason *it cannot be assumed at all times* that the central venous pressure is an accurate measure of either circulating blood volume or cardiac performance. In the normal heart there is little difference between right and left atrial pressures, but in the presence of left ventricular failure and in certain dysrhythmias when atrio-ventricular blood flow is altered there may be a difference of 1.3 to 2.7 kPa (10 to 20 mmHg). In these circumstances it is only possible to assess cardiac performance with information about the filling pressure of the left ventricle. Direct measurement of left atrial pressure is possible during cardiac surgery and is a valuable guide when restoring blood volume or administering inotropic drugs after cardiopulmonary by-pass. However, when direct access to the left atrium is not possible pulmonary artery wedge pressure, which usually *approximates closely* to the left atrial pressure,[4] is a reliable index of left ventricular function. Central venous and pulmonary artery wedge pressure can only be measured by a direct method using an intravascular pressure line.

Indirect measurement of systemic arterial blood pressure is based on inflation and slow release of a cuff or multiple cuffs applied to the arm to permit detection of changes due to blood flow in the brachial artery. Methods of indirect blood pressure measurement have been classified into four types:[5]

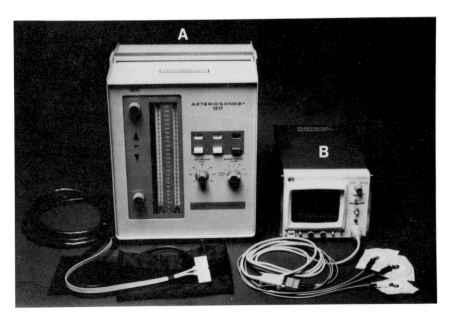

Fig. 8.2   *Non-invasive instruments for monitoring the circulation.* Arteriosonde blood pressure monitor (A) measures blood pressure automatically at intervals pre-set by the user and displays systolic and diastolic pressure as a mercury level in a graduated column. (Roche-Kontron). Cardiac monitor (B) provides continuous display of ECG waveform and heart rate. (Hewlett Packard)

1. Oscillotonometry in the lumen of the cuff(s)
2. Auscultation of the sounds under the cuff(s)
3. Detection of arterial wall movements under the cuff(s)
4. Detection of the onset of flow beyond the cuff(s).

Most of the indirect methods of measuring blood pressure are satisfactory when making measurements on healthy volunteers but are unreliable when the blood pressure is low and when the patient is restless. A most promising method of indirect blood pressure measurement based on the detection of movement of the brachial artery wall using the technique of Doppler ultrasound (Fig. 8.2) has been introduced in recent years. This method is particularly useful in the management of infants and neonates and also in situations when the blood pressure is very low. Blood pressures measured by this method tend to underestimate systolic pressure and to exceed diastolic pressure by 0 to 1.3 kPa (0 to 10 mmHg) when compared with direct intra-arterial pressure measurements[6] and whilst the method is susceptible to artefacts due to muscle movement it is often reliable even under difficult conditions.

Direct blood pressure measurement is accomplished by the introduction of a cannula or catheter into the appropriate position in the circulation and connecting it to a *calibrated* pressure measuring system. The development of reliable low displacement transducers has made it possible to obtain satisfactory pressure measurements through small bore fluid filled lines which can be introduced into the circulation without causing significant damage to blood vessels or the surrounding tissues. Systemic arterial pressure is normally measured through a short cannula located in a radial artery; central venous pressure is measured through a cannula introduced into the circulation via a basilic, subclavian, or internal jugular vein, when the tip is located in the superior vena cava in the region of the right atrium; and pulmonary artery wedge pressure is measured through the main lumen of a flow-directed balloon-tipped pulmonary artery catheter when the tip is located in a wedge position. With practice, systemic arterial and central venous pressure lines can be introduced percutaneously in the majority of patients, including small children. However, the flow-directed balloon-tipped pulmonary artery catheter is a somewhat different proposition and whilst it can be introduced with comparative ease using a modified Seldinger technique many are deterred from using it because of its size.

The most useful version of the flow-directed balloon-tipped pulmonary artery catheter is the *triple lumen monitoring catheter*.[7] The main lumen terminates at the catheter tip, the second lumen communicates with the balloon, and the third lumen terminates either 20 or 30 cm proximal to the tip depending on the model. The balloon when fully inflated has a capacity of 1.5 ml and a diameter of 13 mm. The introduction of the catheter and placement of the tip must be carried out with continuous display of the ECG and dynamic pressure waveform. The widest diameter of this catheter when the balloon is deflated is 2.6 mm and it can be readily introduced into the circulation via a vein normally used for inserting central venous pressure lines using a 3 mm percutaneous catheter introducer. When the catheter tip is in the vicinity of the right atrium the balloon is inflated to the recommended volume and the catheter is then advanced through the right heart and pulmonary artery following its progress by observing the pressure waveform display. Once a satisfactory wedge position is achieved the balloon is deflated and *only* reinflated during measurement of pulmonary artery wedge pressure (Fig. 8.3). Particular care should be taken when reinflating the balloon because if wedging occurs before the recommended volume of gas is introduced the catheter has probably advanced into a smaller vessel and needs to be repositioned. This catheter when correctly positioned can be used to provide continuous *display of right atrial and pulmonary artery pressure*, for *measurement of pulmonary artery wedge pressure*, and for the *withdrawal of samples of mixed venous blood* from the pulmonary artery. When it is not possible to obtain a satisfactory wedge position pulmonary artery end-diastolic pressure which approximates closely to mean left atrial pressure, provided that pulmonary vascular resistance is not raised, is a reliable index of left heart performance.[8,9] Complications associated with this procedure include pulmonary artery thrombosis[10,11,12] and the use of this catheter should be restricted to the acute phase of treatment.

The greatest amount of information is obtained from blood pressure monitoring when measurements are made with *calibrated* transducers connected to pressure monitors and an oscilloscope. Such systems display measurements as meter readings and dynamic pressure waveforms which can provide valuable information about the functional state of the heart. If there is not sufficient electronic equipment available mean blood pressure measurement can be readily accomplished, once the pressure lines are positioned correctly, using a suitable aneroid gauge connected to the cannula or catheter by means of a sterile hydraulic system. Mean central venous, pulmonary artery, and pulmonary artery wedge pressure can be measured, and often is, using a water manometer connected directly to the pressure line.

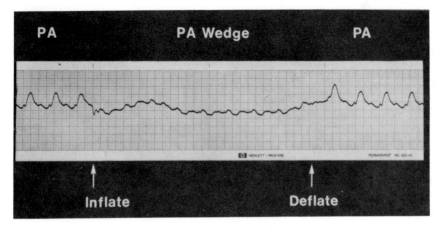

Fig. 8.3   Waveform changes during pulmonary artery wedge pressure measurement

Blood pressure should be quoted in terms of *pressure above the heart.* Zero calibration of transducers and all subsequent pressure measurement should be carried out with the transducer diaphragm set at a fixed reference level, normally taken as the mid-axillary line or 100 mm above the surface of the operating table with the patient supine.[13,14] A similar procedure should be employed when using an aneroid pressure gauge or a water manometer. This can be readily accomplished by attaching the transducer holder, pressure gauge, or water manometer stand, to a pole with a locking clamp to allow the system to be moved up or down as required. Correct alignment can be checked using a joiner's spirit level held between the appropriate point on the measuring system and the reference level or by means of a 'gunsight' device attached to the locking clamp. An alternative arrangement is to use an adjustable transducer holder which can be secured to the operating table (Fig. 8.4). Transducers need to be calibrated before use preferably by the application of a known pressure to the pressure measuring system. The quality of pressure measurements depends on the avoidance of leaks or air bubbles in pressure lines, intermittent flushing of arterial cannulae with *small* volumes of heparinised Ringer-lactate solution, and continuous *slow* infusion of heparinised 5 per cent dextrose in water through centrally placed pressure lines. Damping of arterial pressure waveform due to arterial spasm may be eliminated by injection of small volumes (0.5 ml up to a total of 2 ml) of papaverine (30 mg diluted in 5 ml of Ringer-lactate solution) through the arterial line.

Patient safety. Patient safety during continuous direct pressure measurement depends on an awareness of the possible complications associated with the long term use of intravascular pressure lines, which may be divided into those related to the patient connection and mishaps which result from harmful effects of electrically operated equipment. The main problems associated with the patient connection are:

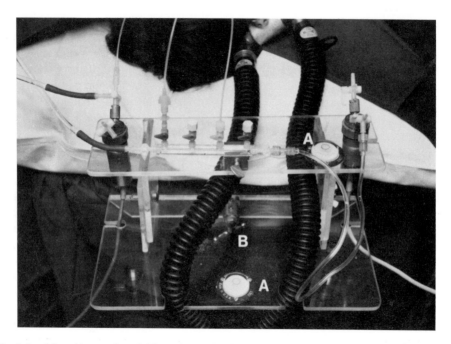

Fig. 8.4 *Adjustable transducer holder and tap table.* The transducer holder is secured to a two-section base plate held between the mattress and table top which permits height adjustment and correction for rotation of the operating table. Alignment of the transducers to the reference point is carried out when the spirit levels (A) indicate that the operating table and transducer holder are both horizontal. Correction for lateral tilting of the patient during the operation can be made by releasing locking clamp (B) and restoring the transducer heads to the horizontal plane

1. Infection resulting from careless technique during insertion of pressure lines and from their prolonged use
2. Embolism due to thrombus, air, or severed portions of pressure lines
3. Cardiac depression or arrest due to administration of cold blood or injection of undiluted drugs through central venous pressure lines
4. Tissue necrosis following arterial cannulation.

The harmful effects arising from the use of electrical equipment are electrocution, surface burns, and ventricular fibrillation due to mains leakage currents.

Complications arising from the patient connection can be kept to a minimum by taking meticulous care during the insertion and subsequent management of intravascular pressure lines. The cannulae or catheters should be introduced under *aseptic* conditions, and in the case of centrally placed pressure lines or when insertion is to be performed using a cut-down technique the procedure should be carried out with full sterile precautions. Once the pressure line is correctly placed it should be secured to the skin with a stitch and after the application of an aerosol preparation containing neomycin to the puncture site the area should be covered with a sterile dressing which should be changed daily. The position of the tip of centrally placed pressure lines should be checked by chest X-ray as soon as possible after insertion so that adjustment can be carried out if necessary, and to exclude complications such as pneumothorax and haemothorax. Blood sampling should be performed through a tap situated clear of dressings applied to the puncture site. When it is proposed to use central venous pressure lines for administration of blood, fluids, or drugs, a short extension with a two way tap should be included in the line to enable connection of infusion sets and injection of drugs to be carried out away from the region of the puncture site. Tissue necrosis can be largely avoided when arterial cannulation is carried out *only* if it can be established that there is a satisfactory collateral blood supply to the area distal to the proposed puncture site and by restricting the use of these pressure lines to the acute phase of treatment.

The harmful effects arising from the use of electrical equipment can be largely avoided by ensuring that instruments are in a safe condition to use and when maintenance is carried out by electronics technicians employed by the hospital. Arrangements should be made for *regular safety testing* along the lines set out in the DHSS Safety Code for Electro-Medical Apparatus.[15] Also, because of the risk of ventricular fibrillation being caused by currents of less than 100 μA when there is a direct connection to the heart via a catheter,[16] it is essential to ensure that the patient connection in mains powered apparatus is *earth free* when possible. Ideally electrical apparatus which is connected to patients should have built in warning devices to draw attention to high mains leakage currents and to faults in the isolation circuit. On those occasions when earth free connection is not possible all electrical apparatus connected to the patient should share a common earth to which the patient is also linked through the indifferent electrode of the diathermy apparatus. If only one instrument is to be connected to the patient ideally this should be battery operated.

Cardiac output
The recent introduction of the flow-directed balloon-tipped thermodilution pulmonary artery catheter and thermodilution cardiac output computers (Fig. 8.5) removed the main problems associated with the determination of cardiac output in everyday clinical situations.

Determination of cardiac output by the thermodilution method[7] is based on the injection of a known volume of cold indicator (10 ml of 5 per cent dextrose in water) into the right atrium and measurement of the blood-indicator temperature in the pulmonary artery. The whole procedure from injection of indicator to the display of the calculated cardiac output takes 15 to 20 seconds. The accuracy of this method is determined by the accuracy with which the volume and temperature of the indicator is known and the temperature of the blood-indicator mixture in the pulmonary artery which may be influenced by variations in the temperature of the blood returning to the heart. The main factor giving rise to variations in the temperature of blood reaching the heart which may affect the results of cardiac output determination by this method is fluctuation in venous return from different parts of the body due to changes in intrathoracic pressure associated with respiration. Studies comparing the thermodilution method with the Fick method and the dye dilution method of determining cardiac output have demonstrated a statistically significant correlation between these three methods.[17]

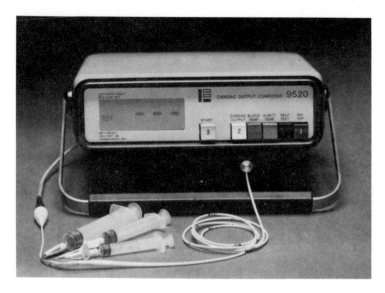

Fig. 8.5 *Instruments for monitoring cardiac output.* Swan Ganz thermodilution catheter (triple lumen flow-directed balloon-tipped pulmonary artery catheter with built-in thermistor located 4 cm proximal to catheter tip) and cardiac output computer. (Edwards Laboratories)

Tissue perfusion

The most useful indicators of tissue perfusion when the patient is unconscious are measurement of urinary output, temperature difference between the core (rectum, oesophagus, and nasopharynx) and a peripheral site (toe or somatic muscle) and brain activity.

There is usually some delay between changes in blood flow and significant alteration in temperature gradients between the core and the periphery, and in the presence of kidney disease measurement of urinary output is only of limited value as an index of tissue perfusion. However, brain activity is both a sensitive and reliable indicator of this function.

The development of the Cerebral Function Monitor (Fig. 8.6) by Maynard[18] has made it possible to obtain a satisfactory *recording of the electrical activity of the brain* without sophisticated equipment and skilled technical help. This instrument detects brain activity by means of two silver/silver chloride surface electrodes or two platinum needle electrodes which are connected to the patient in the

shunt (Qs/Qt) using the shunt equation. Estimation of right to left shunting in the pulmonary circulation can be of considerable help in assessing the need for mechanical ventilation of the lungs, particularly in the management of chest injuries.

Measurement of *expired volumes* can be carried out readily in the intubated patient using an anemometer or a pneumotachograph. Both of these instruments can be influenced by condensation and secretions, and also they need to be checked against known standards from time to time. However, there is an ultrasonic spirometer[22] available which is not affected by condensation or accumulation of secretions, but its calibration is influenced by temperature and alteration in the composition of the gas mixture.

Monitoring metabolism

Monitoring metabolism is based on temperature measurement combined with balance studies and a selection of investigations determined by the condition of the patient. These topics are largely outside the scope of this chapter, but, no account of monitoring would be complete without reference to the importance of keeping accurate records of the volumes and composition of all fluid losses and replacement solutions administered, regular determination of the pH and acid-base status, and assessment of those factors which influence oxygen release to the tissues.

Oxygen availability depends on cardiac output, arterial oxygen content, and the position of the oxyhaemoglobin dissociation curve. Shifts in the position of the dissociation curve may be measured by determining the P50 (the partial pressure of oxygen required for 50 per cent saturation of haemoglobin under standard conditions of temperature, pH, and base excess). A rise in P50 indicates a shift to the right and a fall a shift to the left. A fall in the P50 may occur in association with massive blood transfusion, particularly when acid-citrate dextrose is the preservative, rapid correction of acidosis, phosphate deficient parenteral feeding regimes, and during haemodialysis, due to depletion of 2, 3-diphosphoglycerate.[23] However, changes in P50 are only of limited significance in comparison with changes in arterial oxygen tension and tissue perfusion.

COMPUTERS IN MONITORING

The possible development of computer based monitoring systems was foreseen from the earliest days of medical computing but for a variety of reasons the place of computers in medicine is still very much a subject for debate both in medical circles and also in the Houses of Parliament.[24] There are, however, a number of clearly recognisable areas in which computers can be of assistance in patient monitoring but because of the large capital outlay involved in the purchase of computer based monitoring systems, not to mention the cost of maintenance and servicing, progress is still rather slow.

Computer applications in patient monitoring include:

1. Rapid calculation of indices of function employing programmes based on standard formulae

2. Conversion of analogue signals collected from monitoring instruments into measurements which can be used to assess organ function
3. Data recording and storage[25,26]
4. Control of treatment by means of programmes which regulate the rate of infusions and drug administration using measurements fed directly into the computer from monitoring instruments attached to the patient.[26]

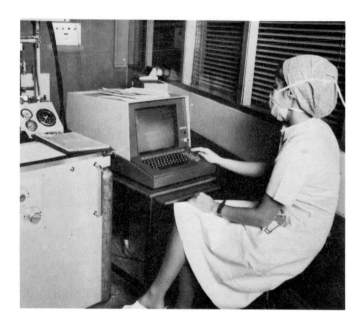

Fig. 8.8   Anaesthetist inspecting patient record at visual display terminal (Grafoskop). Data inspection is carried out by operating computer function keys located immediately below the display screen. The typewriter keyboard is used mainly during entry of patient information into the computer based patient record from this terminal. (Datasaab AB, Sweden)

In planning computer based monitoring it is essential to define the precise function of the proposed system and to establish beyond reasonable doubt that the use of a computer is really necessary. Also, it is important to ensure that the manner in which the proposed system is to be used will be compatible with existing routines and that staff will not have to be retrained.

The use of computers to handle large amounts of information collected during the course of clinical care is not a very big step from a number of established business applications and such systems have been under investigation in a number of centres throughout the world since the middle of the 1960s. Systems for handling clinical data in this way are based on direct linkage to monitoring instruments or the manual entry of measurements using a data entry keyboard and the retrieval of information is carried out by inspection at a visual display terminal (Fig. 8.8) or by obtaining hard copy print out from a high speed printer connected to the computer. Data handling systems which have been tried and tested have been in continuous use for over 99 per cent of the time available on a 24 hours a day basis throughout the year since they were first installed and the most common reason for stoppages is to permit essential maintenance or amendment of programmes in order to introduce new routines.[27]

Experience with these systems has shown that *essential requirements* for computer based patient data handling are:

1. The system should be able to handle large amounts of data in real-time on a 24 hours a day basis throughout the year
2. The information should be at least as readily available to all users as it is in manually kept records
3. The procedures for data entry and inspection should be uncomplicated
4. The format of data presentation should contribute to the decision making process
5. It should be possible to carry out planned maintenance and revision of programmes with the minimum amount of inconvenience to the users
6. A suitable emergency electricity supply must be included in the installation to cover the possibility of mains failure.

The *benefits* of such systems over manual techniques in those situations which generate large amounts of information such as in the period associated with open heart operations and the management of patients undergoing treatment in intensive care units are:

1. Staff are able to devote themselves more fully to the job of caring for patients because less time is spent performing clerical tasks
2. Time taken over decision making is reduced because information is frequently more readily available than it is in manually kept records, particularly when the results of laboratory investigations can be entered directly into the patient record using a data entry keyboard (Fig. 8.9) at the workbench or a visual display terminal located nearby
3. Doctors are in a position to contribute to the care of patients in any of the areas covered by the system without having to leave the immediate vicinity of patients under their care at the time.[27] Also, experience gained with systems employing on-line entry of measurements from monitoring instruments has made it possible to identify more clearly groups of patients who are most likely to benefit from monitoring.[28]

THE WAY AHEAD

The future development of monitoring will inevitably continue to depend to a degree on economic considerations. However, the wider application of methods of monitoring blood flow through the heart and aorta based on the technique of Doppler ultrasound[29,30,31] point to the possibility of, at least in part, reducing the need to carry out invasive procedures to monitor the circulation. Also, refinement of the technique of transcutaneous measurement of the arterial Po_2[32] may remove the need for blood sampling to make this measurement in newborn infants. At the same time investigations into a transcutaneous method for measuring electrolyte levels[33] could provide the means of obtaining valuable new information about the adequacy of tissue perfusion and intracellular function. The place of computers will, it is hoped, become clearer once it is seen whether the potential of the recently introduced micro-computer systems can be realised.

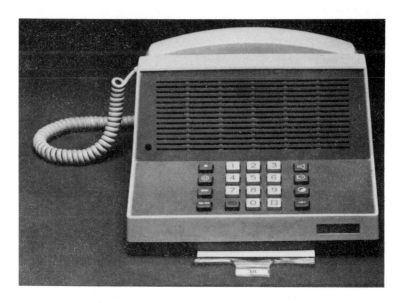

Fig. 8.9 *Data entry keyboard.* The keyboard of the intercom set is used for manual entry of numerical values of physiological measurements and the results of laboratory investigations into the computer based patient record using a two digit code to identify the various parameters being recorded. (Datasaab AB, Sweden)

It certainly seems likely that clinically orientated systems will be used to fulfil a more dedicated role in the future either dealing with a single activity such as dysrhythmia monitoring in a coronary care unit or handling all of the data for one patient using many of the routines developed for use in the existing computer based patient data handling systems.

REFERENCES

1. Swan, H. J. C., Ganz, W., Forrester, J. S., Marcus, H., Diamond, G. & Chonette, D. (1970) Catheterisation of the heart in man with the use of a flow-directed balloon-tipped catheter. *New England Journal of Medicine*, **283,** 447–451.
2. Forrester, J. S., Diamond, G., McHugh, T. J. & Swan, H. J. C. (1971) Filling pressures in the right and left sides of the heart in acute myocardial infarction. *New England Journal of Medicine*, **285,** 190–192.
3. Weisse, A. B., Narang, R., Haider, B. & Regan, T. J. (1973) Right and left heart pressures in acute myocardial infarction. *Cardiovascular Research*, **7,** 251–260.
4. Kaltman, A. J., Herbert, W. H., Conroy, R. J. & Kossman, C. E. (1966) The gradient in pressure across the pulmonary vascular bed during diastole. *Circulation*, **34,** 377–384.
5. Crul, F. J. & Payne, J. P. (1970) *Patient Monitoring*, p. 75. Amsterdam: Excerpta Medica.
6. Sheppard, L. C., Johnson, T. S. & Kirklin, J. W. (1971) Controlled study of brachial artery blood pressure measured by a new indirect method. *Journal of Association of Advanced Medical Instrumentation*, **5,** 297–301.

7. Swan, H. J. C. & Ganz, W. (1975) Use of balloon flotation catheters in critically ill patients. *Surgical Clinics of North America*, **55**, 501–520.

8. Jenkins, B. J., Bradley, R. D. & Branthwaite, M. A. (1970) Evaluation of pulmonary artery end-diastolic pressure as an indirect estimate of left atrial mean pressure. *Circulation*, **42**, 75–78.

9. Bouchard, R. J., Gault, J. H. & Ross, J. Jr. (1971) Evaluation of pulmonary arterial end-diastolic pressure as an estimate of left ventricular end-diastolic pressure in patients with normal and abnormal left ventricular performance. *Circulation*, **44**, 1072–1079.

10. Lipp, H., O'Donoghue, K. & Resnekov, L. (1971) Intracardiac knotting of a flow-directed balloon catheter. *New England Journal of Medicine*, **284**, 220.

11. Foote, G. A., Schabel, S. I. & Hodges, M. (1974) Pulmonary complications of the flow-directed balloon-tipped catheter. *New England Journal of Medicine*, **290**, 927–931.

12. Frederick, H. & Yorr, A. (1974) Massive thrombosis associated with use of Swan Ganz catheter. *Chest*, **65**, 682.

13. Latimer, R. D. (1971) Central venous catheterisation. *British Journal of Hospital Medicine*, **5**, 369–376.

14. Debrunner, F. & Buhler, F. (1969) 'Normal central venous pressure' significance of reference point and normal range. *British Medical Journal*, **3**, 148–150.

15. Department of Health and Social Security (1969) *Hospital Technical Memorandum No. 8: Safety Code for Electro-Medical Apparatus.* London: H.M.S.O.

16. Dornette, W. H. L. (1973) An electrically safe surgical environment. *Archives of Surgery*, **107**, 567–573.

17. Vincur, V., Artz, J. S. & Sampliner, J. E. (1975). *Application of a Critical Care Monitoring Programme in the Diagnosis and Management of Critically ill Patients*, p. 6. Cleveland, Ohio: Department of Surgery, Case Western Reserve University School of Medicine.

18. Maynard, D. E., Prior, P. F. & Scott, D. F. (1969) Device for continuous monitoring of cerebral activity in resuscitated patients. *British Medical Journal*, **4**, 545–546.

19. Branthwaite, M. A. (1975) Prevention of neurological damage during open heart surgery. *Thorax*, **30**, 258–261.

20. Wilson, R. S. (1976) Monitoring the lung: mechanics and volume. *Anesthesiology*, **45**, 135–145.

21. West, J. B. (1977) *Ventilation/blood flow and gas exchange*, 3rd edition, pp. 97–98. Oxford: Blackwell.

22. Jacovitch, T. & Eberhart, R. C. (1971) The Doppler principle applied to respiratory flow measurement. *Proceedings of San Diego Biomedical Symposium*, **10**, 47.

23. MacDonald, R. (1977) Red cell 2,3-diphosphoglycerate and oxygen affinity. *Anaesthesia*, **32**, 544–553.

24. House of Commons (1976) *Sixth Report from the Committee on Public Accounts*, Session 1975–76, para, 105–118. London: H.M.S.O.

25. William-Olson, G., Norlander, O. P., Norden, I. & Patterson, S. O. (1969) A patient monitoring system with display terminals. *Opuscula Medica*, **2**, 39–46.

26. Sheppard, L. C. & Kouchoukos, N. T. (1976) Computers as monitors. *Anesthesiology*, **45**, 250–259.

27. Franklin, C. B. (1976) Living with someone else's computer. In *Real-Time Computing in Patient Management*, ed. Payne, J. P. & Hill, D. W., pp. 119–129. England: Peter Perigrinus.

28. Conway, C. M. (1977) Diagnostic and therapeutic instrumentation. In *The Management of the Acutely Ill*, ed. Payne, J. P. & Hill, D. W., pp. 131–134. England: Peter Perigrinus.

29. Light, L. H. (1976) Transcutaneous aortovelography. A new window on the circulation? *British Heart Journal*, **38**, 433–442.

30. Buchtal, A., Hanson, G. C. & Peisach, A. R. (1976) Transcutaneous aortovelography. Potentially useful technique in management of critically ill patients. *British Heart Journal*, **38**, 451–456.

31. Wexler, L. F. & Pohost, G. M. (1976) Haemodynamic monitoring: noninvasive techniques. *Anesthesiology*, **45**, 156–183.

32. Huch, R., Lubbers, D. W. & Huch, A. (1974) Reliability of transcutaneous monitoring of arterial Po_2 in newborn infants. *Archives of Disease in Childhood*, **49**, 213–218.

33. Kessler, M., Höper, J. & Krumme, B. A. (1976) Monitoring of tissue perfusion and cellular function. *Anesthesiology*, **45**, 184–197.

9. Postoperative care

R. S. Atkinson

This chapter considers selected aspects of post-operative patient care which are of particular interest to the anaesthetist. The problem is not one of simple recovery. Observation is the key to early recognition of difficulties and complications and an understanding of the changes occurring in the patient allows intelligent application of therapeutic measures at an early stage.

THE POST-OPERATIVE OBSERVATION WARD

In recent years there has been an increase of interest in the achievements of these units, though regrettably the sound arguments put forward for their establishment over 20 years ago by Jolly and Lee[1] have not been universally accepted and applied.

The nursing of all post-operative patients in a special ward or room adjacent to the theatre complex allows a concentration of nursing expertise and the proximity of the anaesthetist and surgeon allows the patient to be closely observed during the dangerous period of recovery from the effect of anaesthetic drugs and surgical trauma. Early warning is obtained of complications and pain relief can be tailored to suit the individual patient.

It is now generally accepted that *recovery rooms* should be incorporated whenever theatre suites are planned. The writer prefers the term *post-operative observation ward*, believing it to be more descriptive of the function of such a unit. This should be part of the theatre complex, but with access both from the 'sterile' areas and the outside corridors; this facilitates both routeing of patients and visits by medical staff throughout the 24 hours. While primarily for post-operative patients it can be used as a reception area when major accidents are admitted for immediate surgery. The main function of the unit is *observation*. Simple observations of arterial pressure, pulse rate and respiration are often all that is required, but there should also be provision for use of the electrocardiogram, central venous pressure monitoring and simple measurement of respiratory volumes. It is observation which gives warning of impending catastrophe, and this is hard to maintain continuously on a busy general ward, especially during the night hours. The unit should be a *ward* and not a room or recovery bay. The implication is that there must be a ward sister in charge aided by staff nurses with the help of students who should be on a rota so that they can receive instruction in this very important facet of nursing expertise. The nursing staff require special training and this is quite different from that appropriate to nurses working in the theatre itself. It is now being recognised that nurses in such a unit should be administered by a clinical nursing officer independent of the theatre team.[2]

The equipment required in the post-operative ward need not be elaborate or expensive. The main requirement is *space*, space to accommodate all the patients required during the busiest time of the week and space to enable access for medical staff all round the bed or trolley. The space required will vary according to the nature of the surgery carried out, but the average district hospital will require 2 to 3 bed spaces per theatre with additional room for trolleys when a large number of short cases pass through.

Equipment must be available for simple monitoring, oxygen therapy, intravenous therapy, cardiac resuscitation, tracheal intubation and intermittent positive pressure ventilation.[1]

The post-operative ward should be staffed 24 hours a day, 7 days a week. This is not possible in many hospitals and the undesirable practice of taking post-operative patients to the main intensive care unit is accepted as a compromise. Transfer to such a unit, even for a short time, is often difficult due to bed shortages and may involve transfer of the unconscious patient along corridors and even in lifts. The dangers of cross-infection are also significant when traffic flow through the intensive care unit is increased.

It is difficult to quantify the value of the post-operative ward in terms of saving in mortality and morbidity, but early reports[3,4] suggested that a significant number of preventable deaths occurred when patients were returned immediately to the general ward. All those who have worked in post-operative wards will appreciate that findings such as hypotension, bradycardia and respiratory inadequacy occur more frequently than is generally realised. Presumably many of these abnormalities cease spontaneously without therapy, but 'unexplained' cardiac arrest and death still occur sometimes when supervision has been less than perfect and it seems clear that only vigilant observation and prompt therapy will prevent such disasters. Such measures can be taken more swiftly in the theatre complex than in the general ward.

RECOVERY FROM ANAESTHESIA

Modern anaesthetic techniques are associated with a rapid return of consciousness, though this itself carries some disadvantages as phenomena such as shivering and the early return of pain sensation are more frequent than if patients awake gradually.

Post-operative shivering has been reported when a variety of anaesthetic agents have been administered, but the incidence following halothane supplementation of nitrous oxide and oxygen has been quoted as approaching 30 per cent of patients.[5] Shivering has been correlated with a fall in core temperature[6] and this has been supported by a recent study in which administration of warmed humidified gases throughout surgery maintained normothermia and eliminated the complication of post-operative shivering.[7]

Day case surgery

Early recovery of consciousness together with rapid return of complete mental orientation and cerebral activity is important when patients return home the day that operation and anaesthesia are carried out. Many anaesthetists prefer to use drugs that are rapidly metabolised or eliminated rather than those which are redistributed to other body tissues as recovery occurs. Agents such as Althesin are often preferred to barbiturates for the intravenous induction of anaesthesia, though the absence of side effects with the latter combined with the long experience of their safe clinical use make methohexitone and also thiopentone worthy of consideration provided dosage is not excessive. Various workers have studied the period of recovery from intravenous anaesthetic agents by a series of tests involving mental activity,[8-11] but these techniques are not readily adaptable to the screening of patients before travelling home. An interesting method which has recently been tried out for this latter purpose is stabilometry;[12] the patient stands on a platform and changes in the activity of postural muscles are recorded, indicating whether or not the patient has full conscious control of his limb movements. There may be a place for a simple screening device in clinical practice, but the present policy of assuming that the patient requires an escort home and is unable to drive a car, operate machinery or cook has much to recommend it.

The anaesthetic technique used has considerable bearing on the rapidity of recovery. Premedication is generally unnecessary; anaesthesia should not be induced until the surgeon and his equipment is ready; minimal intravenous dosage is the order of the day and this can be supplemented by inhalation agents which are rapidly eliminated such as nitrous oxide, halothane and enflurane. The last named agent avoids the repeated use of halothane as, for example, in day case cystoscopy.

Long acting agents such as ketamine and non-depolarising relaxants are to be avoided. It has been shown that disturbances of vision can exist for many hours following administration of non-depolarising relaxants.[13] Suxamethonium is also a problem drug because of the high incidence of post-operative muscle pains following its use. The incidence of pains is related to the rate of firing of motor unit potentials as recorded electromyographically and not to the visible fasciculations.[14] It can be reduced markedly by the prior administration of a non-depolarising relaxant, tubocurarine 3 mg or gallamine 20 mg administered 3 minutes before suxamethonium to allow significant amounts of the drug to reach receptors, or by a larger dose, tubocurarine 10 mg or gallamine 60 mg 1 minute previously. Suxamethonium has advantages when tracheal intubation is required as it avoids the need for deep anaesthesia. Intubation of the trachea is however associated with a considerable incidence of sore throat, particularly when a pharyngeal pack is used. The technique should therefore be reserved for those day cases who cannot be safely managed using a facemask.

Regional blocks have a distinct place in day case surgery. Post-operative problems can however arise due to remaining analgesia which can occasionally persist for a long period[15] and care must be taken to avoid skin damage as a result of trauma. Pneumothorax as a complication of brachial plexus block may not become apparent for some hours post-operatively. The technique of intravenous regional analgesia has considerable advantages for minor surgical procedures on the upper limb. Sensation returns soon after release of the tourniquet and the writer finds it the method of choice for minor orthopaedic procedures on the forearm, wrist and hand.

POST-OPERATIVE PAIN

It is the anaesthetist's duty to relieve pain, if only for humanitarian reasons. Pain does have adverse effects on morale, but also on respiratory and sometimes on cardiovascular function.

Post-operative analgesia is often prescribed on an empirical basis, a standard dosage at standard time intervals, but this clearly does not suit all patients. Adequate pain relief depends upon good prescribing and intelligent interpretation by the nursing staff. Standards are not easily maintained when junior medical staff are inexperienced and nurses qualified to check drugs in scarce supply, a situation not uncommon during the night hours in hospital. Apparatus for the self-administration of pethidine during labour has been evaluated with encouraging results[16] and such a technique might also have a place in the post-operative period, though clearly adequate supervision is still necessary. Interest has also extended to the use of longer acting analgesics which would reduce the need for frequent administration and a greater likelihood that analgesia would last until the next dose could be given. A number of new analgesic drugs have recently been investigated.

Butorphanol

This is a synthetic analgesic with a benzomorphan nucleus, closely related in chemical structure to pentazocine.[17] Its potency is 5 times that of morphine and 20 times that of pentazocine with a similar duration of action. Like pentazocine it has both agonist and antagonist properties. Any reversal of effect is best achieved using the pure antagonist, naloxone. It is claimed that the incidence of respiratory depression is low and that it will not cause addiction. A recent clinical trial suggests that a dosage of 1 to 2 mg is safe and effective in the relief of post-operative pain.[18]

Buprenorphine

This drug is a synthetic analgesic drug which has high potency and a long duration of action. It was synthesised in Britain in 1966 and is a thebaine derivative, related in structure to morphine.[19] Clinical studies have been carried out in Belgium,[20] Canada[21,22] and South Africa[23] as well as in Britain.[24] This drug also shows both agonist and antagonist activity. Respiratory depression can be reversed by naloxone. Buprenorphine is about 35 times as potent as morphine and has about half the potency of fentanyl. The only significant side effect reported is drowsiness. Favourable results have been reported in dosages of 0.2 and 0.4 mg and the commercial preparation (Temgesic) contains 0.3 mg per ml. The drug may be given intramuscularly or by slow intravenous injection. The effect lasts up to 6 hours and serious cardiovascular and respiratory depression has not so far been reported. The prolonged action of buprenorphine is an attractive feature as a single dose may produce a long period of sleep undisturbed by pain.

Post-operative respiratory depression

Respiratory depression in the immediate postoperative period may be due to a variety of causes including central depression produced by opiates, barbiturates and volatile agents and peripheral abnormalities as in the case of inadequate reversal of muscle relaxants and reduction in chest wall compliance.[25] The role of potent analgesic drugs used during surgery may be important, especially when large doses are used in an effort to obtund autonomic responses.[26] There is evidence that a biphasic response occurs when fentanyl is administered, as measured by the rebreathing carbon dioxide response curve.[27] It is likely that fentanyl, as is the case with pethidine, is sequestered in the stomach during operation and is later re-absorbed to the circulation. Delayed respiratory depression after the use of fentanyl has been described recently[28] and this phenomenon is potentially dangerous when the supposedly short-acting agent is used in day case surgery. It should also be noted that naloxone has a shorter period of action than many potent analgesics and that repeated doses can cause nausea and vomiting.[29] Other writers[30,31] have condemned the use of morphine and papaveretum for premedication when fentanyl is to be used during anaesthesia, believing that untoward depression will not occur when the latter is the sole agent used.

Doxapram
Doxapram has been advocated as a respiratory stimulant to counteract postoperative respiratory depression and thereby to reduce the incidence of postoperative chest complications.[32] The drug may be given as a single dose, 1 to 1.5 mg/kg, or in an intravenous infusion, 250 mg in 5 per cent dextrose. Doxapram has also been used for arousal from anaesthesia after day case surgery. In a recent study,[36] waking from halothane anaesthesia occurred some 3 to 4 minutes earlier than when it was not administered, probably because the increased alveolar ventilation resulted in quicker elimination of the volatile agent. The advantage of doxapram over other respiratory stimulants lies in the fact that it does not antagonise the analgesic actions of the opiate. However, studies in small mammals[37] sound a note of warning. Analeptic agents have a low therapeutic index and there is evidence that in the rabbit and mouse, doxapram reverses the respiratory depressant action of morphine. However, a number of mice used in the studies died later. The LD_{50} for doxapram in the presence of morphine was much less than that for either doxapram or morphine alone. Moreover the mode of death was different. The tendency to use larger doses of opiates with doxapram in clinical situations must therefore be viewed with reserve until further information is available.

Other new analgesics
New agents are constantly being synthesised and undergoing trials, but few offer advantages over those in present use. Some of those undergoing evaluation at the present include nefopam,[38] a non-narcotic analgesic of heterocyclic chemical structure and meptazinol,[39,40] a hexahydroazepine derivative, while anidoxime has been tried as an oral medicant.[41]

Opiates and endorphins
Major developments in our understanding of the action of narcotic analgesics on the brain have demonstrated that physiological substances exist which have

actions similar to that of morphine.[42] It has even been suggested that acupuncture techniques result in the release of these endorphins since the analgesia produced is antagonised by naloxone.[43] Increasing knowledge of the physiological mechanisms of analgesia may well lead to the development of better methods of post-operative analgesia in the future.

Ketamine

Ketamine has been used in sub-anaesthetic doses to provide analgesia.[44] The absence of respiratory and cardiovascular depression when ketamine is administered suggest that it might be an attractive drug in the post-operative period, always supposing that hallucinatory phenomena are not produced. Ketamine has been successfully used as a 0.1 per cent solution in 5 per cent dextrose as a continuous slow intravenous infusion.[45] The drip rate can be adjusted to relieve pain but at the same time to maintain consciousness and communication with the patient. The technique may be useful in elderly and debilitated patients and in those admitted to an intensive care unit. Single doses of 30 mg ketamine have also been shown to be effective, though when combined with pethidine it had little advantage over pethidine alone.[46]

Nitrous oxide

Nitrous oxide in the form of Entonox, premixed 50 per cent nitrous oxide and 50 per cent oxygen in the same cylinder, is a useful analgesic agent in many circumstances.[47] Inhalation is useful prior to physiotherapy and as an aid to expectoration. Entonox, however, contains rather too much nitrous oxide for continuous administration since 25 per cent is regarded as roughly equivalent to 10 mg morphine.[48] Entonox may be diluted by use of an MC (Mary Catterall) or Edinburgh mask with air dilution[49,50] and may be used for a period up to 24 hours without risk of bone marrow depression. When elective ventilation of the lungs is used in the immediate post-operative period, Entonox can be added to the inspired gases to provide analgesia without cardiovascular depression.

Regional analgesia

Continuous extradural blockade after insertion of a catheter in the thoracic region affords post-operative analgesia of excellent quality. Bupivacaine is the drug of choice and provided dosage is minimal cardiovascular depression does not occur. The initial enthusiastic reports[51] have not resulted in widespread adoption of the technique. This may be partly due to the fear of serious complications in a small percentage of patients,[52] but it also results from the logistic implications of supervision of top-ups were the technique to be adopted as a general routine. There may even be psychological problems when the catheter technique is discontinued. The very superior quality of analgesia may make the patient dissatisfied when it is withdrawn. This is the time when the patient who has had conventional opiates finds discomfort getting easier. There is no doubt, however, that it is an excellent method for selected patients with borderline respiratory function in whom failure to expectorate post-operatively might be disastrous. Extradural block is superior to morphine in terms of lung function post-operatively.[53] The fall in functional residual capacity and the arterial hypoxaemia which occur after abdominal surgery is reversed better by extradural block than by opiate analgesia, though recent work has failed to confirm that extradural block prevents a fall in functional residual capacity after lower abdominal surgery.[54]

Sacral block is useful following circumcision,[55] posterior vaginal repair and haemorrhoidectomy.[56]

Block of peripheral nerves is not as widely used as it deserves. Several hours of pain relief can be obtained by intelligent use of bupivacaine, for example in iliac crest block after appendicectomy or herniorrhaphy. Intercostal block is effective in relieving somatic, though not visceral, pain after thoracotomy and upper abdominal surgery,[57] though care must be taken to avoid inadvertent pneumothorax. The intercostal nerves can also be blocked as they enter the abdominal wall below the costal margin and a modification of abdominal field block [58] is worthy of consideration in thin subjects. Rectus sheath block[58] has also been used in poor risk cases and it can be maintained by intermittent injection through a small plastic catheter placed in the sheath during closure of the abdomen.

Transcutaneous nerve stimulation

The gate control theory of pain[59] suggests that relief may be obtained by transcutaneous stimulation.[60] Its use for post-operative pain relief has been studied by various workers.[61-64] The technique works in a proportion of cases, though evaluation of relief of post-operative pain is notoriously difficult. It has, however, the enormous advantage that it is a simple technique without side effects and there is no contraindication to the use of pharmacological methods if it proves unsatisfactory in a particular patient. Indeed it has been suggested that pain should be treated initially with placebos, then with stimulation techniques, and with systemic analgesics only when the simpler methods have failed.[65]

Organisation of pain relief

The provision of post-operative analgesia is more than a straightforward pharmacological problem. Individual requirements vary considerably and the placebo effect is often marked. It is clear that psychological factors are important.[66-69] Emotional stability is important and the neurotic patient is more likely to suffer impaired vital capacity, subjective pain and chest complications post-operatively than his more phlegmatic counterpart. In this group of patients pre-operative encouragement as a result of the anaesthetist's pre-operative visit may be particularly helpful.[70] The techniques used during surgery also have an effect on pain in the post-operative period. Supplementation by agents such as phenoperidine gives rise to less pain, less impairment of vital capacity and better arterial oxygen tension values than when agents such as halothane are used.[71]

The individual patient will receive good pain relief if he is closely observed by a competent medical and nursing team. This in turn will mean intelligent administration of analgesic drugs, whether by the intramuscular, intravenous or oral route, with a reduction in chest complications and a smoother transition to convalescence. There may be a place for a doctor-nurse team to supervise all patients with post-operative pain within a hospital.[71a]

OXYGEN THERAPY

Post-operative arterial hypoxaemia

It has been recognised for some years that arterial hypoxaemia occurs following major surgery.[72] The aetiology is multifactorial,[73] but one very important mechanism is the changing relationship of functional residual capacity to airways closure in the post-operative period. Functional residual capacity falls following laparotomy[74,75] and also after operations on the limbs.[76] Spasm of the expiratory muscles may contribute to the fall in functional residual capacity and this may be minimised or abolished if adequate analgesia is provided.[53] The closing volume of the lungs increases as age advances and when the patient adopts the recumbent as opposed to the erect posture.[77,78] Closing volume exceeds functional residual capacity after the age of about 60 years, with resultant changes in ventilation-perfusion relationships and arterial hypoxaemia. When the supine position is assumed these changes occur from the age of about 44 years. As many hospital patients are elderly and are nursed in the horizontal position after operation it is not surprising that hypoxaemia occurs. To this effect may be added the depressant effects of anaesthetic and analgesic drugs, the difficulty of coughing without pain and the possibility of diffusion hypoxia during the elimination of nitrous oxide.

Changes in the pulmonary circulation are also important. A fall in cardiac output not only results in reduced oxygen availability to the tissues, but the associated diminution in pulmonary blood flow may be at the expense of the apical areas of the lungs which become relatively underperfused with resultant changes in ventilation-perfusion relationships.[73]

The pulmonary circulation also filters blood aggregates which may enter the circulation when stored blood is transfused.[79] If this occurs to a significant extent the effect is one of an increase in physiological dead space. The use of blood filters is therefore recommended when large volumes of blood are given.[80,81,82]

Pulmonary oedema, should it arise from any cause, is associated with marked deterioration of pulmonary function. Compliance is decreased, airway resistance is increased, and the distribution of alveolar ventilation and pulmonary blood flow may show considerable change. Appropriate treatment must be applied to correct these abnormalities.

Oxygen administration

Cyanosis is not easy to detect in patients who have less than 5 grams per cent of reduced haemoglobin in the circulating blood. This corresponds to an oxygen saturation of about 75 per cent in the patient with a normal haemoglobin value, or a Pao_2 of about 5 kPa (37 mmHg). It is therefore not easy to detect arterial hypoxaemia of the order commonly encountered in the post-operative period and the policy of routine oxygen administration to patients who have undergone major surgery or who are elderly is to be recommended.

The inhalation of 30 to 40 per cent oxygen is satisfactory for the majority of patients and can be maintained for a period of 24 to 48 hours.[83] The 35 per cent Venturi-type mask is satisfactory for the majority of patients,[84-86] though a few severe hypoxaemic patients may require higher concentrations. Oxygen can also be administered by nasal cannula or catheter.[87] The nasal catheter has the advantage of simplicity. A flow rate of 2 litres per min will produce an inhaled concentration of 30 to 35 per cent.[88] A safety blow-off can be incorporated, using a T-connection and a side tube dipping 5 cm under water to prevent undue pressure build-up.

On the other hand, administration of oxygen in the early post-operative period can lead to respiratory depression and carbon dioxide narcosis in susceptible individuals. There is therefore a sound case for the more widespread use of measurement of oxygen tension in arterial and mixed venous blood combined with the accurate prescription of oxygen administration using devices of the 'high air flow with oxygen enrichment' design such as the Ventimask series.[89] Even so, it has been pointed out that the oxygen concentration in the trachea is likely to be up to 5 per cent less than that supplied by the Ventimask,[90] probably due to addition of water vapour, and in the case of the 35 per cent mask possibly because peak inspiratory flow rate can exceed 32 litres per min, the flow supplied by the apparatus.

Elective ventilation of the lungs

Experience of management of patients in intensive therapy units has demonstrated the value of intermittent positive pressure ventilation in the maintenance of gas exchange in critically ill patients. It is therefore logical to continue to control ventilation for the first 12 to 24 hours following major surgery or in patients with minimal respiratory reserve. Controlled ventilation is discussed fully in Chapters 3 and 7. It may be combined with intravenous or intramuscular narcotic analgesics for post-operative pain or Entonox may be introduced to the inspired gases. Intermittent positive pressure helps to prevent hypoxaemia and can be discontinued on the morning following operation if the patient's condition is satisfactory.

INTRAVENOUS THERAPY

The effect of surgery on renal function is to cause a reduction in the excretion of water and sodium. The hormonal response to the stress of surgery and anaesthesia is complex.[91] The increased secretion of steroids from the adrenal cortex and of antidiuretic hormone from the pituitary may be accompanied by the production of hormones within the kidney itself. The clinical anaesthetist must distinguish between the reduced urine output associated with these factors and the changes which indicate renal failure. A urine flow of less than 20 ml per hour for two hours or more suggests renal failure when kidney function has been previously normal, but a urine flow higher than this does not exclude it.

Renal failure occurs when renal blood flow is inadequate or when the renal tubules are affected by hypoxia or toxic substances. These latter may become concentrated when urine volumes are reduced. Renal protection can be afforded by the use of diuretics such as frusemide, while mannitol has been recommended for the jaundiced patient.[92] A rapid infusion of 100 ml 15 per cent mannitol or the administration of 80 mg frusemide have been recommended when the patient becomes oliguric after an unexpected stress has been placed on the kidney, such as a period of hypotension as a result of blood loss or a mis-matched transfusion.[91]

Recommendations have been put forward for fluid and electrolytes administration to the otherwise healthy patient during the post-operative period.[93] They must clearly be modified if there has been an imbalance pre-operatively. The modern anaesthetist requires a clear understanding of the fundamentals of osmolality,[94,95] if patients with serious imbalances are to be treated intelligently.[96]

Understanding of the nature of hyponatraemic states has increased in recent years. The 'sick cell syndrome', when sodium ions pass from the extra-cellular to the intra-cellular fluid compartment has been reviewed recently.[97,98] It is unwise to infuse solutions containing sodium to patients with this condition, but rather the underlying cause should be treated vigorously.

REFERENCES

1. Jolly, C. & Lee, J. A. (1957) Post-operative observation ward. *Anaesthesia*, **12**, 49.
2. Andrewes, S. J. (1978) Paper read to Section of Anaesthetics, Royal Society of Medicine.
3. Ruth, H. S., Haugen, F. P. & Grove, D. D. (1947) *Journal of the American Medical Association*, **135**, 881.
4. Lowenthal, P. J. & Russell, A. S. (1951) *Anesthesiology*, **12**, 470.
5. Moir, D. D. & Doyle, P. M. (1963) Halothane and post-operative shivering. *Current Researches Anesthesia Analgesia*, **42**, 423.
6. Jones, H. D. & McLaren, C. A. B. (1965) Post-operative shivering and hypoxaemia after halothane, nitrous oxide and oxygen anaesthesia. *British Journal of Anaesthesia*, **37**, 35.
7. Pflug, A. E., Aasheim, G. M., Foster, S. & Martin, R. W. (1978) Prevention of post-anaesthesia shivering. *Canadian Anaesthetists' Society Journal*, **25**, 43.
8. Carson, I. W. (1975) Recovery from anaesthesia. A review of methods for evaluation of recovery from anaesthesia and a comparative study of the intravenous steroid anaesthetic Althesin (CT1341), with methohexitone and thiopentone. *Proceedings of the Royal Society of Medicine*, **68**, 108.
9. Steward, D. J. (1975) A simplified scoring system for the post-operative recovery room. *Canadian Anaesthetists' Society Journal*, **22**, 111.
10. Kortilla, K., Linnoila, M., Ertama, P. & Hakkinens, S. (1975) Recovery and simulated driving after intravenous anesthesia with thiopental, Methohexital, propanidid or alphadione. *Anesthesiology*, **43**, 291.
11. Korttila, K. (1976) Recovery after intravenous sedation. A comparison of clinical and paper and pencil tests used in assessing late effects of diazepam. *Anaesthesia*, **31**, 724.
12. Steward, D. J. & Volgyesi, G. (1978) Stabilometry. A new tool for the measurement of recovery following general anaesthesia. *Canadian Anaesthetists' Society Journal*, **25**, 4.
13. Hannington-Kiff, J. G. (1970) Residual post-operative paralysis. *Proceedings of the Royal Society of Medicine*, **63**, 73.
14. Collier, C. (1975) Suxamethonium pains and fasciculations. *Proceedings of the Royal Society of Medicine*, **68**, 105.
15. Moraitis, K. (1977) Prolonged action of bupivacaine hydrochloride. *Anaesthesia*, **32**, 161.
16. Evans, J. M., Rosen, M., MacCarthy, J. & Hogg, M. I. J. (1976) Apparatus for Patient-Controlled administration of intravenous narcotics during labour. *Lancet*, **1**, 17.
17. Dobkin, A. B., Eamkaow, S., Zak, S. & Caruso, F. S. (1974) Butorphanol: A double blind evaluation in post-operative patients with moderate or severe pain. *Canadian Anaesthetists' Society Journal*, **21**, 600.
18. Dobkin, A. B., Africa, B. F., Noveck, R. J., Caruso, F. S., Esposito, B. & Simonds, J. (1976) Butorphanol tartrate: 1. Safety and efficacy in multidose control of post-operative pain. *Canadian Anaesthetists' Society Journal*, **23**, 596.

19. Lewis, J. W., Mayor, P. A. & Haddleser, D. I. (1973) Novel analgesics and molecular re-arrangements in the morphine-thebaine group. *J. Med. Chem.*, **16**, 12.
20. Rolly, G. & Versichelen, L. (1976) First experience with a new analgesic drug, buprenorphine. *Acta Anaesthesiol Belg.*, **27**, suppl.
21. Dobkin, A. B. (1977) Buprenorphine hydrochloride: Determination of analgesic potency. *Canadian Anaesthetists' Society Journal*, **24**, 186.
22. Dobkin, A. B., Esposito, B. & Philbin, C. (1977) Double-blind evaluation of buprenorphine hydrochloride for post-operative pain. *Canadian Anaesthetists' Society Journal*, **24**, 195.
23. Downing, J. W., Leary, W. P. & White, E. S. (1977) Buprenorphine? A new potent long-acting synthetic analgesic. Comparison with Morphine. *British Journal of Anaesthesia*, **49**, 251.
24. Hovell, B. C. (1977) Comparison of buprenorphine, pethidine and pentazocine for the relief of pain after operation. *British Journal of Anaesthesia*, **49**, 913.
25. Knill, R., Cosgrove, J. F., Olley, P. M. & Levinson, H. (1976) Components of respiratory depression after narcotic premedication in adolescents. *Canadian Anaesthetists' Society Journal*, **23**, 449.
26. Florence, A. (1978) Neuroleptanaesthesia for surgery of the abdominal aorta. *Anaesthesia*, **33**, 439.
27. Becker, L. D., Paulson, B. A., Miller, R. D., Severinghaus, J. W. & Eger, E. I. (1976) Biphasic respiratory depression after fentanyl-droperidol or fentanyl alone used to supplement nitrous oxide anesthesia. *Anesthesiology*, **44**, 291.
28. Adams, A. P. & Pybus, D. A. (1978) Delayed respiratory depression after use of fentanyl during anaesthesia. *British Medical Journal*, **1**, 278.
29. Longnecker, D. E., Grazis, P. A. & Eggers, G. W. N. (1973) Naloxone for antagonism of morphine-induced respiratory depression. *Current Researches Anesthesia and Analgesia*, **52**, 447.
30. Wright, C. J. (1978) Correspondence. *British Medical Journal*, **1**, 441.
31. Williams, J. H. (1978) Correspondence. *British Medical Journal*, **1**, 441.
32. Gupta, P. K. & Dundee, J. W. (1974) Morphine combined with doxapram or naloxone. A study of postoperative pain relief. *Anaesthesia*, **29**, 33.
33. Lees, N. W., Howie, H. B., Mellon, A., McKee, A. H. & McDairmid, I. A. (1976) The influence of doxapram on postoperative pulmonary function in patients undergoing upper abdominal surgery. *British Journal of Anaesthesia*, **48**, 1197.
34. Gawley, T. H., Dundee, J. W., Gupta, P. K. & Jones, C. J. (1976) Role of doxapram in reducing pulmonary complications after major surgery. *British Medical Journal*, **1**, 122.
35. Downing, J. W., Jeal, D. E., Allen, P. J. & Buley, R. (1977) I.V. doxapram hydrochloride and pulmonary complications after lower abdominal surgery. *British Journal of Anaesthesia*, **49**, 473.
36. Robertson, G. S., MacGregor, D. M. & Jones, C. J. (1977) Evaluation of doxapram for arousal from general anaesthesia in outpatients. *British Journal of Anaesthesia*, **49**, 133.
37. Gregoretti, S. M. & Pleuvry, B. J. (1977) Interactions between morphine and doxapram in the rabbit and mouse. *British Journal of Anaesthesia*, **49**, 323.
38. Tigerstedt, T., Sipponen, J., Tammisto, T. & Turunen, M. (1977) Comparison of nefopam and pethidine in postoperative pain. *British Journal of Anaesthesia*, **49**, 1133.
39. Paymaster, N. Y. (1976) Clinical evaluation of meptazinol, a new analgesic, in postoperative pain. *British Journal of Anaesthesia*, **48**, 599.
40. Paymaster, N. J. (1977) Analgesia after operation. A controlled comparison of meptazinol, pentazocine and pethidine. *British Journal of Anaesthesia*, **49**, 1139.
41. Grainger, D. J., Gawley, T. H. & Dundee, J. W. (1977) Anidoxime: A clinical trial of an oral analgesic agent. *British Journal of Anaesthesia*, **49**, 257.
42. Norman, J. (1977) Editorial. Opiates, receptors and endorphins. *British Journal of Anaesthesia*, **49**, 523.
43. Pomeranz, B. (1977) Brain's opiates at work in acupuncture? *New Scientist*, **73**, 12.
45. Ito, Y. & Ichiyanagi, K. (1974) Postoperative pain relief with ketamine infusion. *Anaesthesia*, **29**, administered in subdissociative doses. *Current Researches Anesthesia and Analgesia*, **50**, 452.
45. Ito, Y. & Ichiyanagi, K. (1974) Post-operative pain relief with ketamine infusion. *Anaesthesia*, **29**, 222.
46. Parkhouse, J. & Mariott, G. (1977) Postoperative analgesia with ketamine and pethidine. *Anaesthesia*, **32**, 285.
47. Baskett, P. J. F. & Bennett, J. A. (1971) Pain relief in hospital: the more widespread use of nitrous oxide. *British Medical Journal*, **2**, 509.
48. Parbrook, G. D., Rees, G. A. D. & Robertson, G. S. (1964) Relief of postoperative pain: comparison of 25 per cent nitrous oxide and oxygen mixture with morphine. *British Medical Journal*, **2**, 480.
49. Parbrook, G. D. (1967) Techniques of inhalational analgesia in the postoperative period. *British Journal of Anaesthesia*, **39**, 730.

50. Parbrook, G. D. (1972) Entonox for postoperative analgesia. *Proceedings of the Royal Society of Medicine*, **65**, 8.
51. Simpson, B. R., Parkhouse, J., Marshall, R. & Lambrechts, W. (1961) Extradural analgesia and the prevention of postoperative pulmonary complications. *British Journal of Anaesthesia*, **33**, 628.
52. Dawkins, C. J. M. (1969) An analysis of the complications of extradural and caudal block. *Anaesthesia*, **24**, 554.
53. Spence, A. A. & Smith, G. (1971) Postoperative analgesia and lung function. A comparison of morphine with extradural block. *British Journal of Anaesthesia*, **43**, 144.
54. Drummond, G. B. & Littlewood, D. G. (1977) Respiratory effects of extradural analgesia after lower abdominal surgery. *British Journal of Anaesthesia*, **49**, 999.
55. Kay, B. (1974) Caudal block for post-operative pain relief in children. *Anaesthesia*, **29**, 610.
56. Watt, M. J., Ross, D. M. & Atkinson, R. S. (1968) A clinical trial of bupivacaine. A preliminary report on a new local analgesic agent in extradural analgesia. *Anaesthesia*, **23**, 2.
57. Moore, D. C. (1975) Intercostal nerve block for post-operative somatic pain following surgery of thorax and upper abdomen. *British Journal of Anaesthesia*, **47**, 284.
58. Atkinson, R. S., Rushman, G. B. & Lee, J. A. (1977) A Synopsis of Anaesthesia. 8th Edition, Wrights, Bristol, p. 401.
59. Melzack, R. & Wall, P. D. (1965) Pain mechanisms: a new theory. *Science N. Y.*, **150**, 971.
60. Melzack, R. (1975) Prolonged relief of pain by brief, intense transcutaneous somatic stimulation. *Pain*, **1**, 357.
61. Vanderark, G. D. & McGrath, K. A. (1975) Transcutaneous electrical stimulation in treatment of postoperative pain. *American Journal of Surgery*, **130**, 338.
62. Hymes, A. C., Raab, D. E., Yonehiro, E. G., Nelson, G. D. & Printy, A. L. (1973) Electrical surface stimulation for control of acute postoperative pain and prevention of ileus. *Surgical Forum*, **24**, 447.
63. Cooperman, A. M., Hall, B., Mikalacki, K., Hardy, R. & Sadar, E. (1977) Use of transcutaneous electrical stimulation in the control of postoperative pain: Results of a prospective, randomized, controlled study. *American Journal of Surgery*, **133**, 185.
64. Pike, P. M. H. (1978) Transcutaneous electrical stimulation. Its use in the management of postoperative pain. *Anaesthesia*, **33**, 165.
65. Modell, J. H. (1977) Editorial comment. *Survey of Anesthesiology*, **21**, 460.
66. Dalrymple, D. G., Parbrook, G. D. & Steel, D. F. (1973) Factors predisposing to postoperative pain and pulmonary complications. *British Journal of Anaesthesia*, **45**, 589.
67. Parbrook, G. D., Steel, D. F. & Dalrymple, D. G. (1973) Factors predisposing to postoperative pain and pulmonary complications. A study of male patients undergoing elective gastric surgery. *British Journal of Anaesthesia*, **45**, 21.
68. Dalrymple, D. G. & Parbrook, G. D. (1976) Personality assessment and postoperative analgesic. A study in male patients undergoing elective gastric surgery. *British Journal of Anaesthesia*, **48**, 593.
69. Boyle, P. & Parbrook, G. D. (1977) The interrelation of personality and postoperative factors. *British Journal of Anaesthesia*, **49**, 259.
70. Egbert, L. D., Battit, G. E., Welch, C. E. & Bartlett, M. K. (1964) Reduction of postoperative pain by encouragement and instruction of patients. *New England Journal of Medicine*, **270**, 825.
71. Henderson, J. J. & Parbrook, G. D. (1976) Influence of anaesthetic technique on postoperative pain. A comparison of anaesthetic supplementation with halothane and with phenoperidine. *British Journal of Anaesthesia*, **48**, 587.
71a. Knight, C. L. & Mehta, M. (1978) Perioperative care. Postoperative pain relief. *British Journal of Hospital Medicine*, **19**, 462.
72. Nunn, J. F. & Payne, J. P. (1962) Hypoxaemia after general anaesthesia. *Lancet*, **2**, 631.
73. Hewlett, A. M. & Branthwaite, M. A. (1975) Postoperative pulmonary function. *British Journal of Anaesthesia*, **47**, 102.
74. Beecher, H. K. (1933) Effect of laparotomy on lung volume. Demonstration of a new type of pulmonary collapse. *Journal of Clinical Investigation*, **12**, 651.
75. Alexander, J. I., Horton, P. W., Millar, W. T., Parikh, R. K. & Spence, A. A. (1972) The effect of upper abdominal surgery on the relationship of airway closing point to end-tidal position. *Clinical Science*, **43**, 137.
76. Alexander, J. I., Spencer, A. A., Parikh, R. K. & Stuart, B. (1973) The role of airway closure in postoperative hypoxaemia. *British Journal of Anaesthesia*, **45**, 34.
77. Leblanc, P., Ruff, F. & Milic-Emili, J. (1970) Effects of age and body position on 'airways closure' in man. *Journal of Applied Physiology*, **28**, 448.
78. Editorial (1974) New problems for old in the respiratory system. *British Journal of Anaesthesia*, **46**, 467.

79. Mosely, R. V. & Doty, D. B. (1970) Changes in the filtration characteristics of stored blood. *Annals of Surgery*, **171**, 329.
80. Reul, G. J., Beall, A. C. & Greenberg, S. D. (1974) Protection of the pulmonary microvasculature by fine screen blood filtration. *Chest*, **66**, 4.
81. James, O. (1977) The use of blood microfilters. *British Journal of Clinical Equipment*, **2**, 199.
82. Buley, R. & Lumley, J. (1975) Some observations on blood microfilters. *Annals of the Royal College of Surgeons*, **57**, 262.
83. Sub-Committee of the Standing Medical Advisory Committee, Scottish Home and Health Department (1969) Uses and dangers of Oxygen Therapy. Edinburgh, H.M.S.O.
84. Drummond, G. B. (1975) Postoperative hypoxaemia and oxygen therapy. *British Journal of Anaesthesia*, **47**, 491.
85. Drummond, G. B. & Wright, D. J. (1977) Oxygen therapy after abdominal surgery. *British Journal of Anaesthesia*, **49**, 789.
86. Drummond, G. B. & Milne, A. C. (1977) Oxygen therapy after thoracotomy. *British Journal of Anaesthesia*, **49**, 1093.
87. Tantum, K. R. (1969) Comparison of nasal catheter and nasal cannula in patients recovering from general anaesthesia. *Anesthesiology*, **31**, 376.
88. Sykes, M. K., McNicol, M. W. & Campbell, E. J. M. (1976) Respiratory Failure. 2nd edition. Blackwell: Oxford, London, Edinburgh, Melbourne.
89. Leigh, J. M. (1975) Postoperative oxygen administration. *British Journal of Anaesthesia*, **47**, 108.
90. Gibson, R. L., Comer, P. B., Beckham, R. W. & McGraw, C. P. (1976) Actual tracheal oxygen concentrations with commonly used oxygen equipment. *Anesthesiology*, **44**, 71.
91. Bevan, D. R., Dudley, H. A. F. & Horsey, P. J. (1973) Renal function during and after anaesthesia and surgery: Significance for water and electrolyte management. *British Journal of Anaesthesia*, **45**, 968.
92. Dawson, J. L. (1968) Acute post-operative renal failure in obstructive jaundice. *Annals of the Royal College of Surgeons of England*, **42**, 164.
93. Jenkins, M. T., Giesecke, A. H. & Johnson, E. R. (1975) The postoperative patient and his fluid and electrolyte requirements. *British Journal of Anaesthesia*, **47**, 143.
94. Bevan, D. R. (1978) Osmometry 1: Terminology and principles of measurement. *Anaesthesia*, **33**, 794.
95. Bevan, D. R. (1978) Osmometry 2: Osmoregulation. *Anaesthesia*, **33**, 801.
96. Zideman, D. A., Dudley, F. A. H. & Bevan, D. R. (1978) Osmolar output in the peri-operative period. *Anesthesia*, **33**, 788.
97. Flear, C. T. G. & Singh, C. M. (1973) Hyponatraemia and sick cells. *British Journal of Anaesthesia*, **45**, 976.
98. Stoddart, J. C. (1976) Fluid balance and acute cardiovascular failure in 'Recent Advances in Anaesthesia and Analgesia—12' ed. Hewer, C. L. & Atkinson, R. S.; Churchill Livingstone; Edinburgh, London and New York.

10. The anaesthetist and trauma

Donald Campbell

The continuing and proper concern of anaesthetists for their role and function throughout the whole spectrum of management of severely injured patients is evidenced by many recent publications on the subject[1,2,3] and enthusiastic participation in symposia on trauma.[4] This interest reflects the involvement of many anaesthetists for much of their professional careers in some aspect of the management of the appalling number of these patients still admitted to hospital and their recognition of the alarming fatality rate, some 18 000 deaths in England and Wales alone in 1973.[5] Much attention has been given to the organisational aspects of immediate care and to the training of those involved in this work, whether medical or paramedical personnel.[6] The value of accident flying squads for immediate care remains to be proven however in terms of a reduction in mortality and morbidity as measured against the great cost of such services to the community. While the latter point is unresolved, there is little debate now as to the therapeutic objectives in the treatment of the patient with multiple injuries, although the resolution of the many subtle and complex problems encountered may be anything but straightforward. An initially successful resuscitation may produce a critically ill patient with progressive failure of various organ systems and death unless the complications and sequelae of the initial injuries are anticipated, prevented if possible, but certainly aggressively treated. Shoemaker and Bryan-Brown[7] have to this end stressed the advantages of defining in advance the various life-threatening problems likely to be encountered and preparing in advance therapeutic protocols as a guide to management. Provided such protocols are flexibly applied, there is a great deal to be said for this approach, especially from the point of view of training teams of clinicians and other personnel concerned with the management of these patients.

It is not the purpose of this brief review to give a detailed account of all the large amount of recent published work on the subject of trauma and the anaesthetist, beginning with the organisation of immediate care through the definitive anaesthetic and surgical management to ongoing intensive therapeutic support. It would seem more pertinent to highlight a few of the important recent advances in this field which are likely to alter our approach to the complex problems encountered or provide further effective weapons in our therapeutic armamentarium.

BLOOD REPLACEMENT AND THE TREATMENT OF SHOCK

Massive transfusion is relatively commonplace in the initial management of severe trauma with all the well-known attendant hazards. The transfusion in an emergency of the equivalent of one blood volume or more always produces potentially lethal effects on the general metabolism and coagulation system. Miller[8] has described the problems involved ranging from the deleterious effects of cold, acid transfusions to citrate intoxication and deficient oxygen carrying capacity due to decreased concentration of 2:3 diphosphoglycerate (2:3 DPG) in the stored red cells.[9,10] The adult form of the respiratory distress syndrome (shock lung) which may occur following massive transfusion may be caused by the embolisation of the lung with micro-aggregates from the stored blood.[11] It is therefore the increasing practice of many anaesthetists to minimise this risk by the use of micropore filters, preferably of the surface filter type.[12] There is nevertheless a significant practical problem, when most available filters are used, in maintaining an adequately high flow rate where an urgent and massive trans-fusion is indicated. It is hardly surprising that there is considerable interest in the use of plasma substitutes for grave emergency situations where whole blood is not immediately available or ready in sufficient quantity. The most widely used materials are the natural plasma protein solutions or human albumin fraction and the synthetic colloids, namely, the high molecular weight dextrans, gelatin and hydroxyethyl starches. The latter are prepared from animal or plant sources and Moffitt[13] has indicated the ideal properties such synthetic substances should possess. These substances should be capable of (a) maintaining an adequate colloid osmotic pressure for several hours, (b) should be stable and have a long shelf life at a wide range of ambient temperatures, (c) should be free from pyrogens and antigens and (d) should have no adverse metabolic effects on the patient. Table 10.1 lists the origin and characteristics of the various substitutes currently available.[14] Adverse histaminoid and anaphylactic reactions varying from mild to severe have been reported with all these plasma substitutes although the mechanism may vary with different solutions and the real incidence of such reactions is not at all clear. Despite this inherent risk, there can be no doubt that plasma substitutes will continue to play an important therapeutic role in the treatment of the severely injured.

Table 10.1 Production and properties of different colloidal plasma substitutes. Reproduced by kind permission of the authors and the editor of the *British Journal of Anaesthesia.*[14]

Substitute	Production	Types	Mean molec. wt	Intravascular half-life	Indications
Plasma protein	Human plasma, placenta	Serum conserves Human albumin (5% and 20%)	50 000	4–15 days	Volume substitution, hypoproteinaemia, haemodilution
Dextran	B. *Leuconostoc mesenteroids* B512 on agar-sucrose plates	D 60/75 D 40	60 000 40 000	6 h 2–3 h	Haemodilution Microcirculation disturbances (Both:) Volume sub-stitution, throm-bosis prophylaxis
Gelatin	Hydrolysis from animal collagens	Modified gelatin Urea-linked Oxypolygelatin	35 000	2–3 h	Volume substitution
Starch	Acid hydrolysis and ethylene oxide treatment of soya and corn	Hydroxyethylene starch	450 000	6 h	Volume substitution, haemodilution

The role of sympathomimetic amines in the treatment of shocked patients has always been a matter of considerable debate. Their lack of specificity results in a high incidence of unwanted side effects such as impaired myocardial or renal perfusion and serious dysrhythmias.[15] The endogenous catecholamine dopamine,[16] an immediate precursor of adrenaline, and its more recent synthetic analogue dobutamine[17] are currently under critical appraisal in this respect. This drug's apparent advantage to the shocked patient is that it increases myocardial contractility and cardiac output by direct action and also indirectly by releasing endogenous noradrenaline.[18] Equally important in this situation, it increases renal blood flow and the glomerular filtration rate and causes mesenteric vasodilatation. Great care has to be taken in patients with ischaemic heart disease since dangerous tachydysrhythmias may occur and one of the drug's relative disadvantages is that it must be given by continuous infusion due to its short half-life of approximately two minutes. Although continual controlled evaluation of dopamine and its synthetic analogue is necessary, the results so far are encouraging and it may prove to be an important additional supportive measure in the resuscitation of shocked patients following major trauma.

PULMONARY COMPLICATIONS OF TRAUMA

Adult respiratory distress syndrome

One of the dreaded complications of trauma is the gradual development of respiratory insufficiency despite the absence of direct initial damage to the thorax and its contents. The condition has been described as 'shock lung' but as an indistinguishable disturbance can occur in many diverse clinical conditions it is better now referred to as the adult respiratory distress syndrome.[19] The histopathological changes in the lungs have been well described and comprise the development of interstitial oedema, a protein-rich alveolar exudate (hyaline membrane), loss of surfactant and atelectasis, but diagnosis during life rests upon clinical findings such as the onset of dyspnoea, tachycardia and cyanosis. The chest X-ray may be clear initially but subsequently ill-defined opacities develop and may coalesce to give a 'white-out' appearance with only the larger bronchi delineated by air.

Branthwaite in a review of the condition emphasised that the diagnosis is largely presumptive and the treatment empirical.[20] Avoidance of overtransfusion with crystalloid solutions is important in prevention and the use of micropore filters for massive blood transfusion advisable. Treatment is controlled oxygen therapy, avoiding prolonged high inspired concentrations of oxygen, administered in all but the mildest cases by a mechanical ventilator. These patients benefit from the controlled use of a respiratory pattern which includes an end-inspiratory pause and the judicious application of a positive end-expiratory pressure phase. Indiscriminate use of positive airway pressure, however, is hazardous in that reduction in cardiac output with diminished tissue oxygenation may occur despite apparently better oxygenation as judged by arterial oxygen tension alone. Since the mechanism of pulmonary damage seen in shock states may be related to the release of toxins and vasoactive substances,[21] there has been widespread advocacy of the use of steroids in high dosage in these patients. The supportive evidence is mainly from experimental animal models and the value of this therapy in man is highly debatable. Apart from oxygen therapy as described, the most useful adjuncts to treatment would appear to be the avoidance of fluid overload and the use of diuretics where development of pulmonary oedema is detected.

Thermal damage to the airway and lungs

Another form of lung damage associated with trauma and of considerable interest to anaesthetists is where there has been inhalation of smoke or toxic fumes by the patient as a result of the accident. The damage may be difficult to detect or may be entirely overlooked, particularly where there is no other obvious thermal trauma to the body. This is especially true in children. Vivori and Cudmore[22] advocate early intubation with mechanical ventilation and controlled oxygen therapy where respiratory distress appears to be progressive. They also emphasise the need to employ a smaller than usual endotracheal tube to permit an air leak and minimise mucosal damage with the subsequent increased risk of sub-glottic stenosis. It is probably also wise to determine blood carboxy-haemoglobin and cyanide concentrations where possible on admission since many cases suffer from deficiencies in oxygen transport and hypoxic cerebral irritation in addition to the pulmonary complications. Where the diagnosis is suspected fibre-optic laryngoscopy and bronchoscopy may be useful confirmatory procedures since they will reveal oedema of the mucosa and the presence of carbon particles in the lower airway. To assist in the monitoring of pulmonary function in these patients, Armstrong et al[23] advocate the frequent calculation of the virtual shunt[24] and respiratory index as an indication of the clinical trend.

Pulmonary embolism

In patients who have suffered from major trauma there is a considerable risk of embolisation of the lungs from two sources and this complication of injury is potentially lethal and can be difficult to diagnose.

Where long bones have been damaged or there are multiple rib fractures, the fat embolism syndrome is particularly likely to occur but the diagnosis may be missed easily where there is already impaired consciousness and respiratory distress from other causes. Cutaneous petechiae, which in any case are not an invariable accompaniment of fat embolisation, may also be difficult to detect where there are large areas of skin bruising as a result of the initial injury. The detection of non-dietary fat in the urine is of no assistance in diagnosis since it may be present after a simple rib fracture without any clinical evidence of the embolism syndrome. The diagnosis is of necessity presumptive where an injured patient's conscious level deteriorates without other explanation and particularly when this is accompanied by the onset of the respiratory distress syndrome. The treatment is in any case oxygen therapy, intermittent positive pressure ventilation frequently being necessary. There is no firm evidence that heparin, trasylol or steroid therapy in any way reduce morbidity or mortality.

Pulmonary thromboembolic episodes are probably commoner after major trauma than is generally appreciated. The incidence of fatal embolism after major surgery and trauma is of the order of 1 in 200 patients. It is generally accepted that low-dose heparin considerably reduces the development of isotopically diagnosed deep venous thrombosis following elective surgery[25,26] but, of course in injured patients heparin cannot be given prophylactically and the magnitude of the thrombotic challenge is probably greater. There are more serious problems too from haemorrhage in the severely injured patient and heparin should only be administered where the diagnosis is certain. Where the development of thrombi is suspected clinically venography is the most certain method of diagnosing their presence in popliteal, femoral and iliac veins. Pulmonary angiography will demonstrate clearly the presence of a detached embolus in the pulmonary venous system where this is clinically suspected. There are then only two lines of specific therapy open to the clinician apart from full cardio-respiratory supportive measures, the one being anticoagulant therapy with its attendant risk of provoking serious haemorrhage and the other being the surgical removal of thrombus from the pulmonary vasculature on emergency cardio-pulmonary bypass which is a formidable undertaking but may be lifesaving.[27] The use of dextran solutions in all severely injured patients may be the safest method of reducing the incidence of fatal pulmonary embolisation from this cause.

HEAD INJURIES

The patient with multiple injuries and a concomitant head injury is notoriously difficult to manage. This is particularly the case where there is an accompanying crushing injury to the chest. Campbell[28] drew attention to the harmful interaction of these two serious injuries, the mortality for the isolated severe injury to the chest being increased from around 30 per cent to over 50 per cent if a head injury is also present. Rose et al[29] judged that in a series of 116 patients known to have talked before dying from a head injury, 54 per cent had an avoidable factor certainly contributing to death. While in the greater number of these deaths delay in treatment of an intracranial haematoma was the contributing factor, extra-cranial causes such as airway obstruction and hypotension were implicated in a significant number of patients. This finding emphasises yet again the role of the impeccable airway in reduction of mortality emphasised by Lewin[30] in his recent review of the management of head injuries. Assessment of these patients can be much improved if the coma scale devised by Teasdale[31] is used in addition to overall clinical monitoring. Unlike other systems of surveillance devised for such patients, many of which depend on attempts to correlate clinical signs with specific anatomical lesions where there is in fact no such relationship, the coma scale depends on three separate aspects of the patient's responsiveness. These are: the stimulus needed to produce opening of the patient's eyes, the best verbal response and the best motor response. Each can be observed and described by relatively junior medical and nursing staff and together indicate the degree of central nervous system dysfunction. The use of these three responses avoids the need to employ arbitrary and non-standard descriptive terms of the degree of unconsciousness or to assume specific anatomical lesions in the brain. A further advantage of this method of monitoring patients with head injuries is that it facilitates communication between personnel in the accident or intensive care unit with the neurosurgical staff who may be some distance away, although available for telephone consultation.

A recent review[32] firmly underlined the responsibility of the anaesthetist in the care of head injuries and, in addition, where an anaesthetic must be given for urgent surgical treatment of other extracranial injuries, the anaesthetist must be fully alert to the dangers of inducing a 'second accident' by injudicious choice of drugs or technique.[33]

RENAL COMPLICATIONS IN TRAUMA

The anaesthetist should be acutely aware that severely injured patients are in the high risk category so far as the development of renal failure is concerned. Hypovolaemia, whether from loss of whole blood, plasma or fluid, is often accompanied by hypoxaemia and in these circumstances renal function is prejudiced. Furthermore, crushing injuries resulting in high circulatory levels of myoglobin are accompanied by an increased incidence of acute renal failure.[34] It must not be forgotten that direct damage to the kidneys or urinary tract is also likely to occur in multiple injuries and cystoscopy and radiography may be required early in management to eliminate these possibilities. Unavoidable emergency surgery and anaesthesia may further embarrass renal function since they frequently result in oliguria in normal circumstances by diminishing renal perfusion and the glomerular filtration rate and increasing tubular reabsorption and ADH and aldosterone secretion.

No one test of incipient renal failure can be relied upon and Lee[35] recommends that the following criteria should be met before diagnosis can be established with confidence:

1. A urine/plasma (U/P) urea ratio of less than 10 to 1
2. A U/P osmolality of less than 1.1
3. A urine flow of less than 20 ml/h
4. A urinary sodium of greater than 10 mmol/litre
5. The exclusion of pre-existing chronic renal failure or obstruction to the urinary tract.

The correction of any deficit in circulatory volume and any hypoxaemia during early resuscitation may be sufficient to reverse the trend to established renal failure and this is facilitated by adequate monitoring of the patient in the usual way with the importance of central venous pressure and continuous urine flow measurements not being forgotten. If these essential basic measures do not result in an immediate improvement, then aggressive treatment is indicated. It is most important to embark upon treatment early since if the situation is allowed to persist beyond 48 hr results are poor. The treatment of choice is the intravenous infusion of 20 g of 20 per cent mannitol over a period of 30 minutes to one hour. If urine flow does not increase within four hours, this dose of osmotic diuretic should be repeated.

In the elderly or where there is evidence of myocardial insufficiency, the patient must be very carefully observed since a sudden increase in extracellular fluid volume may precipitate congestive cardiac failure. If mannitol fails to produce an improvement, it is probably worth while administering an intravenous infusion of 0.25 to 0.5 g of frusemide over a period of 20 minutes. Failure to respond to this regimen indicates that renal failure is established and appropriate measures such as peritoneal or haemodialysis will be required.

When considering this serious complication of trauma it is salutary to remember that the mortality despite the best management is still high, being around 50 per cent in patients over 50 years of age.[36]

MANAGEMENT OF INFECTION

The risk of bacterial contamination where there has been massive tissue damage is high and gives rise to the vexed question of whether it is justifiable to employ antibiotics prophylactically in these patients. The widespread preventive use of broad-spectrum antibiotics is likely to increase the prevalence of resistant organisms but this risk may be reduced by short-course prophylaxis as proposed for reducing wound sepsis following cholecystectomy.[37] The development of gram-negative infection in traumatised patients is a formidable complication and a potent cause of endotoxic shock. The choice of antibiotic here is of prime importance and the clinician must be aware of the attendant risks in certain circumstances such as nephrotoxicity where an aminoglycoside is given simultaneously with a diuretic such as frusemide. The antibiotic combination of choice where there is a gram-negative infection is probably an aminoglycoside such as gentamicin along with lincomycin, the latter being employed to combat gram-positive as well as gram-negative anaerobic bacteria. New antibiotics are being introduced every year and there are now over 60 systemic antibiotics available to the clinician. Consequently, there is often confusion as to the best choice and relative merits, particularly with regard to potential toxicity. An extremely useful account of the current position has been recently given by McAllister[38] and a brief symposium of recent date is also available for up-to-date guidance in this confusing field of therapy.[39]

Undue reliance on antibiotics when dealing with the problem of infection in severely injured patients is unwise. The anaesthetist must not be blind to the importance of prevention of bacterial invasion by meticulous attention to the more general aspects of patient management which influence the incidence of serious infection. There is evidence, for example, in the treatment of crushing injuries to the chest that a reduction in the number of tracheostomies performed and of patients over-enthusiastically subjected to IPPV might significantly reduce morbidity and mortality in these patients.[40]

The anaesthetist's primary and essential role in the management of severely injured patients remains to ensure adequate resuscitation with preservation of vital functions and to administer a meticulously safe anaesthetic should this be required. The anaesthetist's technical expertise also makes him perculiarly suitable to oversee the conduct of monitoring of vital functions throughout treatment but he has also an important contribution to make in the wider aspects of organisation of immediate care services as well as involvement at all levels of therapy. Many problems remain unresolved in this demanding area of patient care and morbidity and mortality rates following severe trauma are still sufficiently formidable to banish any tendency to complacency despite the undoubted advances of recent years.

REFERENCES

1. Symposium on the management of trauma. (1977) *British Journal of Anaesthesia*, **49**, 643–720.
2. Baskett, P. J. F. & Zorab, J. S. M. (1975) Priorities in the immediate care of roadside and other traumatic casualties. *Anaesthesia*, **30**, 80–87.
3. Finch, P. & Nancekievill, D. G. (1975) The role of hospital medical teams at a major accident. *Anaesthesia*, **30**, 666–676.
4. Faculty of Anaesthetists of the Royal College of Surgeons of England (1977) Symposium on 'Trauma and the Anaesthetist'.
5. Registrar General's Statistical Review of England and Wales for the Year 1973 (1975) Part I (A) Tables, Medical. London: H.M.S.O.
6. Stewart, R. D. (1977) The training of paramedical personnel. *British Journal of Anaesthesia*, **49**, 659–671.
7. Shoemaker, W. C. & Bryan-Brown, C. W. (1973) Resuscitation and immediate care of the critically ill and injured patient. *Seminars in Drug Treatment*, **3**, 249–267.
8. Miller, R. D. (1973) Complications of massive blood transfusions. *Anesthesiology*, **39**, 82–93.
9. Benesch, R. & Benesch, R. E. (1967) The effect of organic phosphates from the human erythrocyte on the allosteric properties of haemoglobin. *Biochemical and Biophysical Research Communications*, **26**, 162–167.
10. Macdonald, R. (1977) Red cell 2,3-diphosphoglycerate and oxygen affinity. *Anaesthesia*, **32**, 544–553.
11. McNamara, J. J., Burran, E. L., Larson, E., Omiya, G., Suchiro, G. & Yamase, H. (1972) Effects of debris in stored blood on pulmonary microvasculature. *Annals of Thoracic Surgery*, **14**, 133–139.
12. Marshall, B. E., Wurzel, H. A., Neufeld, G. R. & Klineberg, P. L. (1976) Effects of Intersept micropore filtration of blood on microaggregates and other constituents. *Anesthesiology*, **44**, 525–534.
13. Moffitt, E. A. (1975) Blood substitutes. *Canadian Anaesthetists' Society Journal*, **22**, 12–19.
14. Doenicke, A., Grote, B. & Lorenz, W. (1977) Blood and blood substitutes. *British Journal of Anaesthesia*, **49**, 681–688.
15. Stoner, J. D. III, Bolen, J. L. & Harrison, D. C. (1977) Comparison of dobutamine and dopamine in treatment of severe heart failure. *British Heart Journal*, **39**, 536–539.
16. Dopamine Hydrochloride. Proceedings of an International Symposium. (1976) *Proceedings of the Royal Society of Medicine*, **70**, Supplement 2.
17. Loeb, H. S., Bredakis, J. & Gunnar, R. M. (1977) Superiority of dobutamine over dopamine for augmentation of cardiac output in patients with chronic low output cardiac failure. *Circulation*, **55**, 375–381.
18. Goldberg, L. I. (1972) Cardiovascular and renal actions of dopamine: potential clinical applications. *Pharmacological Reviews*, **24**, 1–29.
19. Hedley-Whyte, J., Burgess, G. E. III, Feeley, T. W. & Miller, M. G. (1976) Effect of sepsis on respiratory function. In *Applied Physiology of Respiratory Care*, p. 55. Boston: Little, Brown & Co.
20. Branthwaite, M. (1977) Communication on Shock Lung at Symposium on 'Trauma and the Anaesthetist'. Faculty of Anaesthetists of the Royal College of Surgeons of England.
21. Blaisdell, F. W., Lim, R. C. Jr. & Stallone, R. J. (1970) The mechanism of pulmonary damage following traumatic shock. *Surgery, Gynecology and Obstetrics*, **130**, 15–22.
22. Vivori, E. & Cudmore, R. E. (1977) Management of airway complications in burned children. *British Medical Journal*, **2**, 1462–1464.
23. Armstrong, R. F., Mackersie, A. M., McGregor, A. P. & Woods, S. D. (1977) The respiratory injury in burns. *Anaesthesia*, **32**, 313–319.
24. Benatar, S. R., Hewlett, A. M. & Nunn, J. F. (1973) The use of iso-shunt lines for control of oxygen therapy. *British Journal of Anaesthesia*, **45**, 711–718.
25. Nicolaides, A. N., Desai, S., Douglas, J. N. et al (1972) Small doses of subcutaneous sodium heparin in preventing deep venous thrombosis after major surgery. *Lancet*, **2**, 890–893.
26. International Multicentre Trial (1975) Prevention of fatal postoperative pulmonary embolism by low doses of heparin. *Lancet*, **2**, 45–51.

27. Price, D. G. (1976) Pulmonary embolism: Prophylaxis, diagnosis and treatment. *Anaesthesia*, **31**, 925–932.
28. Campbell, D. (1977) Immediate care of the injured. *British Journal of Anaesthesia*, **49**, 673–679.
29. Rose, J., Valtonen, S. & Jennett, B. (1977) Avoidable factors contributing to death after head injury. *British Medical Journal*, **2**, 615–618.
30. Lewin, W. (1976) Changing attitudes to the management of severe head injuries. *British Medical Journal*, **2**, 1234–1239.
31. Teasdale, G. (1976) Assessment of head injuries. *British Journal of Anaesthesia*, **48**, 761–766.
32. Horton, J. M. (1976) The anaesthetist's contribution to the care of head injuries. *British Journal of Anaesthesia*, **48**, 767–771.
33. Greenbaum, R. (1976) General anaesthesia for neuro-surgery. *British Journal of Anaesthesia*, **48**, 773–781.
34. Crush injuries. Leading article (1977) *British Medical Journal*, **2**, 1244.
35. Lee, H. A. (1977) The management of acute renal failure following trauma. *British Journal of Anaesthesia*, **49**, 697–705.
36. Lindsay, R. M. (1974) The prognosis of acute renal failure. In *Acute Renal Failure*, ed. Flynn, C. I., p. 103. Lancaster: M.T.P. Co. Ltd.
37. Strachan, C. J. L., Black, J., Powis, J. A. et al (1977) Prophylactic use of cephazolin against wound sepsis after cholecystectomy. *British Medical Journal*, **1**, 1254–1256.
38. McAllister, T. A. (1976) Recent advances in antibiotics. *Scottish Medical Journal*, **21**, 210–217.
39. Newer Antibiotics: a Symposium. (1977) Chairman, Geddes, A. M. *Prescribers' Journal*, ed. Hunt, J. L. Leeds: John Blackburn Ltd.
40. Trinkle, J. K., Richardson, J. D., Franz, J. L., Grover, F. L., Arom, K. V. & Holmstrom, F. M. G. (1975) Management of flail chest without mechanical ventilation. *Annals of Thoracic Surgery*, **19**, 355–363.

11. Poisoning

J. Krapez

Suicide and attempted suicide seem to be an integral part of human behaviour. The Japanese have made it into a near-religion, and while Westerners prefer slightly less spectacular methods than ritual disembowelling, their more mundane approach to the choice of agent is made up for by the large numbers involved. Over 96 000 cases of self-poisoning were admitted to hospital in the UK alone in 1974,[1] and the figure has almost certainly risen since then.[2] Indeed such is the size of the epidemic that the majority of young women admitted to medical wards have taken an overdose[2] and, in the absence of trauma, acute poisoning is the commonest cause of impaired consciousness in anyone aged 15–50.[3]

The situation may however be improving. Holding et al[4] recently reported that the rate of increase in admissions had fallen, and data from other workers[5] supports this heartening trend. There has also been a decrease in the number of successful suicides, the total falling by approximately 10 per cent between 1972 and 1974.[1] Nearly 70 per cent of this reduction is admittedly due to the widespread introduction of natural gas, but there has also been a fall in the number of deaths from drug overdoses. How much of this is due to altered prescribing habits (in particular the substitution of 'safer' drugs—e.g. benzodiazepines—for barbiturates) or simply to improved patient care is not clear. Patients do however ingest those drugs which are available, and it is a sobering thought for the medical profession that up to 90 per cent of overdose cases have taken drugs issued on prescription.[6]

The management of the acutely poisoned patient is essentially simple, requiring techniques which are second nature to anaesthetists. The vast majority of patients can be successfully treated with a combination of accurate assessment followed by good supportive therapy. It is unusual for antidotes and more specialised techniques to be required, although in a few instances (e.g. cyanide, iron and insecticide poisonings) the rapid use of the appropriate antidote may be life-saving. Some cases of severe poisoning may also benefit from the use of more active methods of drug removal, e.g. haemoperfusion, but such techniques if they are to be of value must be supplementary to a well-planned system of basic care.

ASSESSMENT

The essential elements in assessing the acutely poisoned patient are as follows:

Assessment of coma

Most drugs when taken in excess produce coma, and its depth provides a good guide to the patient's progress. Several schemes for grading coma have been proposed, but the following one, suggested by Matthew and Lawson,[7] has the virtue of being simple and provides useful results.

Grade 1.   Drowsy but responds to vocal command.
Grade 2.   Unconscious but responds to minimal stimuli.
Grade 3.   Unconscious and responds only to maximal painful stimuli.
Grade 4.   Unconscious and totally unresponsive.

Observations of limb reflexes, pupil size or corneal reaction are of little value, and may actually provide misleading data. Rubbing the patient's sternum with a clenched fist provides an excellent 'maximal painful stimulus'. The progress of Grade 4 patients may be followed by the use of the electroencephalogram (EEG)[8,9] and the cerebral function monitor (CFM),[10] lightening of coma being signalled by increasing EEG activity and a rising voltage on the CFM. It is important to note that a 'flat' EEG for as long as 28 hours has been associated with complete recovery.[11]

Assessment of respiratory function

Death from acute poisoning is most commonly due to respiratory complications. Assessment should include the patency of the airway, the gag and cough reflexes, cyanosis, respiratory rate, tidal volume and arterial blood gases. Tidal volume is best measured using a Wright's respirometer and anaesthetic face mask, inadequate tidal exchange probably being present if the minute volume is less than four litres. Any doubts about the efficacy of ventilation should prompt the measurement of arterial blood gases. It is impossible to make hard and fast rules, but artificial ventilation is likely to be required with a $Paco_2$ above 7.5 kPa (55 mmHg) and a Pao_2 below 8.0 kPa (60 mmHg).

Admission is not synonymous with improvement and it is of the utmost importance that observations should be continued after the patient has reached the ward.

Assessment of cardiovascular function

Tissue perfusion, pulse rate and rhythm, systemic blood pressure and central venous pressure are the factors which must be considered. Tissue perfusion is the most important of these. The well perfused patient will be warm, pink and will have a good urine output (> 30 ml/hr) without the need to resort to diuretics. Systemic blood pressure measurements can provide misleading information but are not entirely without value. A blood pressure below 80 mmHg (or 90 mmHg in those over 50) is likely to be associated with impaired tissue perfusion. An increasing base deficit can also provide presumptive evidence of poor perfusion, but it should be remembered that metabolic acidosis may be produced by the agent ingested (e.g. aspirin, phenformin). Temperature monitoring (vide infra) can also aid in assessing tissue perfusion.

Pulse rate and rhythm are likely to be abnormal when drugs such as digoxin and tricyclic antidepressants have been taken, and continuous ECG monitoring will be particularly relevant in these cases.

Systemic blood pressure is low following overdosage with most drugs, particularly when intoxication is severe,[12] but hypertensive crises may be produced by some drugs, especially monoamine oxidase inhibitors.

Clinical evidence of heart failure should be sought and central venous pressure monitoring carried out via an indwelling catheter as necessary. This is also of value in elderly patients and when employing forced diuresis.

Assessment of body temperature
Hypothermia (core temperature below $36°C$) is common, being present in nearly 50 per cent of serious overdoses.[12] Its detection requires the use of low reading mercury or electrical thermometers. The latter may be inserted into the rectum and attached to the skin of the leg, allowing continuous monitoring of core and peripheral temperature. This will also provide evidence of circulatory efficacy, a falling peripheral temperature with a constant or a rising central temperature being indicative of failing tissue perfusion.

Determination of the ingested agent
It is worth attempting to discover which poison(s) the patient has ingested, but time spent on inquiries should not be allowed to detract from the patient's basic care. Samples of blood, urine and gastric contents should be sent to the pathology laboratory and/or the Regional Poisons Centre for analysis. Information concerning the likely nature of the agent responsible may be obtained from eye witnesses, empty drug containers and recovered tablets. It may be worth asking the patient what has been taken, but any answers should be accepted with reservations since the patient's account is notoriously unreliable. Mixtures of drugs are being used with increasing frequency, and alcohol is often taken in addition.

CONSERVATIVE MANAGEMENT

The adoption of conservative techniques of management, otherwise known as 'the Scandinavian method'[13] has been the single most important factor in reducing the mortality from acute poisoning to its present value of less than 1 per cent.[7] The basic principles involved are the care of respiratory and cardiovascular function, correction of altered physiology and removal of ingested poison from the body.

Respiratory system
The maintenance of a clear airway is essential. Vomit, saliva and dentures should be removed and the patient positioned on his left side with an oropharyngeal airway in place. If there is any doubt concerning the patency of the airway then tracheal intubation should be carried out using a Portex tube fitted with a low-pressure cuff. The use of suxamethonium and cricoid pressure has been recommended for patients who react too strongly to the laryngoscope,[14] but such a manoeuvre should not be lightly undertaken.

Oxygen therapy is often required to correct hypoxia. We have not found it necessary to use 24 per cent Ventimasks,[15] and would recommend a 'shell' type with an initial flow rate of four—five litres of oxygen per minute. This can be altered subsequently in the light of arterial blood gas estimations.

The decision to institute artificial ventilation should be based on clinical grounds in combination with arterial Po_2 and Pco_2 levels. The choice of ventilator is immaterial, but it should be borne in mind that the institution of intermittent positive pressure ventilation (IPPV) in these patients can precipitate marked falls in cardiac output, and rapid therapy with intravenous fluids and/or vasopressors may be required. Inspired gases should always be warmed and humidified.

Bronchial toilet will be required in the intubated patient, and it is vital that an aseptic technique be used. Suction should only be applied for short (< 10 seconds) periods to avoid exacerbation of airways collapse and hypoxia. It is unusual for tracheostomy to be necessary, particularly with the use of non-irritant tracheal tubes, which can be left in place for several days. When tracheostomy is indicated it should always be carried out as an elective procedure.

Cardiovascular system

A relative degree of hypovolaemia due to expansion of the microcirculation is the usual cause of a reduced cardiac output.[16] Elevation of the legs is a useful short-term measure to improve venous return. For subsequent therapy the choice lies between vasoconstrictors and intravenous fluids. While Matthew[17] makes a case for vasopressors we would favour the use of plasma expansion, preferably using Plasma Protein Fraction (PPF), or if this is not available, Haemacel or Dextran 70. This avoids the risk of renal and hepatic ischaemia from the use of vasoconstrictors.

Dysrhythmias can be produced by ingestion of some drugs. Their therapy is discussed under the individual agents concerned.

Water and electrolyte balance do not normally present major problems. Infusion of dextrose (4.8 per cent) and saline (0.18 per cent) (isotonic in combination) according to urine output and insensible loss is usually all that is necessary. Occasionally more marked alterations of fluid balance and biochemistry occur, and these require appropriate therapy in the light of clinical examination and serum electrolyte and acid-base measurements.

Removal of poison

The majority of drugs will have left the stomach four hours after ingestion (either by being absorbed or by passing into the small intestine). Hence there is no point in attempting to empty the stomach when this length of time has elapsed. Aspirin, anticholinergics and tricyclic antidepressants are an exception to this rule since they pharmacologically delay gastric emptying. The time limit may thus be extended for these drugs, particularly aspirin. Emesis and lavage should not be carried out following ingestion of petrochemicals because of the risk of aspiration pneumonitis. *Emetics must never be administered in the presence of impaired consciousness.*

Induced emesis with syrup of ipecacuanha is now generally considered to be the treatment of choice in children.[18] Gastric lavage in children is at best ineffective[19] and may be extremely traumatic for all concerned. The dose of the syrup is 15–30 ml, and provided that this amount is not exceeded, cardiotoxicity due to the contained emetine is extremely unlikely.[20] Emesis will occur within 30 minutes in nearly 90 per cent of patients.[21] Saline, apomorphine and copper sulphate have also been recommended as emetics. Saline is not only a poor emetic[20] but has also been responsible for several deaths due to hyper-natraemia.[22,23] Apomorphine acts rapidly and is as effective as ipecacuanha,[24] but the depression of consciousness it produces and the fact that it must be given parenterally make it less desirable. Copper sulphate is quick-acting but its use is associated with a significant rise in serum copper level[25] and at least one death due to copper poisoning has been reported.[26] Mechanical induction of vomiting by inserting a finger into the pharynx is certainly non-toxic, but it has a high failure rate and the recovery of gastric contents is poor. It may also be hazardous for the operator!

Gastric emptying in adults is probably best accomplished by using lavage. This technique should also be used to recover stomach contents in all unconscious patients. It is however a procedure not devoid of risk. All patients with impaired laryngeal reflexes must be intubated in order to minimise the danger of aspiration. Patients should be positioned head-down on their left sides and as large a gastric tube as possible (30 f.g. in adults) should be used to ensure that the maximum number of undissolved tablets are retrieved. Water should be used in adults and normal saline in children. It is important that as much of the lavage medium as possible is recovered, since fluid overload can otherwise be produced. Sharman et al[27] demonstrated that drug removal is incomplete, even with careful lavage, and recommended continued drainage of stomach contents via a nasogastric tube. The stomach should be left empty afterwards to minimise the risk of aspiration.

General nursing care

A high standard of nursing care is mandatory if morbidity and mortality are to be kept to a minimum. In addition the careful recording of the patient's vital functions by the nursing staff is an essential prerequisite for soundly-based medical decisions. The role of the intensive care unit has been examined by Piper and Griner[28] who concluded that intensive care resulted in lower mortality, shorter stay in hospital and fewer complications with no increase in expenditure.

Urine output

This provides such a useful indicator of tissue perfusion that, as far as possible, diuretics should be avoided. Where urine output is low it can usually be improved by infusion of fluids to restore the cardiac output. If diuretics are necessary then mannitol 20 per cent 100 ml should be the agent of first choice. Frusemide or bumetamide may be used should this fail to produce the desired result.

Catheterisation should not be employed routinely. Indications for its use include forced diuresis and failure to maintain a good urine output.

Hypothermia

Most patients can be managed by passive methods of rewarming e.g. the use of 'space' blankets. However at temperatures below 30°C the patient becomes increasingly poikilothermic and more active means must be employed. Ventilation via a Water's canister with added CO_2 is a useful method as is immersing the patient's forearm in warm water (ca. 42°C). Heated mattresses may also be utilised, although care must be taken to avoid skin burns. This is best achieved by setting the mattress temperature to 2°C above the patients *skin* temperature (maximum setting 35°C).

Convulsions

While coma is the result of overdosage with most drugs, convulsions are not infrequently produced by some agents (e.g. tricyclic antidepressants). They are best controlled with small intravenous doses of diazepam.

ACTIVE MANAGEMENT

The opportunities for the doctor to display his therapeutic brilliance in managing cases of acute poisoning are severely limited. Effective antidotes are scarce. They are discussed under the relevant drugs at the end of this section. There are none-the-less a number of more active techniques which merit discussion. Such techniques must always be additional to a sound regime of conservative management.

Activated charcoal

There is now a considerable body of evidence to show that activated charcoal will adsorb certain drugs.[29,30] In particular the absorption of aspirin, paracetamol and barbiturates can be reduced. For the best results the charcoal should be administered as a slurry within 30 minutes of ingestion of the drug,[31] although it has been shown that charcoal can 'catch up' drugs within the bowel despite the fact that they may have been swallowed several hours previously.[33] A charcoal: drug ratio of 10:1 is recommended[30] although Corby and Decker[31] consider that, since it is so non-toxic, the maximum amount possible should be used. The charcoal/drug complex is not completely stable, and during its passage down the intestine a proportion of the drug will be released and absorbed. This can be minimised by using an excess of charcoal. The continued absorption of drugs which undergo entero-hepatic circulation (especially digoxin and tricyclic anti-depressants) can be reduced by trapping the drug within the bowel by adsorption on to charcoal.[32]

Analeptics

Loenecken[34] has documented a fall in mortality due to barbiturate overdose from 9 per cent to 2.1 per cent simply by omitting analeptics from the therapeutic regime. There are now virtually no indications for the use of such drugs as nikethamide and picrotoxin in the management of acute poisoning. Dundee et al[35] however have reported that doxapram used as a bolus injection (100 mg) and by infusion (5–10 mg/minute) produced improved respiration and arousal in patients who had taken barbiturate overdoses. Side effects were minimal, one patient becoming restless and two others being confused for a short time.

Forced diuresis

For forced diuresis to be of value certain criteria concerning the ingested agent must be met. Firstly the active drug must be excreted in the urine. It must not be bound to plasma protein to any great extent and must be present in reasonable quantities within the blood stream. Forced diuresis is usually carried out in combination with manipulation of urinary pH in an attempt to 'trap' filtered drug within the tubule by increasing the ionised fraction. Alkaline diuresis is of value in salicylate overdoses[36] and severe phenobarbitone[17] and barbitone[37] poisoning.

Raising urinary pH to 7.5 increases salicylate excretion fivefold[36] and doubles phenobarbitone elimination.[38] Acid diuresis is in practice best reserved for severe amphetamine overdoses.[39] Forced diuresis is contra-indicated in the presence of a persistently low urine output and/or cardiac failure.

Dialysis

The enthusiastic use of dialysis in the fifties and sixties has given way to a more critical approach[40] and there is a growing list of drugs previously thought to be amenable to dialysis where this has been demonstrated to be untrue.[41,42] Haemodialysis is quicker and more efficient than peritoneal dialysis, but the latter has the advantages of simplicity and ease of management.

Haemoperfusion

This involves the passage of blood over an adsorbing agent, either charcoal or a synthetic resin. The agent is packed into a column and the patient's blood is circulated through this with the aid of a peristaltic pump. Heparinisation is necessary. Marked thrombocytopaenia and charcoal emboli were frequent occurrences when the technique was first introduced, but these have been considerably reduced (although not eliminated) by the use of polymer coating[43,44] and by fixing the charcoal in position.[45] Rosenbaum et al[46] have reported good results with a synthetic resin, Amberlite XAD-4. Haemoperfusion is particularly effective in the treatment of glutethimide, barbiturate and ethchlorvynol overdoses[47] but since conservative management results in a mortality of less than 1 per cent it is necessary to select cases. Vale et al[45] have set out guidelines recommending its use in severe intoxication, patients who do not respond to conservative management and patients in prolonged coma who develop complications (e.g. pneumonia). They also point out its value in cases where hypoxic brain damage may have occurred. The use of haemoperfusion in this situation can, by shortening coma time, allow for an earlier assessment of any permanent cerebral damage.

SPECIFIC DRUGS

The following list of drugs is by no means exhaustive, nor could it ever hope to be. The size of present day pharmacopoeas is such that the choice available to the would-be suicide case is enormous. Instead a list is given of those drugs for which specific antidotes are available, those necessitating particular techniques in management and those producing unusual effects. It is assumed that in all cases conservative management has already been instituted.

Amphetamine

Symptoms include marked stimulation of the central nervous system, cardiac dysrhythmias and abdominal pain. Since up to 50 per cent of the active drug is excreted in an acid urine,[39] forced acid diuresis is of value.

Scheme

1. Infuse 5 per cent dextrose (one litre) and 0.9 per cent saline (500 ml) with lysine or arginine hydrochloride (10 g) in the first hour.

2. Continue infusion using saline and dextrose at 500 ml/hour, keeping urine pH at 5.5–6.5 with ammonium chloride 4 g two hourly p.o.

Barbiturates

General supportive care only is indicated for the majority of cases, although phenobarbitone and barbitone elimination is aided by the use of forced alkaline diuresis (see under 'salicylates'). Haemoperfusion has been reported to be of value.[44,46]

Benzodiazepines

These have a very good record of safety following overdose. However Rada et al[48] have recently reported two deaths following ingestion of chlordiazepoxide with alcohol. They suggest that there may be a synergistic action between the two agents.

Beat-blockers and anti-dysrhythmics

There are now several reports in the literature of overdose with these groups of drugs.[49,50,51] The main features are profound bradycardia or asystole with no response to isoprenaline or artificial pacing. Mattingly[52] has reported return of cardiac activity after two hours of resuscitation, and concludes that prolonged cardiac massage may eventually result in a successful outcome. Glucagon has also been used with some success.[53]

Bleaches and household chemicals

There are two different groups of bleaches—oxalate (or commercial) bleach and hypochlorite (or household) bleach. The former is less common but more toxic, causing severe and sometimes fatal, hypocalcaemia and renal failure. Treatment consists of oral administration of calcium lactate (100 ml of 1 per cent solution) to bind oxalate within the bowel. Calcium gluconate should also be administered intravenously. The effects of hypochlorite bleach are predominantly caustic, damage being largely confined to the oesophagus and stomach. Chlorine gas can however be produced by a reaction between the bleach and hydrochloric acid in the stomach. Aspiration of this gas may then give rise to chemical pneumonitis. Sodium thiosulphate solution 2.5 per cent used as a lavage fluid will neutralise the bleach. Toxicity has probably been overrated,[54] Pike et al[55] reporting no significant injury in 129 cases of hypochlorite ingestion in children. Supportive therapy alone will therefore suffice in most cases.

Soluble water softeners can produce hypocalcaemia and metabolic acidosis. Treatment is as for oxalate bleach.

Disinfectants and deodorisers are caustic to varying degrees and require treatment as for corrosives. Those containing naphtha or phenol can also produce renal failure and haemolysis. Alkaline diuresis increases naphthalene excretion.

Carbon monoxide

This produces death from hypoxia due to two mechanisms. Conversion of haemoglobin to carboxyhaemoglobin reduces the oxygen carrying capacity. In addition the presence of carboxyhaemoglobin produces a left-shift of the oxyhaemoglobin dissociation curve,[56] thus making oxygen delivery to the tissues more difficult.

Treatment consists of removing the patient from the poisoned atmosphere, and the administration of a high inspired oxygen concentration as rapidly as possible. Artificial ventilation may be required to maintain an acceptable Pao_2. Carbon dioxide/oxygen mixtures are of no value and have largely been abandoned in favour of pure oxygen. Hyperbaric oxygen has theoretical advantages, but difficulties in instituting therapy make it much less valuable in practice. Cerebral oedema due to hypoxia can occur, and mannitol infusion, dexamethasone and artificial ventilation may be used to treat this.

Clonidine

Severe hypertension has been reported following overdose[57] although it is not invariably present and postural hypotension may be the only effect.[58] Hunyor et al[57] successfully used diazoxide to treat the hypertensive effect.

Cyanide (including sodium nitroprusside)

Cyanide poisoning produces rapid death from tissue hypoxia as a result of inactivation of the cytochrome oxidase system. It is one of the few examples of poisoning which require the rapid administration of an appropriate antidote. Excessive infusion of sodium nitroprusside can also produce cyanide poisoning, and deaths have occurred from this.[59,60]

Where inhalation of cyanide as HCN has occurred, the patient should obviously be removed from the contaminated atmosphere, and artificial ventilation instituted if necessary. *It is important not to use expired air (mouth to mouth)* ventilation in any case of cyanide poisoning otherwise the number of patients will increase exponentially.

Neutralisation of cyanide can be produced in three different ways. Inhalation of amyl nitrite converts haemoglobin into methaemoglobin. This then combines with cyanide to form cyanmethaemoglobin, thereby neutralising the poison. Amyl nitrite can produce hypotension.

Sodium thiosulphate when injected intravenously neutralises cyanide by converting it into non-toxic thiocyanate. 25 ml of a 50 per cent solution should be used. Rapid intravenous injection can produce hypotension.

Cobalt edetate chelates cyanide when given by intravenous injection. 600 mg should be given over one minute, followed by a further 300 mg if this proves ineffective. It can produce vomiting and severe abdominal cramps. (See also Chapter 6.)

Digoxin

The major complications of digoxin overdoses are cardiac dysrhythmias and hyperkalaemia. Various degrees of A-V block and supraventricular dysrhythmias are the most common abnormalities of cardiac action. Hyperkalaemia probably arises as a result of poisoning of sodium—potassium ATP-ase[61] and mortality can be related to the initial potassium level.[62]

Atropine can be used to counteract bradycardia, although pacing may be required. Bismuth[62] recommends prophylactic insertion of a pacing wire in patients who have hyperkalaemia when first seen. Dysrhythmias may be treated with intravenous injections of lignocaine, bretylium, procainamide, phenytoin or β-blockers. The latter have been used successfully in the treatment of supraventricular dysrhythmias.[63] Phenytoin would appear to offer particular advantages since it does not impair A-V conduction,[64] and it also suppresses dysrhythmias without abolishing the inotropic effects of digoxin.[65] The toxicity of digoxin is enhanced by hypokalaemia, and potassium should be administered to maintain a normal serum level.

Hyperkalaemia should be treated with insulin and dextrose, but haemodialysis may occasionally be required. Even so, dialysis has been reported to be ineffective in controlling serum potassium in all cases.[66]

Digoxin-specific antibodies are now available, and Smith et al[67] have reported their successful use in a case of severe poisoning.

Glutethimide
Overdose can result in raised intra-cranial pressure presenting as papilloedema and apnoea. Twenty per cent mannitol should be given by infusion to combat this. Martin et al[68] have reported the successful management of severe glutethimide poisoning (cases with an expected mortality of 50–60 per cent) using charcoal haemoperfusion.

Heavy metals
Arsenic
The effects of poisoning include vomiting, severe diarrhoea, coma, renal failure and hepatic failure.

British Anti-Lewisite (BAL, dimercaprol) is the antidote of choice. It should be administered intravenously, 4mg/kg 4 hourly for 12 hours, and subsequently 3 mg/kg 12 hourly for 8 days.

Cadmium
This usually presents as chronic poisoning. Calcium-edetate chelates the metal, the complex being excreted in the urine. The dose of the antidote is 0.5 g two hourly by mouth, and therapy may be required for one–two weeks. Penicillamine and BAL are contraindicated since they enhance deposition of cadmium in the kidneys and increase its toxicity.

Iron
Iron poisoning is most often seen in children as an accidental overdose. There are four phases in poisoning:

Phase 1.   Vomiting and diarrhoea (often blood-stained): onset within 30–120 minutes.

Phase 2.   General condition improves. Mild cases then recover, but sudden deterioration occurs in more severe cases.

Phase 3.   Cardiovascular collapse occurs, often with no warning. Oliguria, convulsions, coma and hepatic failure follow.

Phase 4.   Duodenal stenosis can occur as a late complication following recovery from the acute phases.

Most patients are awake on admission and unconsciousness is a bad prognostic sign. The severity of the overdose can be assessed by measurement of serum iron levels within the first six hours. Levels over 500 μg/100 ml are associated with increasing shock and depression of the central nervous system.

Treatment consists of emesis or gastric lavage and oral administration of sodium bicarbonate 1 per cent solution (to precipitate iron as ferric carbonate). Desferrioxamine is the chelating agent of choice. It can be given intramuscularly (90 mg/kg, 6–12 hourly, three or four doses) or by intravenous infusion (15 mg/kg/hour). Rapid infusion produces hypotension. Oral desferrioxamine is not recommended since it can *increase* iron absorption.[69] Treatment should be continued until iron is no longer present in the urine (colour changes from dark orange-brown to normal) and serum iron is less than total iron binding capacity (usually within 24–48 hours).

Lead
Children are most commonly affected, presenting with anaemia, abdominal pain or mental retardation. The latter may not respond completely to treatment.

Calcium edetate should be administered as an intravenous infusion of 2 g in 500 ml of 5 per cent dextrose at a rate of 1–2 grams 12 hourly for three–five days.

Mercury
Acute poisoning produces nausea, vomiting and renal failure. Chronic ingestion gives rise to Pink's disease. Penicillamine is the antidote of choice.[70] It should be given orally, 250 mg 6 hourly for 10 days. More than one course may be required. BAL may also be used in acute poisoning (see 'arsenic').

Thallium
This is used as a rodenticide. It produces renal failure, convulsions and coma following ingestion.

Colloidal Prussian Blue is the antidote of choice. It should be administered orally, 250 mg/kg/day in four divided doses. Prolonged administration may be required.[71]

Hypoglycaemic agents
These produce severe hypoglycaemia, which can be particularly prolonged in the case of chlorpropamide. Overdose of phenformin has been associated with metabolic acidosis.[72]

Fifty per cent dextrose injection should be given intravenously, followed by a 5 per cent infusion at a rate dependent on blood sugar levels.

Lithium
Effects include hypokalaemia, dysrhythmias, tremor and convulsions. Replacement of intracellular potassium by lithium (with consequent reduction in polarisation) may be responsible for the dysrhythmias.[73] Treatment should be with intravenous potassium, gastric lavage with sodium phosphate (to precipitate lithium phosphate) and dialysis.

Methaqualone

Overdose results in hypertonia, myoclonia, coma and pulmonary oedema. Peripheral neuropathy has also been reported.[74]

Matthew et al[75] report good results from the use of conservative management, and consider forced diuresis (which has previously been recommended) to be contraindicated.

Monoamine oxidase inhibitors

These can produce agitation, convulsions and hyper- or hypotension.

Indirectly acting sympathomimetics are absolutely contra-indicated when treating hypotension as their use may precipitate hypertensive crises. Hypertension should be treated with ganglion blockers e.g. pentolinium.

Opiates

Overdosage results in apnoea, cardiovascular collapse and coma. The former is the usual cause of death, although pulmonary oedema with a mortality of 20 per cent has been reported in up to 50 per cent of drug addicts who have taken overdoses.[76]

Naloxone (0.4 mg intravenously) is the treatment of choice for all opiate overdoses, including related compounds such as propoxyphene,[77] 'Lomotil'[78] and 'Immobilon'.[79] Since naloxone has a short duration of action (20–30 minutes), repeat injections are likely to be required. Nalorphine (10 mg) or levallorphan (1 mg) can also be used as antidotes, but their own significant agonist activity makes them less valuable. Opiate antagonists can precipitate a withdrawal syndrome in drug addicts.

Orphenadrine

This drug produces convulsions, coma and shock when taken in overdose. Marked bradycardia may be a feature. Overdose has unfortunately followed its use in the treatment of Parkinsonian symptoms produced by phenothiazines. Toxicity is high, death having occurred within 30 minutes of ingestion.[80] Physostigmine has been successfully used to treat central nervous system effects,[81] but Sangster et al[82] consider this to be contra-indicated in view of the risk of bradycardia.

Paracetamol

Overdose results in hepatic failure in a proportion of patients. This is most probably due to overloading of the normal glutathione conjugation pathway which neutralises a highly toxic metabolite.[83] Liver failure can take up to five days to develop, earlier onset being associated with a higher mortality.[84] Attempts at early recognition of patients who will go on to develop liver failure have proved difficult. Jones et al[85] found that an aspartate aminotransferase level above 400 units/litre was likely to be associated with severe liver damage. They also concluded that a plasma paracetamol below 100 mg/litre at four hours and 40 mg/litre at 12 hours after ingestion was unlikely to be associated with liver failure, while this was likely if plasma paracetamol was above 300 mg/litre at four hours and 80 mg/litre at 12 hours. However, Gazzard et al[86] found that there was no good, reliable prognostic test, and that 30 per cent of patients will receive unnecessary treatment if therapy is given on the basis of plasma paracetamol levels.

Treatment consists of lavage, administration of activated charcoal and cholestyramine to bind the drug in the bowel. Haemoperfusion, which initially looked promising, has not proved to be of value.[84] Active treatment now centres around either administration of sulphydryl donating drugs—e.g. cysteamine, BAL—or increasing hepatic glutathione content by giving methionine. All antidotes require the first dose to be given within 10 hours of drug ingestion, which reduces the value of half-life measurements (see above). Cysteamine should be given as 2 g intravenously, followed by 1.6 g divided into four doses over the next 24 hours.[87] It is a toxic substance, producing nausea, vomiting, severe abdominal pain and meningism in some patients, and should not be given without first establishing that paracetamol levels are raised. BAL was compared with cysteamine by Gazzard et al,[88] who found it to have a lower incidence of side effects. However more of the BAL-treated patients subsequently developed liver damage.

Methionine is a much less toxic antidote. Crome et al[89] reported no deaths in 30 severely poisoned patients who received methionine (expected mortality would have been 5–10 per cent). No side-effects were seen and where liver damage did occur, its severity was greatly reduced. Methionine is administered orally, 2.5 g 4 hourly to a total dose of 10 g and should be given within 10 hours of paracetamol ingestion as it can produce hepatic encephalopathy in patients with established liver damage. McLean[90] concludes that methionine is superior to cysteamine.

Paraquat

Paraquat is available as a 20 per cent aqueous solution and as granules containing 2.5 per cent paraquat and 2.5 per cent diquat. The majority of reported fatalities have followed ingestion of the aqueous preparation, possibly because the corrosive nature of the poison facilitates absorption. Immediate effects include vomiting, dysphagia and diarrhoea. Renal and hepatic damage may develop within three days of ingestion. Progressive pulmonary fibrosis, which is the usual cause of death, can take up to seven days to appear.

There is no specific antidote, and treatment consists of preventing absorption from the gastro-intestinal tract. Lavage should be performed and 250 ml of adsorbent suspension left in the stomach. Fuller's earth (sub-bentonite) 30 per cent is the preferred adsorbent,[91] although bentonite 7 per cent may be used if this is not available. 12.5 g of magnesium sulphate should be added to the suspension to induce diarrhoea and reduce paraquat absorption. Oxygen therapy should be delayed for as long as possible since it enhances toxicity. Haemoperfusion has produced some encouraging results,[92] although it is still under investigation.[93] Cytoxic drugs, steroids and immunosuppressive agents have also been suggested as treatment, but there is no good evidence to show that they improve survival.

Pesticides

There are three types of insecticide in general use: the organophosphorous compounds (e.g. Malathion), carbamates, (e.g. Carbaryl) and chlorinated hydrocarbons (e.g. DDT).

Organophosphorous poisoning can be produced by ingestion or inhalation of the agent, or by absorption through the intact skin. The most important effects of poisoning are excessive bronchial secretion and respiratory paralysis. The organophosphates are cholinesterase inhibitors, producing both muscarinic and nicotinic effects. They become irreversibly bound to cholinesterase after 24–48 hours, but the initial bond is not so stable. The onset of symptoms can be delayed, and so 24 hours hospitalisation is mandatory.

Gastric lavage should be performed unless the agent is known to be dissolved in a petroleum base. Intubation and IPPV may be required. Atropine antagonises the muscarinic effects and it should be administered in divided doses (up to 25 mg may be required). Full atropinisation should be continued for at least 24 hours.

Pralidoxime is a specific antagonist, but it is only effective if given before the bond has become irreversible. There is little value in its use after 24 hours. The dose is 120 mg/kg by slow intravenous injection. Ganendran[95] has reported the failure of pralidoxime to antagonise all organophosphorous compounds.

Carbamates are also cholinesterase inhibitors, but their action is shorter-lived than the organophosphates. Treatment is as for the latter, with the omission of pralidoxime which is ineffective.

Poisoning with chlorinated hydrocarbons produces gross tremor and convulsions. Treatment is symptomatic using short-acting barbiturates.

Petrochemicals

Most cases are due to accidental ingestion by children. Respiratory complications are the most serious, and are present in 25–40 per cent of patients. Death is usually due to pulmonary damage, which is most probably caused by aspiration.[96] Tachypnoea and tachycardia indicate significant lung involvement. Severe intoxication can produce pulmonary oedema, haemoptysis and cyst formation.

Emesis and lavage are contra-indicated in view of the risk of further aspiration. IPPV carries the risk of pneumothorax following cyst rupture.

Pheniramine and thioridazine

Overdose can give rise to dysrhythmias, both supraventricular and ventricular (including fibrillation).[97,98]

Management should include continuous ECG monitoring. Phenytoin, β-blockers and procainamide are of value in treatment.

Plants and fungi

Gastro-intestinal symptoms usually predominate, with burning of the mouth and throat, colic, vomiting and diarrhoea. Careful control of fluid and electrolyte balance will usually result in a successful outcome. One or two species however produce more serious effects. Emesis should be carried out on all conscious patients. It is probably better than lavage at removing plant particles.[99] Activated charcoal should be administered after the stomach has been emptied.

Digitalis-containing plants (lily-of-the-valley, foxglove, oleander) most commonly produce conduction defects, which can usually be corrected with atropine. Dysrhythmias may be treated with potassium chloride and/or phenytoin.

Atropine-containing plants (e.g. deadly nightshade) produce hyperpyrexia, convulsions and coma. Physostigmine given by intravenous injection (0.5 to 2 mg in children) will antagonise all the effects of the atropine. Neostigmine can also be used but it will not combat the central nervous system effects.

Fungi account for approximately 50 per cent of all childhood plant ingestions. There are two groups of fungi as judged by their clinical effects—those producing symptoms in under six hours and those in whom the onset of effects is delayed beyond this time. The former are the less toxic their effects being confined largely to the gastrointestinal tract, although *A. Muscarina* and a few other fungi in this group contain significant amounts of muscarine. Their ingestion produces para-sympathomimetic activity, with salivation, bradycardia and abdominal colic. Atropine is the specific antidote.

The 'delayed onset' group of fungi e.g. Death Cap (*Amanita Phalloides*) are much more toxic. There is an initial phase of colic and diarrhoea, which may be severe and require energetic fluid therapy. This is followed by an apparent improvement, but three to five days later, hepatic and renal failure develop. Haemodialysis (to remove circulating toxins) may be of value in the early stages, but once 36–48 hours have passed it is of no value. The traditional folk remedy of the ground extract of the livers of a dozen rabbits then offers as much hope as anything.

Salicylates

Salicylate poisoning produces multiple effects on the respiratory system, the clotting mechanism, the gastro-intestinal tract and tissue metabolism. Hyperventilation occurs, initially due to a direct stimulatory action on the respiratory centre, and subsequently as a compensatory response to the metabolic acidosis which ensues. The respiratory alkalosis phase is important in that it reduces the amount of buffer base available to cope with the metabolic acidosis. Gastric bleeding can be severe, and perforation has been reported.[100] Thrombocytopenia, impaired platelet aggregation, capillary fragility, decreased factor VII levels and hypoprothrombinaemia all combine to impair coagulation. The effects on metabolic pathways include hyperpyrexia, hypo- and hyperglycaemia and metabolic acidosis. Salicylates uncouple oxidative phosphorylation and inhibit dehydrogenases.[101] The result is an accumulation of lactic acid and ketone bodies.

Serum salicylate levels are of value in management, a concentration above 70 mg/100 ml denoting a serious overdose.

Treatment consists of emesis or gastric lavage, activated charcoal by mouth, dextrose intravenously to combat hypoglycaemia and bicarbonate to correct metabolic acidosis. Prolongation of the prothrombin time can be treated with vitamin K. Excretion of salicylate should be increased in patients with serum salicylate levels above 50 mg/100 ml by using alkaline diuresis. The patient should be catheterised and saline 0.9 per cent (500 ml), dextrose 5 per cent (500 ml) and sodium bicarbonate 1.4 per cent (500 ml) administered in turn. 10 mmol of potassium chloride should be added to each 500 ml infused. The rate of infusion should be 2 litres/hour for the first three hours and subsequently 1 litre/hour. An infusion rate of 30 ml/kg/hr should be used in children. Forced diuresis should be discontinued when the serum salicylate level is below 35 mg/100 ml. Regular measurements of serum electrolytes are necessary. Infusion should be stopped if urine output is low or if cardiac failure develops. Haemodialysis may then be of value in removing salicylate.

Tricyclic antidepressants

Cardiac dysrhythmias, probably produced by the anticholinergic action of these drugs, are the main concern. They also produce fixed dilated pupils, myoclonus and respiratory depression. Estimation of the plasma drug concentration may be of value in predicting the likelihood of complications and the eventual outcome.[102] Prolongation of the QRS complex is very closely related to the plasma level,[103] and may be used to determine the severity of overdose when biochemical analysis is not available. Spiker and Biggs[104] noted that plasma levels remain above the therapeutic range for several days after an overdose, and point out that this will interfere with psychiatric assessment.

Management should include continuous ECG monitoring. Dysrhythmias may be treated with phenytoin, β-blockade and physostigmine.[42] Physostigmine (2 mg intravenously, repeated as necessary) has the advantage of reversing central as well as peripheral effects, although its use has been criticized by Newton,[105] who reported convulsions, marked salivation and bradycardia in four patients. Atropine should always be available when physostigmine is used. Brown et al[106] reported eradication of dysrhythmias following administration of sodium bicarbonate.

REFERENCES

1. Sharratt, M. (1977) Personal communication.
2. Jones, D. I. (1977) Self-poisoning with drugs: The past 20 years in Sheffield. *British Medical Journal*, **1**, 28–29.
3. Matthew, H., Lawson, A. A. (1975) *Treatment of Common Acute Poisonings* Ch. 4. p. 13. Edinburgh: Churchill Livingstone.
4. Holding, T. A., Burglass, D., Duffy, J. C. & Kreitman, N. (1977) Parasuicide in Edinburgh. *British Journal of Psychiatry*, **130**, 534–543.
5. Christian, M. (1977) Principles of emergency treatment for swallowed poisons. *Proceedings of the Royal Society of Medicine*, **70**, 764–766.
6. Dean, G., Adelstein, A. & Spooner, J. (1976) Suicide and self-poisoning in Great Britain and Ireland. *International Journal of Epidemiology*, **5**, 145–151.
7. Matthew, H. & Lawson, A. A. (1975) *Treatment of Common Acute Poisonings*. Ch. 5. p. 18. Edinburgh: Churchill Livingstone.
8. Sament, S. & Huott, A. D. (1969) The EEG in acute barbiturate intoxication. *Electroencephalography and Clinical Neurophysiology*, **27**, 695.
9. Myers, R. & Stockard, J. (1975) Neurologic and EEG correlates in glutethimide intoxication. *Clinical Pharmacology and Therapeutics*, **17**, 212–220.
10. Krapez, J. R. & Cole, P. V. (1977) The management of acute poisoning. *Anaesthesia*, **32**, 494–498.
11. Haider, I., Oswald, I. & Matthew, H. (1968) EEG signs of death. *British Medical Journal*, **3**, 314.
12. Morgan, E. B. (1975) Severe drug overdose. *Anaesthesia and Intensive Care*, **3**, 131–138.
13. Clemmensen, C. & Nilsson, E. (1961) Therapeutic trends in the treatment of barbiturate poisoning. *Clinical Pharmacology and Therapeutics*, **2**, 220–229.
14. Write, R. C. (1974) A simple plan for the management of drug overdosage. *Anaesthesia and Intensive Care*, **2**, 288–302.
15. Matthew, H. & Lawson, A. A. (1975) *Treatment of Common Acute Poisonings*. Ch. 5 p. 20. Edinburgh: Churchill Livingstone.
16. Shubin, H. & Weil, M. (1965) The mechanism of shock following suicidal doses of barbiturates. *American Journal of Medicine*, **38**, 853–863.
17. Matthew, H. (1975) Barbiturates. *Clinical Toxicology*, **8**, 495–513.
18. Goulding, R. & Volans, G. N. (1977) Principles of emergency treatment for swallowed poisons. *Proceedings of the Royal Society of Medicine*, **70**, 766–769.

19. Boxer, L., Anderson, F. P. & Rowe, D. (1969) Comparison of ipecac-induced emesis with gastric lavage. *Journal of Paediatrics*, **74**, 800.
20. Cashman, T. M. & Shirkey, H. C. (1970) Emergency management of poisoning. *Paediatric Clinics of North America*, **17**, 525–533.
21. Robertson, W. O. (1962) Syrup of ipecac—A slow or fast emetic? *American Journal of Diseases of Children*, **103**, 136.
22. Roberts, C. & Noakes, M. J. (1974) Fatal outcome from administration of a salt emetic. *Postgraduate Medical Journal*, **50**, 513–515.
23. Winter, M. & Taylor, D. J. (1974) Letter: Danger of saline emetics. *British Medical Journal*, **3**, 802.
24. MacLean, W. C. (1973) A comparison of ipecac syrup and apomorphine. *Journal of Paediatrics*, **82**, 121–124.
25. Holzman, N. A. & Haslam, R. H. (1968) Elevation of serum copper following cupric sulphate as an emetic. *Paediatrics*, **42**, 189–193.
26. Stein, R. S., Jenkins, D. & Korns, M. E. (1976) Letter: Death after use of cupric sulphate as emetic. *Journal of the American Medical Association*, **235**, 801.
27. Sharman, J. R., Cretney, M. J., Scott, R. D. & Janus, E. D. (1975) Drug overdoses—Is one stomach washing enough? *New Zealand Medical Journal*, **81**, 195–197.
28. Piper, K. W. & Griner, P. F. (1974) Suicide attempts with drug overdose. *Archives of Internal Medicine*, **134**, 703–706.
29. Activated charcoal in the treatment of acute poisoning. *Drugs and Therapeutics Bulletin*, (1974) **12**, 27–28.
30. Levy, G. & Houston, J. B. (1976) Effect of activated charcoal on acetaminophen absorption. *Paediatrics*, **58**, 432–435.
31. Corby, D. G. & Decker, W. J. (1974) Management of acute poisoning with activated charcoal. *Paediatrics*, **54**, 324–329.
32. Hayden, J. W. & Comstock, E. G. (1975) Use of activated charcoal in acute poisoning. *Clinical Toxicology*, **8**, 515–533.
33. Levy, G. & Tsuchiya, T. (1972) Effect of activated charcoal on aspirin absorption. *Clinical Pharmacology and Therapeutics*, **13**, 317.
34. Loenecken, S. R. (1967) *Acute Barbiturate Poisoning.* p. 66. Bristol: Wright.
35. Dundee, J. W., Gray, R. C. & Gupta, P. K. (1974) Doxapram in the treatment of acute drug poisoning. *Anaesthesia*, **29**, 710–714.
36. Pierce, A. W. (1974) Salicylate poisoning. *Paediatrics*, **54**, 343–346.
37. Lasker, N. (1976) Use of haemodialysis and forced diuresis in the treatment of poisoning. *Annals of Clinical and Laboratory Science*, **6**, 377–380.
38. Bloomer, H. A. (1966) A critical evaluation of diuresis in the treatment of barbiturate intoxication. *Journal of Laboratory and Clinical Medicine*, **67**, 898–905.
39. Yaffe, S. J., Sjöqvist, F. & Alván, G. (1970) Pharmacological principles in the management of accidental poisoning. *Paediatric Clinics of North America*, **17**, 495–507.
40. Sieberth, H. G. (1975) Dialyse Behandlung von Vergiftungen. *Internist*, **16**, 116–122.
41. Tozer, T. N., Witt, L. D., Gee, L., Tong, T. G. & Gambertoglio, J. (1974) Evaluation of haemodialysis for ethchlorvynol overdose. *American Journal of Hospital Pharmacy*, **31**, 986–989.
42. Jefferson, J. W. (1975) A review of the cardiovascular effects and toxicity of tricyclic antidepressants. *Psychosomatic Medicine*, **37**, 160–179.
43. Gazzard, B. G., Langley, P. G., Weston, M. J., Dunlop, E. H. & Williams, R. (1974) Polymer coating of activated charcoal. *Clinical Science and Molecular Medicine*, **47**, 97–104.
44. Vale, J. A., Rees, A. J., Widdop, B. & Goulding, R. (1975) Use of charcoal haemoperfusion in the management of severely poisoned patients. *British Medical Journal*, **1**, 5–9.
45. Barbour, B. H., Lasette, A. M. & Koffler, A. (1976) Fixed-bed charcoal haemoperfusion for the treatment of drug overdose. *Kidney International (Supplement)*, 333–337.
46. Rosenbaum, J. L., Kramer, M. S. & Raja, R. (1976) Resin haemoperfusion for acute drug intoxication. *Archives of Internal Medicine*, **136**, 263–266.
47. Goulding, R. (1976) Experience with haemoperfusion in drug abuse. *Kidney International (Supplement)*, 338–340.
48. Rada, R. T., Kellner, R. & Buchanan, J. G. (1975) Chlordiazepoxide and alcohol: A fatal overdose. *Journal of Forensic Science*, **20**, 544–547.
49. Mackintosh, A. F. & Jequier, P. (1977) Fatal mexiletine overdose. *Postgraduate Medical Journal*, **53**, 134.
50. Kristinsson, J. & Johannesson, T. (1977) A case of fatal propanolol intoxication. *Acta Pharmacologica et Toxicologica*, **41**, 190–192.
51. Khan, A. & Muscat-Baron, J. M. (1977) Fatal oxprenolol poisoning. *British Medical Journal*, **1**, 552.

52. Mattingly, P. C. (1977) Letter: Oxprenolol overdose with survival. *British Medical Journal*, **1**, 776–777.
53. Ward, D. E. & Jones, B. (1976) Glucagon and β-blocker toxicity. *British Medical Journal*, **2**, 151.
54. Done, A. K. (1970) Poisoning from common household products. *Paediatric Clinics of North America*, **17**, 569–581.
55. Pike, D. G., Peabody, J. W., Davis, E. W. & Lyons, W. S. (1963) A re-evaluation of the dangers of 'Clorox' ingestion. *Journal of Paediatrics*, **63**, 303–305.
56. Collier, C. R. (1976) Oxygen affinity of human blood in the presence of carbon monoxide. *Journal of Applied Physiology*, **40**, 487–490.
57. Hunyor, S. N., Bradstock, K., Somerville, P. J. & Lucas, N. (1975) Clonidine overdose. *British Medical Journal*, **4**, 23.
58. Moore, M. A. & Phillipi, P. (1976) Letter: Clonidine overdose. *Lancet*, **2**, 694.
59. Davies, D. W., Kadar, D., Steward, D. J. & Munro, I. R. (1975) A sudden death associated with the use of sodium nitroprusside. *Canadian Anaesthetists' Society Journal*, **22**, 547.
60. Jack, R. O. (1974) Toxicity of sodium nitroprusside. *British Journal of Anaesthesia*, **46**, 952.
61. Nicholls, D. P. (1977) Fatal digoxin overdose. *Postgraduate Medical Journal*, **53**, 280–281.
62. Bismuth, C., Gaultier, M., Bonnet, M. & Pollet, J. (1973) L'Hyperkalémie dans l'intoxication digitalique massive. *Biomédecine Express (Paris)*, **19**, 152.
63. Aranda, J. M., Johnson, C. & Palmieri, M. R. (1973) The use of artificial pacemakers in digitalis toxicity. *Boletin Asociacon Médica de Puerto Rico*, **65**, 85–92.
64. Helfant, R. H., Scherlag, B. J. & Damato, A. N. (1967) The electrophysiological properties of diphenylhydantoin sodium. *Circulation*, **36**, 108.
65. Helfant, R. H., Scherlag, B. J. & Damato, A. N. (1967) Protection from digitalis toxicity with diphenylhydantoin sodium. *Circulation*, **36**, 119–125.
66. Reza, M. J., Kovick, R. B., Shine, K. I. & Pearce, M. L. (1974) Massive intravenous digoxin overdosage. *New England Journal of Medicine*, **291**, 777.
67. Smith, T. W., Haber, E., Yeatman, L. & Butler, V. P. (1976) Reversal of advanced digoxin intoxication with digoxin-specific antibodies. *New England Journal of Medicine*, **294**, 797.
68. Martin, A. M., Mitchell, D. C., Gibbins, J. K., Devapal, D. & Trinder, P. (1975) Letter: Charcoal haemoperfusion in the management of severe poisoning. *British Medical Journal*, **1**, 392.
69. Barker, G. A., Brown, T. C. & Hosking, C. S. (1974) Acute iron poisoning. *Anaesthesia and Intensive Care*, **2**, 345–350.
70. Jones, M. M. & Pratt, T. H. (1976) Therapeutic chelating agents. *Journal of Chemical Education*, **53**, 342–347.
71. Stevens, W., van Petenghem, C., Hendricks, A. & Barbier, F. (1974) Thallium intoxication treated with prussian blue. *International Journal of Clinical Pharmacology, Therapy and Toxicology*, **10**, 1–22.
72. Coronho, V., da Silva, O. A. & López, M. (1976) Acute self-poisoning with phenformin. *Acta Diabetalogica Latina*, **13**, 130–133.
73. Habibzadeh, M. A. & Zeller, N. H. (1977) Cardiac arrhythmia and hypopotassaemia in association with lithium carbonate'overdose. *Southern Medical Journal*, **70**, 628–630.
74. Constantiniois, K. (1975) Severe peripheral neuropathy after mandrax overdose. *British Medical Journal*, **2**, 370–371.
75. Matthew, H., Proudfoot, A. T., Brown, S. S. & Smith, A. C. (1968) Mandrax poisoning. *British Medical Journal*, **2**, 101–102.
76. Neaderthal, R. L. & Calabro, J. J. (1975) Treating heroin overdose. *American Family Physician*, **11**, 141–145.
77. Lattin, D. L. (1976) Treating narcotic overdose. *Journal of the Arkansas Medical Society*, **72**, 465–467.
78. Lovejoy, F. H. (1974) Letter: Indications for naloxone in lomotil poisoning. *Paediatrics*, **54**, 658.
79. Volans, G. N. & Whittle, B. A. (1976) Letter: Accidental injection of immobilon. *British Medical Journal*, **2**, 472–473.
80. Robinson, A. E., Holder, A. T., McDowall, R. D., Powell, R. & Sattar, H. (1977) Forensic toxicology of some orphenadrine-related deaths. *Forensic Science*, **9**, 53–62.
81. Snyder, B. D., Kane, M. & Plocher, D. (1976) Letter: Orphenadrine overdose treated with physostigmine. *New England Journal of Medicine*, **295**, 1435.
82. Sangster, B., van Heijst, A. N. & Zimmerman, A. N. (1977) Letter: Treatment of orphenadrine overdose. *New England Journal of Medicine*, **296**, 1006.
83. Davis, M., Simmons, C. J., Harrison, N. & Williams, R. (1974) Urinary paracetamol metabolites following paracetamol overdose. *Clinical Science and Molecular Medicine*, **47**, 6P.
84. Paracetamol overdose. *Drugs and Therapeutics Bulletin* (1976) **14**, 5–7.

85. James, O., Lesna, M., Roberts, S. H., Pulman, L., Douglas, A. P., Smith, P. A. & Watson, A. J. (1975) Liver damage after paracetamol overdose. *Lancet*, **2**, 579–581.
86. Gazzard, B. G., Widdop, B., Davis, M., Hughes, R. D., Goulding, R. & Williams, R. (1977) Early prediction of the outcome of a paracetamol overdose. *Postgraduate Medical Journal*, **53**, 243–247.
87. Prescott, C., Newton, R., Swanson, C., Wright, N., Forrest, A. & Matthew, H. (1974) Successful treatment of severe paracetamol overdosage with cysteamine. *Lancet*, **1**, 588–592.
88. Gazzard, B. G., Hughers, R. D., Chibber, A. D., Bennett, J. R., Murray-Lyon, I. M., Dorboni, B. & Williams, R. Controlled trial of cysteamine and dimercaprol. *Gut*, **16**, 839.
89. Crome, P., Vale, J. A., Volans, G. N., Widdop, B. & Goulding, R. (1976) Oral methionine in the treatment of severe paracetamol overdose. *Lancet*, **2**, 829–830.
90. McLean, A. E. (1976) Letter: Treatment of paracetamol overdose. *Lancet*, **2**, 362.
91. I.C.I. Publication: The treatment of paraquat poisoning (1977).
92. Okenek, S. (1976) Vergiftung durch Paraquat oder Deiquat. *Medikalische Welt*, **27**, 1401–1404.
93. Vale, J. A. (1977) The immediate care of cases of poisoning. *Anaesthesia*, **32**, 483–493.
94. Zavon, M. R. (1974) Poisoning from pesticides. *Paediatrics*, **54**, 332–336.
95. Ganendran, A. (1974) Organophosphate insecticide poisoning. *Anaesthesia and Intensive Care*, **2**, 361–368.
96. Eade, N. R., Taussing, L. M. & Marks, M. I. (1974) Hydrocarbon pneumonitis. *Paediatrics*, **54**, 351–357.
97. Bobik, A. & McClean, A. J. (1976) Cardiovascular complications due to pheniramine overdosage. *Australian and New Zealand Journal of Medicine*, **6**, 65–67.
98. Hollow, V. M., Clarke, G. M. & Weekes, J. W. (1974) Case report: Thoridazine overdose. *Anaesthesia and Intensive Care*, **2**, 375–379.
99. Lampe, K. F. (1974) Systemic plant poisoning in children. *Paediatrics*, **54**, 347–351.
100. Farrand, R. J., Green, J. H. & Haworth, C. (1975) Enteric-coated aspirin overdose and gastric perforation. *British Medical Journal*, **4**, 85–86.
101. Smith, M. J. & Dawkins, P. D. (1971) Review: Salicylate and enzymes. *Journal of Pharmacy and Pharmacology*, **23**, 729.
102. Petit, J. M., Skier, D. G., Ruwitch, J. F., Ziegler, V. E., Weiss, A. N. & Biggs, J. T. (1977) Tricyclic anti-depressant plasma levels and adverse effects after overdose. *Clinical Pharmacology and Therapeutics*, **21**, 47–51.
103. Spiker, D. G., Weiss, A. N., Chang, S. S., Ruwitch, J. F. & Biggs, J. T. (1975) Tricyclic antidepressant overdose. *Clinical Pharmacology and Therapeutics*, **18**, 539–546.
104. Spiker, D. C. & Biggs, J. T. (1976) Tricyclic antidepressants. Prolonged plasma levels after overdosage. *Journal of the American Medical Association*, **236**, 1771–1772.
105. Newton, R. W. (1975) Physostigmine in the treatment of tricyclic anti-depressant overdosage. *Journal of the American Medical Association*, **231**, 941–943.
106. Brown, T. C. K., Barker, G. A., Dunlop, M. E. & Loughnan, P. M. (1973) The use of sodium bicarbonate in the treatment of tricyclic antidepressant-induced arrhythmias. *Anaesthesia and Intensive Care*, **1**, 203.

Appendix

Some abbreviations used in the text

ADH	Antidiuretic hormone
AFE	Amniotic fluid embolism
ARDS	Adult respiratory distress syndrome
BAL	British Anti-Lewisite (dimercaprol)
CFM	Cerebral function monitor
CPAP	Controlled positive airway pressure
CVP	Central venous pressure
DIC	Disseminated intravascular coagulation
DPG	Diphosphoglycerate
EACA	Epsilonaminocaproic acid
EEG	Electroencephalograph
FRC	Functional residual capacity
HFPPV	High frequency positive pressure ventilation
I:E ratio	Ratio of inspiration to expiration
IMV	Intermittent mandatory ventilation
IPPV	Intermittent positive pressure ventilation
ITU	Intensive therapy unit
MAC	Minimal alveolar concentration
MC	Mary Catterall (face-mask)
MMV	Mandatory minute volume
NEEP	Negative end expiratory pressure
NIST	Non-interchangeable screw thread
PEEP	Positive end expiratory pressure
PPF	Plasma protein fraction
RDS	Respiratory distress syndrome
SNP	Sodium nitroprusside
STPD	0°C, 760 mmHg, dry
TSR	Time to sustained respiration
U/P	Urine/plasma

Index